Immunology

STUDENT
NOTES

Other titles published in the series

Ophthalmology H. B. Chawla
Elements of Medical Genetics A. E. H. Emery & R. F. Mueller
Fractures and Orthopaedics D. F. Paton

Titles planned

Anaesthetics
Bacteriology
Child Health
Dermatology
ENT
Epidemiology
General Medicine
Geriatrics
Neuroanatomy
Neurology
Obstetrics and Gynaecology
Pharmacology
Physiology
Psychiatry
Surgery
Virology

STUDENT NOTES

Immunology

D. M. Weir MD FRCPE
Professor of Microbial Immunology,
Department of Bacteriology,
University of Edinburgh Medical School

SIXTH EDITION

CHURCHILL LIVINGSTONE
EDINBURGH LONDON MELBOURNE AND NEW YORK 1988

CHURCHILL LIVINGSTONE
Medical Division of Longman Group UK Limited

Distributed in the United States of America by
Churchill Livingstone Inc., 1560 Broadway, New
York, N.Y. 10036, and by associated companies,
branches and representatives throughout the world.

First edition 1970
Second edition 1971
Third edition 1973
Fourth edition 1977
Fifth edition 1983
Sixth edition 1988

ISBN 0-443-03916-X

British Library Cataloguing in Publication Data
Weir, D. M.
    Immunology. — 6th ed. — (Student notes).
    1. Immunology
    I. Title   II. Series
    616.07'9   QR181

Library of Congress Cataloging in Publication Data
Weir, D. M. (Donald Mackay)
    Immunology.

    (Student notes)
    Includes bibliographies and index.
    1. Immunology.   I. Title.   II. Series.   [DNLM:
1. Immunity.   QW 504 W425i]
QR181.W392   1988   574.2'9   87-18306

Produced by Longman Singapore Publishers (Pte) Ltd
Printed in Singapore

Preface to the Sixth Edition

Immunology continues to expand with no slackening in pace. The changes in the subject, particularly the contributions from molecular genetics, since the fifth edition of this text appeared in 1983 have necessitated very substantial updating of the material. The book is divided into two main sections: 'Basic immunology' and 'Immunology in action'. The first section contains an outline of the basic sciences of the subject, immunochemistry and immunobiology. In this new edition the chapter on acquired immunity has been extensively reorganized and updated. The second section deals with their application to the understanding of disease states including a much enlarged chapter on infection and immunity; disorders of the immune system; hypersensitivity; autoimmunity, and blood groups; transplantation and tumour immunology. This section is not intended as a comprehensive description of clinical immunology but will provide insight into the way immunological knowledge can help to explain the pathogenesis and origin of many disease states. For more detailed descriptions references are provided to specialist texts and reviews.

This book is written particularly for students new to the subject. There are a large number of new diagrams and tables with the emphasis throughout on simplification of difficult concepts. The format is designed to appeal to those who prefer descriptions in words rather than illustrations. For the latter group there are a number of colourfully illustrated texts now available. The lists of objectives given at the beginning of each chapter are intended to help answer the question *'How much am I expected to know?'*. The ability to achieve the objectives should provide the reader with the vocabularly used in immunology and its fundamental concepts. These serve as a background for pursuing the subject in greater depth, e.g. an honours course in immunology or related disciplines. This approach has shown itself in practice to be much appreciated by students taking coursework in infection and immunity. Postgraduates requiring a revision course in immunology may find these objectives particularly useful.

I am most grateful to my wife, Dr Caroline Blackwell, for help in editing the text and for suggestions for the incorporation of new material, some of which is from our book, *Principles of Infection and Immunity in Patient Care* (Churchill Livingstone, 1981). Once again the publishers have provided invaluable editorial assistance and encouragement at all stages of the preparation

Edinburgh, 1988   D.M.W.

Contents

BASIC IMMUNOLOGY

1 **Immunity**   3
  The scope of immunology
  Recognition
  Immunity
  Antibody specificity
  Self and non-self
  Immunity and molecular genetics
  Technical advances

2 **Innate immunity: non-specific defence mechanisms**   13
  Determinants of innate immunity
  Mechanisms of innate immunity
  Temperature
  The complement system

3 **Antigens**   31
  Antigenic determinants
  Immunogenicity

4 **Acquired immunity**   41
  The response
  Effector mechanisms
  Evolutionary origins of the immune response
  Invertebrate immunity
  Tissues and cells of the immune system
  The cells concerned in the immune response
  Essential steps in the generation of an immune response
  The cellular processes involved in immunity
  The immune response
  The immunoglobulins
  The cell-mediated acquired immune response
  Cell co-operation and the genetic control of the
  immune response

IMMUNOLOGY IN ACTION

5 **Infection, immunity and protection**   119
Evasion
Epithelial attachment and infection
Infection and inflammation
Immunity in infection
Immunity in bacterial infections
Immunity in virus infections
Immunity to protozoa and helminths
Fungal infections
Common vaccination procedures
New developments
Antigens of microorganisms
Routine procedures
Special circumstances

6 **Immunohaematology**   183
Blood groups
Rhesus incompatibility
Maternal responses to other fetal antigens
Other blood group systems
Antigens of blood leucocytes and platelets
ABO blood groups, secretor state and susceptibility to
infection

7 **The immunology of tissue transplantation**   194
Transplantation antigen systems
Mechanisms of graft rejection
Immunosuppression

8 **Malignant disease**   206
Evidence for the role of immune mechanisms
Retroviruses, oncogenes and tumours
Tumour antigens
Implications in cancer therapy
Non-specific immunotherapy
Other forms of immunotherapy

9 **Immunopathology**   221
Hypersensitivity
Immediate and delayed hypersensitivity
Anaphylactic reactions of type 1
Cytolytic or cytotoxic (type 2) reactions

Antibody-dependent cell-mediated cytotoxicity
Toxic-complex syndrome (type 3) reactions
Delayed hypersensitivity (type 4) cell-mediated
hypersensitivity
Immunodeficiency
Defective innate immune mechanisms
Primary defects
Secondary defects
Clinical aspects
Autoimmunity
The recognition of autoimmune disease
Possible mechanisms involved in the development of
autoimmunity
HLA, immune response genes and disease
susceptibility
The pathogenesis of autoimmune disease
Other diseases associated with autoimmune states
Antibodies as a consequence of tissue damage

**10 Interaction of antibody with antigen and applications
in laboratory investigations   268**
Primary interaction and secondary effects
Precipitation
Agglutination
Complement fixation
Antigen-antibody reactions using fluorescent labels
Cytotoxic rests
Radioimmunoussay methods
Immunoassays using enzyme-linked antibody or
antigen
Some common diagnostic applications of antigen-
antibody reactions in medical microbiology
Laboratory investigations in clinical immunology
Investigation of hypersensitivity states
Antibodies to inhaled organic material
Antibodies against self-constituents (autoantibodies)
Immune deficiency states
Other tests
Summary of clinical applications
Diagnosis of infection

Index   303

Basic Immunology

1

Immunity

THE SCOPE OF IMMUNOLOGY

The tissues and cells capable of exhibiting what is now recognized as an adaptive immune response have an evolutionary history of some 400 million years and the forms taken by the response during this period have maintained a remarkable constancy both at the molecular and at the functional level. The basic pattern of the protein molecules involved has been retained, with the diversification that has occurred through evolutionary selective pressures being superimposed on this basic pattern.

Recognition

Immune phenomena as expressed in the higher animals have evolved from **recognition mechanisms** that enabled a multicellular primitive animal to distinguish between itself and other foreign species. This idea of **self-non-self discrimination** lies at the foundation of immunological theory. Self recognition mechanisms appear very early in evolution and can be seen in marine organisms, such as sponges. Reaggregation of dispersed colonies is regulated by species-specific surface glycoproteins. Failure of adhesion of unrelated species amounts to a primitive form of graft rejection. The cells lining the cavity of sponges are able to capture microorganisms present in the water drawn into the cavity, and phagocytosis (p. 21) plays a role in the metamorphosis of insects in removing dead and disintegrated tissue.

An important recognition phenomenon occurs in the interaction between pollen grains and plant stigma, which appears to depend on the nature of surface proteins. Pollination and germination only occur if the pollen and stigma are genetically compatible and self-fertilization is prevented.

Primitive marine species, such as sea stars and corals, appear to be able to reject grafts of unrelated forms. Self-non-self discrimination enables the maintenance of **specific partnerships** between cells of a multicellular organism and provides an organism with the additional benefits of recognizing and excluding changed self-constituents and potentially harmful parasitic organisms, such as fungi and bacteria. The particular cell surface molecules that are recognized and determine foreignness are often carbohydrates or glycoproteins. The recognition factors themselves are proteins and it is interesting to note that the production of one of the recognition proteins (immunoglobulin M, p. 99) of the higher vertebrates is specifically stimulated by carbohydrate molecules. Immunoglobulin M is believed to represent the precursor of all the other forms of **immunoglobulin** and has its origin in the most primitive vertebrate fishes.

This had led to the view that there is a continuity between the primitive ability to recognize carbohydrates of foreign cell surfaces and the highly developed recognition factors found in higher vertebrates, which are able to discriminate between a variety of organic molecules of carbohydrate and non-carbohydrate nature.

Immunity

The meaning of the term 'immunity' as it is used today derives from its earlier usage referring to exemption from military service or paying taxes. It has long been recognized that those who recovered from epidemic diseases such as smallpox and plague were exempt from further attacks and such immune individuals were often used in an epidemic to nurse those suffering from active disease. Immunization against smallpox, by the process of variolation using material from mild cases of smallpox (variola), was recorded as being practised in China in about AD 590 and was also practised in India in ancient times. Dried crusts from the pustules of sufferers from the disease were either inhaled into the nose or cotton pledgets that had been stored for a year after infection with smallpox matter, were placed over scratches on the skin. The procedure was introduced into England from Turkey in the reign of George I by Lady Mary Wortley Montagu the wife of the British Ambassador to Constantinople. The matter from smallpox lesions was introduced on the point of a large needle into the vein of a recipient. The procedure was not without hazard and if the recipient did not develop the disease itself there was the danger of transmission of other infections such as leprosy or syphilis. George I was persuaded to allow the inoculation of two of his grandchildren and variolation became widespread throughout the country. The practice had been used on a small scale even at the end of the previous century in the Scottish Highlands and Wales and was introduced into America by immigrant Negro slaves at the beginning of the eighteenth century.

Despite the hazards associated with variolation, smallpox was so widespread and feared that the small percentage of persons who developed the disease after inoculation was accepted as a worthwhile risk. In England at the time of George I 60 of every 100 persons were likely to develop the disease and of these more than half would die. The efficacy of variolation in preventing the death of young children and women at childbirth is believed to have been largely responsible for the great increase in population in the early part of the eighteenth century. The Edinburgh physician Francis Home, who was familiar with the procedure of variolation, in 1758 applied the same principle to inoculate against measles. Home carried in his pocket book pieces of cotton soaked in the tears, blood or tissue fluid taken from an incision into the rash of a patient. The pieces of cotton were placed over an incision in a recipient and in seven of 15 persons immunized in this way mild measles developed after an incubation period of about nine days.

Edward Jenner, towards the end of the eighteenth century, was the first to indicate the scientific approach to immunization. He took up observations that had passed into folklore, made 20 years earlier by a Dorchester farmer Benjamin Jesty, that persons exposed or deliberately innoculated with cowpox were protected against smallpox. Jenner not only established the value of immunization with cowpox but was able to transmit the cowpox infection from one person to another.

The difficulties Jenner faced in gaining acceptance of vaccination are fully and fascinatingly described in *Victory with Vaccines* (H J Parish). Jenner's paper of 1798, giving the results and conclusions of his investigation, was refused by the Royal Society and he was subjected to crude criticisms and caricatures including cartoonist's representation of vaccinated individuals being transformed into cows. In 1802 and 1807 he was given a parliamentary grant (less deductions for taxes and fees). Surprisingly, variolation was not made illegal until 1840. Two years after Jenner's paper was finally published, Dr Benjamin Waterhouse of Harvard obtained supplies of the vaccine and its use became widespread in America. Napoleon had his troops vaccinated and the first child to be vaccinated in Russia was named Vaccinof.

The foundations for an understanding of immunity were laid by the invention of the microscope by Leenwenhoek, the recognition of microorganisms and the advent of Pasteur's **germ theory of disease**. Pasteur's chance observation that aged cultures of chicken cholera bacillus would not cause the expected disease in chickens led to the development of methods for reducing the virulence of pathogenic microorganisms called **attenuation**. The protection given to animals by preinoculation of such attenuated organisms led to the widespread use of the method for immunization purposes.

Robert Koch developed staining techniques and, later, the fixation of organisms on slides. His work on anthrax showed that the disease could be transferred from animal to animal by pure cultures. He went on to describe tubercle bacilli and the phenomenon of delayed hypersensitivity or **cell-mediated immunity** as it is known today. Immunology as a science began with the demonstration by von Behring and Kitasato at the Koch Institute in Berlin in 1890 of an antibacterial substance or factor in the blood of animals immunized against tetanus and diphtheria organisms. The neutralizing ability of such blood serum for the bacterial toxins was the first demonstration of the effect of what is now recognized as antibody globulin.

The part played by **phagocytic cells** in clearing away and destroying bacteria was recognized by Metchnikoff, a Russian biologist working in France. Later the helpful effect of antibody (called opsonins by Almroth Wright) in encouraging phagocytosis became apparent, thus reconciling two opposing schools of thought on immune mechanisms — one believing the process to be brought about completely by blood factors and the other upholding an entirely cellular viewpoint.

Pfeiffer and Bordet demonstrated the activity of a serum factor called **complement**, which participates with antibody in the destruction of bacteria and has now been shown to have a wide variety of important biological activities. Paul Ehrlich proposed the first theory of antibody formation — **the side chain theory**. This proposed the existence of receptors on the surface of cells that could be released into the blood and neutralize bacterial toxins.

Antibody specificity

The specificity of antibody for the agent (i.e. the antigen) which induced its formation led to the use of antibody as an analytic tool. Thus the antigenic characters of bacterial and non-bacterial substances could be worked out and systems of classification of microorganisms were developed on this basis. Landsteiner used antibody-antigen interaction to define the **ABO blood group system** on the basis of antigenic differences in red cell membranes, and was also responsible for performing the ground work on the chemical basis of antigenic specificity.

Self and non-self

In more recent years, with increasing knowledge of the molecular processes underlying the functioning of cells, it became possible to formulate theories on the mechanisms whereby the tissues and cells responsible for producing antibody performed this function. The need for such theories became apparent with the recognition of human diseases where the immune mechanisms had become deranged and were treating the individual's own tissues as if they were foreign antigens. Thus the question of how the immune system distinguished between what was foreign and what was part of self became important and resulted in the formulation of new theories to explain these phenomena, notable among which was the **clonal selection** theory of Burnet. These attempted to define the scope and limitation of Ehrlich's 'contrivances by means of which the immunity reaction . . . is prevented from acting against the organism's own elements and so giving rise to autotoxin'. The advances made in this area gave a new dimension to the science of immunology which until then was devoted almost exclusively to the prevention of infectious disease by vaccination and immunization. This new field of study — **immunobiology** — has drawn the attention of biologists to the apparantly central importance of immune mechanisms in the evolution of multicellular animals.

The cells of the immune system are probably derived from the primitive cellular defence mechanism that arose with the evolution of the invertebrates. This is manifested by the engulfment and walling off of foreign particles. The phagocytic cells responsible for this do not respond by proliferation so that the animal does not become better adapted to deal more effectively with the foreign material (p. 47). It is doubtful if the immune response, as it is recognized today, first appeared with the need for protection from parasitic microorganisms but evolved in the primitive vertebrates as a way of protecting themselves from their parasitic relatives. In the absence of such protection the parasite could attach itself to a host and because the tissues of the two animals were so similar the host would be unable to react against the parasite which would thus be accepted rather like a piece of successfully grafted compatible tissue (Ch. 7). Burnet, who was one of the main exponents of this view, has suggested that the mechanism that underlies the protective response to parasites depended on the host making its own tissues antigenically different from the parasite so that the parasite could be recognized as foreign. The evolution of a defence mechanism able to resist parasitic invasion would have the added advantage of treating in the same way any tissues of the animal that changed their cell surface antigens. This, as will be discussed later (Ch. 8), is a characteristic of many tumour cells and the employment of the immunological defence mechanisms to rid the body of such cells would confer a clear evolutionary advantage to the species.

Immunity and molecular genetics

Knowledge of the genetic control of protein synthesis is likely to make considerable advances as a result of the study of the synthesis of immunoglobulins. The concept that **two genes** may code for a **single polypeptide chain** and that groups of closely linked genes may be basic units of mammmalian genomes have emerged from studies on immunoglobulin synthesis.

It is now recognized that interaction between different cell types may exert control over protein synthesis, affecting for example the particular class of immunoglobulin being manufactured by a lymphocyte (Ch. 4). The study of immunoglobulin structure has shown that in the human there are at least 10 different types and that each type contains an enormous number of variants differing slightly from each other in amino acid sequence.

The gene complex of the mouse that controls the cell surface antigens important in transplantation (graft) rejection has proved to be an invaluable general model for the study of the **major transplantation antigen systems** of higher vertebrates. More recently the small segment of chromosome 17 that contains this gene

Table 1.1 Development of immunology

	Immunity	
Late eighteenth century	Smallpox vaccination — Jenner	
Late nineteenth century	Germ theory of disease, attenuated and killed vaccines — Pasteur Tubercle bacillus and cell-mediated immunity — Koch Antitoxins against diphtheria and tetanus — von Behring, Kitasato Complement activity — Pfeifer, Bordet Agglutination of bacteria — Durham Side chain theory of immunity — Ehrlich Phagocytosis and cellular immunity — Metchnikoff	
	Immunochemistry	**Immunobiology**
Mid-twentieth century to present day	Blood groups — Landsteiner Antigenic determinants — Landsteiner, Heidelberger, Marrack Electrophoretic separation of gamma globulin — Kabat, Tiselius Structural analysis of antibody molecule — Porter, Edelman	Antiglobulin test — Coombs, Mourant, Race Recognition of autoimmunity Clonal selection theory of immunity — Burnet (Jerne) Immunological tolerance — Medawar, Owen (Glenny) Transplantation immunology, tumour immunology, Rhesus immunization, Deficiency states, role of the thymus
	Relationship between structure and biological activities of immunoglobulin molecule and genetic control mechanisms Determinants of immunogenicity of antigen molecule	Immunogenetics and evolution of immune system Lymphocyte activation and products, cell cooperation Role of macrophages — antibacterial, and cytotoxic effects Monoclonal antibodies — Milstein and Kohler
	Synthesis of determinants for vaccines Vaccine production by genetic engineering	Flow cytometry and cell sorting Recombinant DNA technology Cloning of Lymphocytes Transfection of Lymphocytes

complex has evoked considerable interest among geneticists and immunologists. They have recognized that in addition to controlling cell surface antigens, there are closely linked genes that determine differences in level of antibody responses to many antigens, differences in susceptibility to tumour viruses and a number of other important immunological traits (Ch. 9). This gene complex is now the most thoroughly and extensively characterized segment of chromosome in any mammalian species and as such it consitutes a very valuable model for studies of gene evolution, gene action and organization.

Recent advances in recombinant DNA technology have had a major impact on the understanding of the molecular basis of the immune response. In particular, the advances in DNA sequencing, isolation of restriction enzymes and the construction of vectors for cloning and amplifying defined DNA sequences, with important implications in, for example, vaccine production. Monoclonal cell lines, such as plasmacytomas and lymphomas, have provided the basis for many of the recent advances in the field. Protein structural analysis has shown the immunoglobulin molecule to be a heirarchical organization of fragments and molecular immunology has provided answers to the problems of the evolution of the large library of different structures within the immunolobulin molecule, how they are joined together and how combinatorial diversity has been created.

Investigation in vivo of the function of cloned genes has become possible by injecting the genes into mouse embryos and tracing the expression of the genes in these 'transgenic mice'. This approach is likely to lead to a better understanding of gene expression in cells of the immune system so that, for example, the function of cell surface molecules can be identified; disease-prone animals can be generated and studied, or gene therapy can be attempted on pre-existing models.

The way that the immune response is regulated by feedback effects of antibodies, by T suppressor cells and by the variety of mediators and growth factors — cytokines and interleukins — has been one of the most significant advances in the last few years. There are also the beginnings of an understanding of the roles of hormones in immune regulation, particularly the role of neuroendocrine peptides in immunosuppression, and the hope is that these advances will throw light on stress-related immune depression.

Technical advances

Modern biochemical techniques have helped to add precision and sensitivity to immunological methods. These include the use of radioisotopes to measure accurately the primary binding of antibody with antigen and to demonstrate the metabolic acitivity of cells engaged in antibody production. Protein fractionation techniques and peptide analysis of the antibody molecule have thrown light on the chemical basis of specificity of the molecule and the relationship of structure to function, as well as confirming a genetic basis for antibody formation and providing factual limitations on earlier theories of antibody formation.

The understanding of immunological processes underlying the reaction of the body to tumours, to transplanted tissues and organs and to infectious agents has gained much ground as the result of these advances in immunochemical techniques. Clinical developments have included the recognition of **autoimmune** and **immunological deficiency** diseases and the feasibility of **organ transplantation**. Technical advances in the study of the in vitro behaviour of cells of the immune system and in the quantitation of serum proteins have provided valuable diagnostic help in the recognition and management of these clinical situations. Phylogenetic studies have stimulated investigations into the development and control of the lymphoid tissues leading, for example, to a new understanding of the role of that previously enigmatic organ, the thymus.

Probably the most important development in the last few years has been the emergence of techniques that come under the heading of 'genetic engineering'. The technique having a very considerable impact in many areas of the biological sciences is **monoclonal antibody production**, introduced by Milstein and Kohler. The method described on page 79 has led to the production of unlimited quantities of highly specific antibody to a large variety of biologically important antigens. This will revolutionize radioimmunoassay techniques (p. 287), analysis of at present ill-defined tissue and cell antigens (e.g. those of neurological tissues), treatment of tumours and autoimmunity.

The ability to introduce genetic information into bacteria and yeasts by genetic engineering techniques, leading to the production of therapeutic agents such as insulin or important viral antigens (e.g. hepatitis B antigen), is likely to have important applications over the next few years.

In the last few years immunologists are beginning to recognize the existence of a wide variety of colony stimulating factors and cytokines that enable the survival, proliferation and differentiation of cell populations as well as controlling their functional activity. These growth factors are likely to become increasingly important not only in understanding regulation of the immune response but also in their effects on a variety of different cell types including neoplastic cells.

Thus it can be seen that immunity in its original meaning, referring to resistance to parasitic invasion by means of a specific immune response, is only one activity of a cellular system in animals. The total activity of the cellular system is concerned with mechanisms for preserving the integrity of the individual with far-reaching implications in embryology, genetics, cell biology, tumour biology and many non-infective disease processes.

FURTHER READING

Brock T (ed) 1961 Milestones in microbiology. III. Immunology. Prentice-Hall, Englewood Cliffs, N J, p 121–144

Burnet F M 1969 Changing patterns, Elsevier, New York

Foster W D 1970 A history of medical bacteriology and immunology. Heinemann, London

Good R A 1976 Runestones in immunology: inscriptions to journeys of discovery and analysis. Journal of Immunology 117:1413

Herbert W J, Wilkinson P C, Stott D I 1985 Dictionary of immunology, 3rd edn. Blackwell Scientific Publications, Oxford

Mc Neill W H 1976 Plagues and peoples. Basil Blackwell, Oxford

Parish H J 1965 A history immunization. Livingstone, Edinburgh

2

Innate immunity: non-specific defence mechanisms

Objectives

On completion of this section the reader will be able to:

1. Describe three host determinants of innate immunity
2. Describe with the aid of a diagram the innate immune mechanism of the skin and mucous membranes.
3. Give two examples of the way the normal flora prevent infection by pathogenic microorganisms.
4. Define phagocytosis and list the three essential features of the process.
5. Give two examples of intracellular killing mechanisms.
6. Define opsonin.
7. Describe in outline the differences between complement activation by the classical and alternate pathways; give three examples of the biological activities of complement activation products.
8. Describe the three main features of an inflammatory response and give two examples of endogenous mediators of inflammation.

The healthy individual is able to protect himself from potentially harmful microorganisms in the environment by a number of very effective mechanisms, present from birth, which do not depend upon having previous experience of any particular microorganism. The innate immune mechanisms are **non-specific** in the sense that they are effective against a wide range of potentially infective agents. The main determinants of innate immunity seem genetically controlled, varying widely with species and strain and to a lesser extent between individuals. Age, sex and hormone balance play lesser roles. In comparison, acquired immune mechanisms, discussed below, depend upon the development of an immune response to individual microorganisms that is specific only for the inducing organism.

13

Determinants of innate immunity

Species and strain

Marked differences exist in the susceptibility of different species to infective agents. The rat is strikingly insusceptible to diphtheria whilst the guinea-pig and man are highly susceptible. The rabbit is particularly susceptible to myxomatosis and man to syphilis, leprosy and meningococcal meningitis. Susceptibility to an infection does not always imply a lack of resistance because, although man is highly susceptible to the common cold, he overcomes the infection within a few days. Dogs in contrast are not susceptible to the virus agents responsible for the common cold in man. In some diseases, although a species may be difficult to infect (i.e. insusceptible), once established the disease can progress rapidly (i.e. lack of resistance). For example, rabies, although common to both man and dogs, is not readily established as the virus does not easily penetrate healthy skin. Once infection is established, however, the resistance mechanisms in both species are not able to overcome the disease. Marked variations in resistance to infection between different strains of mice have been noted.

Table 2.1 Determinants of innate immunity

Specific host determinants	Physical determinants	Active antimicrobial determinants
Species and strain	Skin and mucous membrane barrers, moist surfaces	Antibacterial and antifungal secretions of skin — sweat and sebaceous secretions
Individual genetic factors	Anatomical traps, e.g. nasal cavity	Antibacterial and antiviral secretions of mucous membranes
Age	Mechanical cleansing, e.g. cilia	Antimicrobial substances of tissue fluids, e.g. lysozyme, basic polypeptides Phagocytosis and digestion
Hormonal balance		

In man the habits and environment of a community affect his ability to resist particular infections by acquired immune mechanisms developing early in life. This environmentally determined type of resistance is easily confused with the genetically controlled innate immunity and makes it difficult to ascertain differences in innate immunity in different communities. It is, however, fairly clear that the American Indian and the Negro are more susceptible to tuberculosis than are Caucasians. It seems reasonable to assume that certain interspecies and interstrain differences have arisen by a process of natural selection.

Individual differences and influence of age

The role of heredity in determining resistance to infection is well illustrated by studies on tuberculosis infection in twins. If one homozygous twin develops tuberculosis, the other twin has a three to one chance of developing the disease compared to a one in three chance if the twins are heterozygous. Sometimes genetically controlled abnormalities are an advantage to the individual in resisting infection, as for example in a hereditary abnormality of the red blood cells (sickling) which are less readily parasitized by *Plasmodium falciparum*, thus conferring insusceptibility to malaria. Infectious diseases are more severe at the extremes of life, and in the young animal this appears to be associated with immaturity of the immunological mechanisms affecting the ability of the lymphoid system to deal with and react to foreign antigens. In the elderly, on the other hand, physical abnormalities (e.g. prostatic enlargement leading to stasis of urine) are a common cause of increased susceptibility to infection (see also p. 192).

Nutritional factors and hormonal influences

The adverse effect of poor nutrition on susceptibility to infectious agents in usually not seriously questioned. Experimental evidence in animals has shown repeatedly that inadequate diet may be correlated with increased susceptibility to a variety of bacterial diseases and this has been associated with decreased phagocytic activity and leucopenia. Studies in Scotland, for example, have shown that sheep (particularly those grazing on hill farms) can have a deficiency in the trace element copper. This results in a decrease in their leucocyte microbicidal activity, an increased susceptibility to bacterial challenge and enhanced inflammatory reactions. In the case of infective agents such as viruses which depend upon the normal metabolic function of the host cells, malnutrition, if it interfered with such activities, would be expected to hinder proliferation of the potentially infective agent. There is experimental evidence in support of this view in a number of animal species, which when undernourished were less susceptible to a variety of viruses including vaccinia virus and certain neurotropic viruses. The same may be true of malaria infections in man. The parasite requires para-amino benzoic acid for multiplication and this may be deficient when a low level of nutrition exists. The exact role of nutritional factors in resistance to infectious agents in man is difficult to determine by epidemiological data. Poor diet is often associated with poor environmental conditions and increased incidence of infection can correlate with poor sanitary conditions.

There is decreased resistance to infection in diseases such as diabetes mellitus, hypothyroidism and adrenal dysfunction. The reasons for this have yet to be elucidated in detail, but, in the case of adrenal dysfunction, it is known that the glucocorticoids are anti-inflammatory agents, decreasing the ability of phagocytes to digest ingested material (probably by stabilizing the lysozomal membranes).

Mechanisms of innate immunity

Mechanical barriers and surface secretions

The intact skin and mucous membranes of the body afford effective protection against non-pathogenic organisms and a high degree of protection against pathogens (Fig. 2.1 and Table 2.2). The skin is the more resistant barrier because of its outer horny layer. The damp surface of the mucous membranes of the respiratory tract acts as a trapping mechanism and, together with the action of the hair-like processes or cilia, sweeps away foreign particulate material so that it passes into the saliva and then is swallowed. Various physical, chemical and microbiological agents can be toxic to cilia. Respiratory viruses, particularly influenza, and pathogenic *Mycoplasma pneumoniae* interfere with ciliary activity.

There are no cilia in the gastrointestinal tract but the layer of mucus can trap organisms and the effect of peristalsis prevents bacterial overgrowth. Slowing of normal intestinal mobility is likely to lead to increased numbers of gut bacteria and, if the mucosal barrier is damaged, leakage of microorganisms can occur with potentially serious results.

On reaching the stomach the acid gastric juices destroy any microorganisms present. Nasal secretions and saliva contain mucopolysaccharides capable of inactivating some viruses and the tears contain lysozyme active against Gram-positive bacteria. The seb-

SKIN

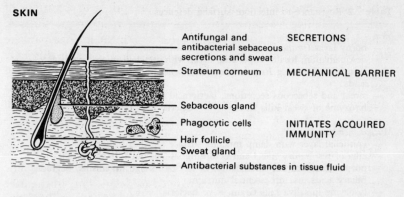

RESPIRATORY MUCOUS MEMBRANE

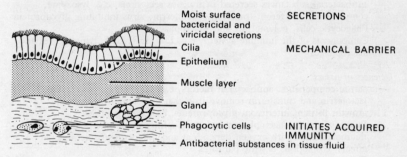

Fig. 2.1 Innate immune mechanisms

aceous secretions and sweat of the skin contain bactericidal and fungicidal fatty acids and these constitute a very effective protective mechanism against potentially pathogenic microorganisms. The antimicrobial substances include the sweat gland secretions: lactic acid, amino acids, uric acid, and ammonia (the acidity of sweat, pH 5.5, has a microbicidal effect); the sebaceous secretions: triglycerides, free fatty acids and wax alcohols; substances derived from the cornification process: steroids, amino acids, pentoses, phospholipids, and complex polypeptides. Certain areas of the body such as the soles of the feet are deficient in sebaceous glands and this explains in part why such areas are susceptible to fungal infection. These are sometimes referred to as alkaline gaps. The protective ability of these secretions varies at different stages of life and it is known that fungal 'ringworm' infection of children disappears at puberty.

Table 2.2 Resistance to infection: surface defences

Skin
— horny layer (*stratum corneum*) mechanical barrier
— desquamation; loss of superficial layer with attached microorganisms
— skin microflora; e.g *Proprionobacterium acnes* produces antibacterial fatty acids
— sweat and sebaceous secretions, lactic acid and fatty acids lower pH of skin, lysozyme of sweat kills Gram + ve bacteria

Mucous membranes
— epithelial layer with damp mucous surface attaches bacteria
— cilia of respiratory tracts and coughing sweeps out foreign particles
— normal flora prevent colonization of gut by foreign organisms, degrade biliary acids, use up essential nutrient
— lysozyme in saliva kills Gram + ve bacteria
— acid production by lactobacilli in vagina — antibacterial
— flow rate of fluids over mucous membranes, e.g. keeps urinary tract sterile
— antibacterial substances secreted in mucous secretions, e.g. lysozyme, complement, interferon, transferin, lactoferrin, virus inhibiting glycoproteins
— Phagocytic cells, polymorphs and macrophages
  Components of the immune system, e.g. IgA, IgG, IgM, lymphocytes and macrophages

Defences of tissues
— serum components, antibacterial factors, e.g. complement, lysozyme, lactoferrin and transferrin remove iron that is essential for bacterial growth; β-lysin, interferon, glycoproteins, basic polypeptides
— Phagocytic cells, macrophages and neutrophil polymorphs phagocytose microorganisms with oxygen dependent and independent microbicidal effects, eosinophils destroy parasites
— Components of the immune system. Humoral and cell-mediated immunity

General influences
— Nutritional, endocrine and metabolic factors
— Age and genetic factors

Areas where there is a high flow rate of secretions such as the urinary tract, biliary tract and lower respiratory tract are generally sterile in contrast to areas where the flow rate is slower, such as the oropharynx and the large bowel. Interference with flow rate in the urinary tract or biliary tract will lead to infection.

Bactericidal substances of the tissues and body fluids

Lysozyme. This is a low molecular weight basic protein found in relatively high concentration in polymorphonuclear leucocytes as well in most tissue fluids except c.s.f., sweat and urine. It functions as a mucolytic enzyme, splitting sugars off the glycopeptides of the cell wall of many Gram-positive bacteria, resulting in their lysis. Lysozyme may also play a role in the intracellular destruction of some Gram-negative bacteria. This antibacterial agent was described by Fleming who, in 1922, was able to measure its effect on a particular Gram-positive organism, *Micrococcus lysodeikticus*. Human tears contain a large quantity of lysozyme and egg white is a rich commercial source.

Lysozyme is synthesized in the parotid gland, in the mucosa of the respiratory and gastrointestinal tracts and in the spleen and lymph nodes. Mononuclear phagocytes make lysozyme and polymorphonuclear granulocytes contain lysozyme but do not synthesize it. Thus protection by lysozyme is brought about by its local synthesis and release into the mucous secretions and by mononuclear phagocytes that infiltrate a tissue during an inflammatory response and release it at that site. The release of lysozyme from the breakdown of granulocytes has the same effect. The importance of lysozyme in phagocytic cells in protection from pathogenic microorganisms is indicated by a reported defect in bacterial killing by leucocytes from a person in whom lack of lysozyme was demonstrated. The possibility has been suggested, on the basis of in vitro work with tumour cells exposed to lysozyme, that lysozyme secreted locally by macrophages may play a role in the prevention of tumour growth. Macrophages are known to be a prominent cell in the inflammatory response associated with tumours.

Basic polypeptides. A variety of basic proteins, derived from the tissue and blood cells damaged in the course of infection and inflammation, have been found in the tissues of animals. This group includes spermine and spermidine, which kill tubercle bacilli and some staphylococci, and the arginine- and lysine-containing basic proteins protamine and histone. The ability of these basic polypeptides to destroy bacteria probably depends on the ability of the NH_2 groups to react non-specifically with the nearest acidic substance.

Humoral factors and phagocytes

A number of other so-called 'acute phase' materials are present in the blood and increase in level in the inflammatory response: C-reactive protein, $\alpha 1$-antitrypsin, $\alpha 2$-macroglobulin, fibrinogen, and ceruloplasmin, and certain complement components. The increase in level of these proteins appears to be mediated by a protein termed leucocytic endogenous mediator that is released by phagocytes. The role of many of these acute phase substances is not clear, but C-reactive protein and microorganisms can activate complement by the classical pathway. There is also evidence that C-reactive protein can bind to both human and mouse T lymphocytes, resulting in the reduction of their activity in certain immune functions. In such a situation, interference with normal immune mechanisms would be expected. Some of the other acute phase substances may also interfere with immunoregulatory mechanisms, and as indicated in Chapter 5, may account for some aspects of the immunosuppression noted in various infections (see Table 5.2).

Normal bacterial flora and protection from infection

The normal bacterial flora of the skin may itself produce various antimicrobial substances such as bacteriocines, and acids. At the same time the normal flora compete with potential pathogens for essential nutrients.

There are a very large number of microorganisms that live in close association with man — around 10^{12} bacteria on the skin and about 10^{14} in the gut (see p. 121–123, Figs. 5.1–5.3). Probably the most valuable function these 'commensal' organisms serve is the exclusion of other microorganisms. Other functions include the degradation of bile acids as well as providing stimulation of the immune system to microbial antigens. The latter role is illustrated by the observation that germ-free animals make only about 1/50th as much immunoglobulin as conventional animals. If the commensal organisms of the gut are removed by antibiotics, pathogenic organisms can readily gain a foothold. Experiments with mice have shown after sterilization of the gut with streptomycin the animals can be killed with 1/10 000 the dose of *Salmonella typhimurium* required to kill the untreated animals. Guinea pigs given penicillin undergo a profound change in the microbial content of the bowel. Such organisms may then get into the bloodstream and kill the animal. The lactobacilli of the vagina ferment glycogen and reduce the pH to about 4. If this flora is disturbed by antibiotics, other bacteria, yeasts or parasites can become established.

These observations point to the importance of not disturbing the relationship between host and its indigenous flora. Damage to the respiratory mucosa, for example by smoking, is likely to be followed by alteration in the normal flora and replacement by pathogenic organisms. Commensal organisms from the gut can cause infection in an area that they do not normally populate. An example of this is urinary tract infections resulting from the introduction of *E. coli* by means of a urinary catheter. These commensals that are given the circumstances in which to cause infections are called 'opportunistic pathogens'. Infections with these opportunists are quite widespread, often appearing as a result of medical or surgical treatment (see the compromised host, p. 120).

Phagocytosis and the inflammatory response

Microorganisms or inert particles such as colloidal carbon entering the tissue fluids or bloodstream are very rapidly engulfed by various circulating and tissue-fixed phagocytic cells. These cells are of two types, the **polymorphonuclear** leucocytes of the blood — or microphages as they are sometimes called — and the **mononuclear** phagocytic cells distributed throughout the body, both **circulating** in the blood and **fixed** in the tissues. The latter cells make up the cells of the reticuloendothelial system or RES and are given the generic name macrophages. Macrophages in the blood are known as monocytes, those in the connective tissues as histiocytes, those in the spleen, lymph nodes and thymus as the sinus-lining macrophages (sometimes called reticulum cells).

It is now established that the macrophages of connective tissues are derived from the peripheral blood monocytes as are the Kupffer cells of the liver, the alveolar macrophages of the lungs, and the free macrophages of the spleen, lymph nodes and bone marrow. In the spleen and lymph nodes, both free and fixed macrophages occur in close association with the reticular cells, which act as a framework for the macrophages. The reticular cells themselves, although able to ingest particulate material, are not regarded as mononuclear phagocytes, nor are the dendritic cells (p. 58) of the follicles of the spleen and lymph nodes. The term **mononuclear phagocyte system** describing actively phagocytic cells is now widely accepted as more satisfactory description of the function, origin and morphology of phagocytes than the older RES classification, which included actively and poorly phagocytic cells.

The three essential features of these phagocytic cells are (i) that they are actively **phagocytic**, (2) that they contain **digestive enzymes** to degrade ingested material and (3) that the macrophages are an important **link** between the innate and the acquired immune mechanisms, partly by passing on antigens or their products to the lymphoid cells and partly by retaining antigens to ensure that lymphoid cells are not overwhelmed by excess antigen (p. 45).

The process of phagocytosis is undoubtedly one of the earliest accomplishments of living cells. At the beginning of the century Metchnikoff in Russia first appreciated the continuity of this function through evolution and the important role of this activity in resistance to infectious agents.

The role of the phagocyte in innate immunity is to engulf particulate (phagocytosis) or soluble material (pinocytosis) and either to digest it or if indigestible to store it away so that it no longer serves as a local irritant, e.g. carbon particles from a polluted atmosphere.

The macrophages of the mononuclear phagocyte system serve a very important role in clearing the bloodstream of foreign particulate material such as bacteria. The efficiency of this process can be dramatically illustrated by injecting colloidal carbon into the circulation of a mouse. Samples of blood taken at short intervals thereafter show a very rapid removal of most of the particles within a few minutes after injection and the blood is completely cleared by 15 to 20 minutes. Dissection of the animal will show massive localisation of the carbon particles, particularly in Kupffer cells of the liver, of the spleen sinus-lining macrophages and in the macrophages of the lungs. This system of phagocytic cells has an enormous capacity to take up material from the blood and the finding of free microorganisms in the bloodstream usually means that there is a continued release of organisms from an abscess or from the bacterial 'vegetation' found in bacterial endocarditis.

There are many examples of the ability of the phagocytic cells of animals to ingest and dispose of different kinds of microorganisms. The destruction of phagocytic cells by chemical agents in the rabbit results in the animal losing resistance to a normally avirulent pneumococcus. The enhanced ability of macrophages from animals infected with tubercle bacilli or listeria to resist these and other infective agents is discussed on page 140. Some microorganisms, such as brucellae and streptococci, can resist intracellular digestion (p. 126).

The way in which phagocytes **recognize, bind** and **ingest** particulate materials such as microorganisms is only beginning to be understood. Initial adherence depends on two distinct mechanisms.

1. Relatively non-specific binding that appears to depend, as shown by work in the author's laboratory, on cell surface glycoproteins of the phagocyte binding to cell wall carbohydrates of the microorganism. This ability is probably derived from the recognition abilities found in primitive species discussed in Chapter 1 and has been retained during evolution.

2. More recently evolved mechanisms that utilize receptors in the phagocyte cell membrane for a part of the antibody molecule (Fc component, p. 94) and for a component of the complement system C3b, p. 29). Microorganisms coated with antibody and complement thus adhere to the phagocyte and can then be ingested. Antibodies can markedly enhance the activities of phagocytic cells and even improve intracellular digestion. Such antibodies are known as **opsonins** (p. 103).

Injury to tissue excites an inflammatory response. Three major changes are associated with the inflammatory response to invading microorganisms:

1. Changes in vascular calibre and blood flow.

2. Increased permeability in the walls of arterioles, capillaries and venules leading to fluid exudation and swelling.

3. Passage of leucocytes through the blood vessel walls via the interendothelial junctions into the surrounding tissues (diapedesis).

These changes are brought about mainly by chemical mediators with a minor role played by nerve impulses. There are two types of mediator, exogenous and endogenous. Bacterial products can act as exogenous mediators and can be directly responsible for increased vascular permeability and leakage of fluid and leucocytes. Such products can also attract leucocytes to the site of infection by a process known as chemotaxis. Endogenous mediators (Table 2.3) are of more importance in inflammation and can be classified into two major groups — those from the blood and those from the tissues.

Table 2.3 Endogenous mediators of inflammation

	Main source
Histamine	Mast cells or basophils
Kinins (eg. bradykinin kallidin leucokinins)	From blood precursors by proteases and leucocytes
Prostaglandins (E_1 and E_2) and acidic lipids	Polymorphonuclear leucocytes, monocytes and eosinophils
Slow reacting substances	Mast cells and basophils
Complement components (anaphylatoxin chemotaxins)	Derived by activation of classical or alternative pathways (Fig. 26)
Components of clotting system and their degradation products (fibrinopeptides)	Blood and tissue fluids
Cytokines (chemotactic factors, macrophage activating factors, mitogenic factors, etc. p. 110)	Lymphocytes and macrophages

Antimicrobial activities of phagocytes

Phagocytes, as noted above, can bind microorganisms by various membrane receptors. The organism is phagocytosed and taken into a phagocytic vacuole (a phagosome) that then fuses with an enzyme-containing lysosomal granule. The formation of this phagolysosome usually results in the destruction of the micro-organism. There are two main systems involved: the oxygen-dependent one and the oxygen-independent one, the former being the most powerful. In the **oxygen-dependent system** (the peroxi-dase-myeloperoxidase-halide system), phagocytosis is followed by an increase in hexose monophosphate shunt activity. This leads to conversion of oxygen to superoxide anion, hydrogen peroxide, single oxygen and hydroxyl radicals. These are all able to destroy microorganisms. Myeloperoxidase generates free halide ions that have powerful bactericidal and viricidal activities. The **oxygen-independent agents** include low pH, lysozyme, lactoferrin, leukin, phagocytin and a variety of hydrolytic enzymes that damage bacterial cell walls and result in digestion of the microbe.

In general, neutrophils generate more toxic oxygen components than monocytes and macrophages and are more effective at rapid killing of microorganisms. Macrophages are more versatile than the polymorphs and are crucial to the elimination of a variety of chronic infective agents as well as participating in a number of immunoregulatory processes.

Many successfully infective microorganisms resist killing and digestion in phagocytic vacuoles and certain organisms are adapted to growing in phagocytes. Specific examples will be found in Chapter 5. With increasing age there appears to be a change in the population of neutrophil polymorphs, some of which seem to show a defect in their phagocytic ability.

Phagocytin. Extracts of the cytoplasm of polymorphonuclear leucocytes from several species have been found to contain an acid-soluble protein bactericidal for Gram-negative bacteria and also for a few Gram-positive organisms. Phagocytin is present together with other antibacterial substances in the granules of polymorphs.

Temperature

The temperature dependence of many microorganisms, is well known and tubercle bacilli, pathogenic for mammalian species, will not infect cold-blooded animals. Hens, which are naturally immune to anthrax, can be infected if their temperature is lowered.

Gonococci are readily killed at temperatures over 40°C and fever therapy was a common treatment of gonococcal infection before the introduction of antibiotics.

It is therefore apparent that temperature is an important factor in determining the innate immunity of an animal to some infective agents and it seems likely that the **pyrexia** which follows so many different types of infection can function as a **protective** response against the infecting microorganisms. Recent evidence shows that human lymphocytes cultured at 39° and 41°C show enhanced responsiveness to plant haemagglutinins (p. 106) and streptococcal products.

The complement system

The existence of a heat-labile serum component with the ability to lyse red blood cells and destroy Gram-negative bacteria has been known for the last 50 years or so. The chemical complexity of the phenomenon was not initially appreciated by early workers who ascribed the activity to a single component — **complement**. Complement is an extremely complex group of serum proteins, present in low concentration in normal serum, consisting of at least 20 plasma glycoproteins. These include 13 components of the classical and alternative pathways and 7 control proteins. Because of its broad range of biological effects, complement activation has been implicated in a variety of physiological situations. Complement activation may be linked to other humoral mediators of inflammation including the kinin and clotting systems. In model systems, one of the components, C3, seems to play a role in the development of immunological memory (p. 44) and the switch from IgM to IgG in the primary immune response (p. 78) to certain types of an antigen.

Complement components have the characteristic of interacting with certain antibody molecules once these have combined with antigen. These components are best known for their ability to combine with anti-erythrocyte antibody attached to the red cell membrane, the effect of complement being to bring about lysis of the red cell by what appears to be enzymic digestion of small areas of the cell membrane. Much of what is known today about the complement system comes from studies of immune haemolysis.

Complement, together with the blood clotting, fibrinolytic and kinin generating systems, are triggered enzyme cascade systems. The first three complement components, C1, 4 and 3, circulate in an inactive form as proenzymes and are converted to their active form by their predecessors in the cascade. Complement components are not all synthesized by a single type of cell and are all fairly large proteins, C3 being the most abundant with a concentration of about 1200 μg/ml serum. The intestinal epithelium, macrophage, liver and spleen are the main sources of the components.

It is now established that the system can be activated in two different ways, the classical pathway and the alternative pathway. The events proceed in a sequential fashion by conformational changes in a protein complex by breaking peptide bonds to release fragments of the original molecule. These fragments are given small letters, the major fragments being assigned the letter b, e.g. C3b, and the smaller peptides usually given an a, e.g. C3a. In both the classical and alternative pathways C3 activation is the common central event. The **classical pathway** in typically initiated by complexes of antibody and antigen in solution or on the surface of a cell. IgM, IgM_1, IgG_2 and IgG_3 subclasses in particular are complement-activating, whereas IgG_4, IgA, IgD and IgE are not (p. 95).

An outstanding feature of the activation of the classical complement pathway is the fragmentation or cleaving of individual components into **large** fragments, which enter into combination with other complement components, and **small** fragments, which have other biological activities described later.

Classical pathway

1. The first component C1 is a complex of three subcomponents q, r and s. C1q is made up of six subunits with globular heads connected to a collagen-like stem and interacts with the second constant domain of the antibody molecule.

2. C1s then acts on the C2 and C4 glycoproteins resulting in a complex called C3 convertase (C4bC2a).

3. The convertase acts on C3 and splits it into a small C3a and a large C3b subunit.

4. C3a is released into the body fluids and acts as an anaphylatoxin that contracts smooth muscle, increases vascular permeability and releases histamine.

5. C3b, in association with its activating enzyme, forms another enzyme, C5 convertase that acts on C5 to produce a small fragment C5a that acts as an anaphylatoxin and chemotaxin (see below) and a large fragment C5b that remains bound to the activating complex.

6. This leads to the incorporation of the remaining complement components C6 to C9. The complex is able to bring about the formation of transmembrane channels in the walls of antibody coated cells like erythrocytes or bacteria, leading to lysis.

Alternative pathway

1. This starts at the C3 step missing out the C1, C4 and C2 components.

2. Initiation depends on aggregated immunoglobulins, various polysaccharides including endotoxin, zymosan and agar that take up C3b that is believed to be continuously formed in small amounts.

3. These substances in the presence of magnesium ions convert a beta-globulin of 100 000 molecular weight called factor B into a C3 activator that splits C3 as in the classical pathway.

4. There is a positive feedback system in which a split product of C3 (C3b) interacts with factor B and other factors to amplify the stimulus leading to increased C3 cleavage.

5. Activation of this pathway can occur in the absence of antibody and thus help in the first line of defence against microorganisms and mediate inflammatory changes.

Regulation of the complement system

1. Uncontrolled activation of the system is avoided in part by the lability of the activated components and by several serum proteins that limit activation. These include a C1 esterase inhibitor and C3b inactivator (factor 1). Factor 1 helped by factor H attacks free C3b in solution or on the surface of cells and cleaves the molecule to non functional products.

2. Red cells have receptors for complement components that bind active components for degradation by inactivating enzymes.

3. Human serum also contains an anaphylatoxin inactivator that destroys C3a, C4a and C5a.

Figure 2.2 shows the biological effects of activation products of the complement system.

Red cell lysis, whilst the most intensively studied complement activity, is by no means the only role played by the complex. Complement action is of some considerable importance because of its ability to neutralize various types of cell such as human cells or Gram-negative bacteria after they have interacted with antibody.

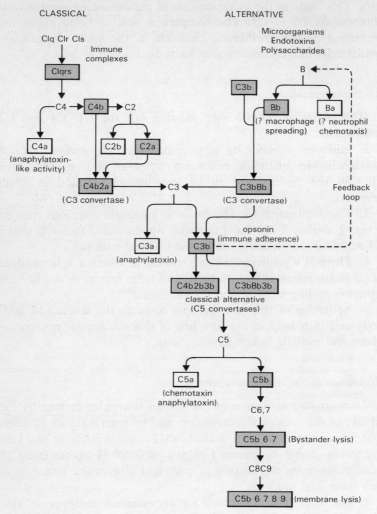

Fig. 2.2 Simplified view of activation of complement pathways and activities of components. Shaded boxes indicate components involved in completion of cascade. The C3 convertases 'decay' by release of C2a or Bb accelerated by control proteins C4BP and factor H.

Complement appears to render the bacteria susceptible to lysozyme. Tumour cells for example can survive indefinitely in the presence of antibody but on the addition of complement the cells develop blebs in the membrane, become fragile and lose many of their intracellular constituents, leading to death of the cell. Another extremely important role of complement is in the attraction of polymorphonuclear phagocytes to sites of antigen-antibody inter-action. This important step in the inflammatory process is known as **chemotaxis** and appears to depend on the components C5, 6 and 7 interacting with the C1, 4, 2, 3 complex. C5a itself has a chemotactic effect. In hypersensitivity states (Ch. 9) complement activation is responsible for the formation of substances known as **anaphylatoxins,** three of which are identifiable by molecular weight differences (7500, 8500 and 10 000). They arise after C3 and C5 activation and are responsible for bringing about the release of histamine leading to increased vascular permeability and smooth muscle contraction. The formation of the plasma kinins, e.g. C-kinin, which are active in hypersensitivity states, also appears to depend upon complement activation. Complement components C1–C3 are concerned in promoting phagocytosis and act as **opsonins** (p. 103). Table 2.4 shows some of the biological effects of activation products of the complement system.

Many cells of the lymphoid system have receptors for complement components. Macrophages and B lymphocytes (p. 71), for example, react with split products of C3 (C3b), which may play

Table 2.4 Biological effects of activation products of complement system

Complexes and components involved	Activities
C1,4	Neutralization of herpes simplex virus together with IgM
C1,4,2	Possible generation of kinins, increase in vascular permeability
C3b	Immune adherence, C3b on rbc[1], wbc[2] or platelet adheres to normal rbcs — agglutination in vitro
	Viruses coated with Ig and complement adhere to platelets or rbcs resulting in removal by phagocytes
C3a	Anaphylatoxin (contraction of smooth muscle, increased vascular permeability and histamine release)
C3e[3]	Mobilization of leucocytes (leucocyte promoting factor)
C3b, C5a	Stimulation of oxidative metabolism of phagocyctes
C5a	Leucocyte chemotaxis
	Anaphylatoxin
	Adherence of leucocytes to vascular endothelium
C5–9	Lysis of susceptible bacteria or cells
C8, 9	Cytotoxic effect

[1] red blood cell. [2] white blood cell. [3] C3e appears to be derived from C3c by proteolytic cleavage which is itself derived from C3b by the action of β1H globulin and the C3b inactivator. Many of the biological effects are mediated by a variety of cellular receptors such as the C3b/C4b (CRI) receptor.

a part in triggering the activation of the lymphocyte and in phagocytosis by macrophages of antigen-antibody complexes with
bound complement.

Complement deficiencies

Normal human serum, as noted above, contains an inhibitor (an
α_2-neuraminoglycoprotein) of C1 esterase. This inhibitor may be
quantitatively or qualitatively deficient and lead to the condition
known as hereditary angioneurotic oedema. The effects are probably due to the formation of anaphylatoxins with the consequent
release of histamine. Complement deficiencies are rare, but hereditary deficiencies of the C1 and components, C2 and C4 are
accompanied in many cases by a variety of chronic diseases,
including recurrent infections and renal disease.

Deficiencies of the later complement components C5 to C9 are
associated with recurrent or disseminated gonorrhoea and meningococcal infections. Deficiency of C2 is associated with a number
of disease states including systemic lupus erythematosus, poly-
myositis and glomerulonephritis. Deficiency of any of the early
components C1 to C4 is associated with immune complex disease
(Ch. 8). In laboratory practice complement lysis tests have wide
and important applications (p. 279).

FURTHER READING

Bacteriological Reviews 1960 Symposium on mechanisms of non-specific
  resistance to infection. Bacteriological Reviews 24:1
van Furth R 1975 Mononuclear phagocytes in immunity. Blackwell, Oxford
Howard J. G. 1963 Natural immunity. In: Cruickshank R (ed) Modern trends in
  immunology I. Butterworth, London
Lachmann P. J, Peters D. K. 1982 Clinical aspects of immunology, 4th edn.
  Blackwell, Oxford
Mackaness G. B., Blanden R. V. 1967 Cellular immunity. Progress in Allergy
  11:89
Müller-Eberhard H. J. 1975 Complement. Annual Review of Biochemistry 44:697
Nelson D. S. 1976 Immunobiology of the macrophage. Academic Press, New
  York
Schur P. H., Austen K. F. 1968 Complement in human disease. Annual Review
  of Medicine 19:1
Vogt W 1974 Activation, activities and pharmacologically active products of
  complement. Pharmacological Reviews 28:125

3

Antigens

Objectives

One completion of this section the reader will be able to:
1. Define immunogen and hapten.
2. Describe the concept of 'foreign' in terms of the immune system.
3. List three important determinants of antigenic specificity.
4. List three molecular requirements for immunogenicity.

Antigens are substances of various chemical types capable of stimulating the immune system of an animal to produce a response specifically directed at the inducing substance and not other unrelated substances. The specificity of the immune response for chemical structures (antigenic determinants) of the antigen molecule is an important characteristic. An antibody directed against an antigenic determinant of a particular molecule will react only with this determinant or another **very similar** structure. Even minor chemical changes in the determinant with the resulting change in shape will markedly alter the ability of the determinant to react with antibody. The term antigen, referring to substances capable of acting as specific stimulants of the immune response or reacting with antibody in an in vitro serological tests, is used rather loosely by immunologists.

Immunogens and haptens

Substances which de novo are capable themselves of inducing an immune response are sometimes referred to as **immunogens** and are usually large molecules. In contrast, substances (often simple chemicals) incapable alone of inducing an immune response are termed **haptens**. To induce an immune response the hapten requires to be attached to a carrier molecule (usually a serum protein such as albumin). The hapten molecule then acts as a

31

determinant of antigenic specificity and is referred to as an **antigenic determinant**. Immunogens also have antigenic determinants which are simply particular chemical groupings within the macromolecule and are referred to as epitopes. Their study has been greatly aided by the advent of monoclonal antibodies (p. 79) that are directed against individual epitopes within complex macromolecules.

Specificity and cross-reactions

It is important at this point to distinguish clearly between structural specificity of an antigenic determinant and its distribution specificity. For example, the ubiquitous nature of the glucose molecule — present in many different types of macromolecule — must be distinguished from its specific chemical structure. An immune response against a glucose determinant in antigen AG would be likely to react also with glucose in antigen BG provided the two determinants are equally accessible. The antibody directed against the glucose determinant is not, as is sometimes thought, a non-specific type of antibody but is simply reacting with an identical chemical determinant in another antigen molecule. A typical cross-reaction is with pneumococcal polysaccharide type S-VIII which has a tetrasaccharide repeating unit containing cellobiuronic acid alternating with an isomer of lactose. Antisera to such a structure will cross-react with oxidized cotton cellulose containing cellobiuronic acid residues.

Heterophile and Forssman antigens

In laboratory serological practice, **cross-reactions** are a common source of difficulty, and cross-reactivity is often found between antisera to certain bacterial antigens and antigens present in cells such as erythrocytes. Antigens shared in this way are known as **heterophile antigens** and antisera to these will cross-react with cells or fluids of many different species of animal and with various microorganisms. The chemical determinants responsible for this cross-reactivity are not known but are presumed to be similar or identical groupings possibly mucopolysaccharides and lipids present in large structural molecules. The best known of the heterophile antigens is the **Forssman** antigen which is present in the red cells of many species as well as in bacteria such as pneumococci and salmonellae. Another heterophile antigen is found in

E. coli and human red cells of group B. Another important example is the cross-reaction between *Treponema pallidum* and an extract of mammalian heart — **cardiolipin**. The common shared antigenic structures are phosphatidylglycerols differing only in their fatty acid side groups. Cardiolipin, being more readily available than *Treponema pallidum*, serves as a useful antigen in the serological test for syphilis (p. 279).

Carbohydrate, lipids, nucleic acids and protein antigens

It is common to classify antigens as proteins, polysaccharides or lipids; this is, however, an oversimplified view. Although many molecules of entirely protein, polysaccharide or lipid nature are antigens, it is also not infrequent to find carbohydrate moieties as determinants on protein or lipid macromolecules or peptide units as determinants on polysaccharide macromolecules.

Carbohydrate determinants are commonly found in the cell wall of bacteria, and antibodies to these determinants are used for grouping the organisms. Streptococcal cell walls contain such antigens, and group A organisms have N-acetylglucosamine as the predominant determinant. In contrast group C streptococci have N-acetylgalactosamine as the main determinant. Pneumococci also contain polysaccharide in their capsules and the biological importance of these is discussed in Chapter 5.

Lipids and nucleic acids in purified form are not good at inducing an immune response and have to be complexed with a larger molecule or altered in some way before they do so. For example, nucleic acids conjugated to methylated bovine serum albumin can induce antibody formation. Nucleic acids as antigens are of some interest to immunologists as antinucleic acid antibodies are found in patients with the disease systemic lupus erythematosus (p. 253).

Proteins are highly complex molecules and have featured prominently in immunological studies because of their wide distribution in nature and their ready availability in highly purified form. Unfortunately, in the present state of knowledge of the antigenic determinants of protein molecules, so little information is available about the precise nature of the peptides acting as determinants in different protein macromolecules that immunologists still describe antigens in terms of the whole molecule, e.g. bovine serum albumin (BSA), rather than the individual determinants of specificity within the macromolecule.

Antigenic determinants

Degradation, chemical modification and synthesis of determinants

The number of determinants or epitopes (sometimes referred to as its valency) in a molecule like BSA is probably in excess of 18 although only about 6 of these are exposed in the native intact molecule. The other (hidden) determinants can be identified only when the molecule is broken down by, for example, enzyme hydrolysis. Antibody produced in response to injection of the whole molecule appears to be able to react with the fragments produced by hydrolysis, and it therefore appears that the molecule is broken down into similar fragments after injection. This might be brought about by the digestive enzymes in phagocytic cells (p. 22 and also 73).

Attempts to identify the chemical nature of antigenic determinants have used this type of degradation procedure with some degree of success and some insight has been gained into the size and other features of the determinants. Two other approaches have also been used — chemical modification of known determinants and synthesis of polyamino acid and polysaccharide antigens. The use of monoclonal antibodies referred to above (p. 79) is a recent valuable development in the analysis of the epitopes in macromolecules.

Degradation studies have been carried out on silk fibrin, a linear polypeptide chain of molecular weight between 50 000 and 60 000. The determinant site capable of reacting with antibody appears to consist of between eight to 12 amino acids 270–440 nm with the C terminal tyrosine making a considerable contribution to the site. The important role of **tyrosine** is further supported by the finding that the poor antigen gelatin can be made antigenic by the addition of tyrosine, in which the native molecule is very deficient. The possibility that tyrosine confers rigidity on the gelatin molecule has been suggested (see also p. 38).

The protein coat of tobacco mosiac virus consists of identical subunits (approx. 2000) each with a molecular weight of about 16 500 consisting of 158 amino acids. The antigenic determinant site is present in the chain between position 108 and 112 and, unlike fibrin, contains no aromatic amino acids. The hydrophobic nature of leucine appears to be an important characteristic of this particular determinant site.

The blood group substances are large molecules consisting of about 75% polysaccharide and 25% polypeptide. Degradation studies have shown that the substances owe their specificity to groups at the end of the carbohydrate chains, for example, A substances specificity is determined by α-N-acetylgalactosaminoyl-(1–3)-galactose.

Foreignness

A substance which acts as an antigen in one species of animal may not do so in another because it is represented in the tissues or fluids of the second species. This underlines the requirement that an antigen must be a **foreign** substance to elicit an immune response. For example, it follows that egg albumin, whilst an excellent antigen in the rabbit, fails to induce an antibody response in a fowl. The more foreign a substance is to a particular species the more likely it is to be a powerful antigen. A good antigen need not contain different building blocks, e.g. amino acids of a protein, but their arrangement should be such that at least part of the surface of the molecule present a configuration which is unfamiliar to the animal. Since macromolecules have a three-dimensional structure, it is easy to visualize how they could become unfolded by denaturation so as to present new and unique surface arrangements.

Foreignness can be a property which depends on chemical groupings which are entirely unfamiliar to the animals. Arsonic acid, for example, can be introduced by diazotization into a protein molecule. Such a group is known as a **hapten** and acts as the **determinant** of the **antigenic specificity** of the molecule, the protein to which the hapten is attached functioning simply as a **carrier molecule**.

Karl Landsteiner in the early part of this century carried out very extensive studies on the antigenic specificity of such hapten chemical determinants resulting in a new appreciation of how critical and precise was the fit between antibody and an antigenic determinant. Landsteiner's work with, for example, the arsonic acid determinant (AsO_3H_2) showed that changes, even as minor as the replacement in the benzine ring, of the AsO_3H_2 group by a COOH or a SO_3H group (Fig. 3.1) was sufficient to affect substantially the ability of azoproteins containing the determinant to react with antibody against the unchanged hapten.

The influence of changes in shape brought about without the removal or substitution of groups is shown by studies with stereoisomers of macromolecules containing tartaric acid where the antibody to L-tartaric acid fails to combine with its isomer D-

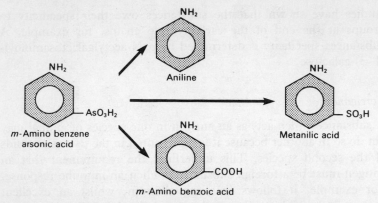

Fig. 3.1 Rabbit antisera to azoproteins containing any of the above acid radicals as antigenic determinants react only with the inducing azoprotein and not with any of to others. Even azoproteins obtained by changing the — COOH of *m*-amino benzoic acid or the — SO₃H of metanilic acid to the ortho or para positions do not react with antisera to the original determinant. Methyl and halogen radicals substituted in the benzene ring instead of the acid radicals shown in the figure are less effective as determinants of specificity and considerable cross reactions are found in precipitin tests

tartaric acid. It was concluded from studies of this type (a) that **acidic** and **basic** groups are very important in regulating the specificity of an antigenic determinant, (b) that **spatial** configuration of haptens is important, (c) that **terminal** group in an antigen are often important determinants of specificity and (d) that **interchange** of non-ionic groups of similar size had little effect on specificity of a determinant.

It became clear from studies of this type that a very slight variation in the chemical constitution or even shape of a molecule could substantially affect the ability of antibody to combine with it. Despite this knowledge immunologists even today are still far from understanding the chemical nature of the determinant groups in complex proteins and polysaccharides. Studies by Sela in Israel with synthetic polypeptides show that the **surface arrangements** of the amino acids in a branched polyamino acid structure are critical as determinants of antigenic specificity (Fig. 3.2).

If the three-dimensional structure of a protein is altered by heating or other form of denaturation, it is no longer able to combine as effectively with antibody to the original native molecule. Enzymes act as antigens and RNase molecules after oxidation became unfolded and the change in shape prevents the interaction of the molecule with antibody to native RNase.

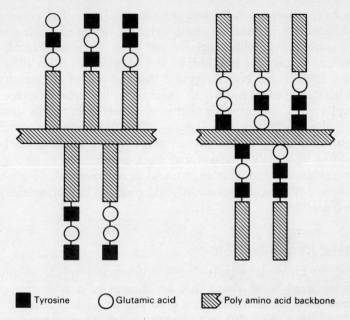

■ Tyrosine   ◯ Glutamic acid   ▧ Poly amino acid backbone

Fig. 3.2 The amino acids, tyrosine, glutamic acid can convert a non-antigenic polyamino acid branched structure (polyalanine and polylysine) into an antigen provided they are attached to the outer end of the branches (left); if attached at the inner end of the branches (right) the complex is not antigenic.

Immunogenicity

Molecular size

For a substance to be antigenic in its own right (i.e. an immunogen) without the need to be attached to a carrier molecule, requires that it has certain properties which have not yet been fully defined. Amongst these is the fact that **high molecular weight** materials are better antigens than those of low molecular weight but above a certain threshold it does not appear to be a determining factor. A substance below a molecular weight of about 5000 is not likely to be a good antigen. This phenomenon may be partly explained by the presence in a larger molecule of repeating antigenic determinant groups, and in a complex molecule of a large variety of potential determinants, one or more being capable of preferentially stimulating an immune response.

Large molecular size alone is not sufficient to confer antigenicity on a substance. Synthetic polymers of many types can be built up into large macromolecules and are non-antigenic. The polyamino acid backbone (polyalanine and polylysine) of the molecule shown in Figure 3.2 is non-antigenic and only becomes capable of inducting an immune response by the addition of further different amino acids. It has been suggested that the lack of antigenicity of synthetic polymers is due to their lack of internal molecular complexity. Thus the antigenicity of naturally occurring macromolecules may be due to their many different low molecular weight constituents giving complexity to the molecule. Tyrosine has been found to be a helpful constituent for a polypeptide to be a good immunogen although this amino acid is not essential. In general, aromatic amino acids consistently enhance the immunogenicity of a polypeptide.

Physical state, shape and charge

Some low molecular weight chemical substances appear to contradict the need noted above that an antigen be a large molecule. Among these are included picryl chloride, formaldehyde and drugs such as aspirin, penicillin and sulphonamides. These substances are highly antigenic, particularly if applied to the skin. The reason for this appears to be that such materials form **complexes** by means of covalent bonds with tissue protein, and the complex of these substances, acting as haptens with tissue protein carrier, forms complete antigen. This has important implications in the development of certain types of hypersensitivity states (p. 231).

The physical state of a protein antigen can affect its antigenicity. The same substance, e.g. the serum protein BSA, in aggregated and aggregate-free form can show wide divergence in ability to stimulate immunity, the aggregated form being strongly antigenic in the rabbit while the aggregate-free form induces a specific state of unresponsiveness (immunological tolerance, p. 45). This knowledge of the influence of **particle size** has been applied to production of antisera to snake venoms. The venom (neurotoxin) of low molecular weight and thus poor immunogenicity was linked to carboxymethylcellulose resin. The toxin-resin complex was non-toxic and highly immunogenic in rabbits.

Some molecules carry what is sometimes called 'built-in-adjuvanticity', which means that they have the capacity to stimulate the cells of the antibody system in a non-specific manner so that they are able to handle antigen more effectively. Bacterial endotoxin produces this effect as also do *Bordetella pertussis* organisms; these materials can enhance the antigenicity of a weak antigen if administered at the same time. The effect seems likely to be due to a powerful 'triggering' effect by bacterial endotoxin on a particular lymphocyte population (B cells, see p. 63) responsible for making antibody. In human immunization the efficacy of the 'triple vaccine', diphtheria, pertussis, tetanus, is partly due to the effect of *B. pertussis* (p. 173).

Polysaccharide antigen, for example dextran of molecular weight (mol.wt) 600 000, is a good antigen, whereas a dextran of mol.wt 100 000 is not. There is no obvious reason for this as the two materials are made up of identical building blocks and do not differ as far as the type of antigenic determinant is concerned.

The effect of electric charge of a molecule on its immunogenicity has been studied and found to be unrelated to its ability to induce an immune response. Polypeptides in which the net charge was zero elicited comparable amounts of antibody as charged polypeptides.

The shape of a polypeptide molecule does not affect its ability to elicit an antibody response and linear polypeptides which have no organized conformational structure can be potent immunogens.

Persistence of antigen

The ability of an animal to **degrade** a polysaccharide antigen can affect its immune reactivity to the antigen. Some pneumococcal polysaccharides appear to be resistant to digestion in the mouse and in sufficient dose are able to mop up antibody as it is made, resulting in the absence of detectable antibody in the serum. The same effect can be produced if the antigen is protected in some way from the tissue fluids and inflammatory cells. This can occur if the material is incorporated in oil as an emulsion (see p. 91) or is walled off by fibrous tissue. The antigen dose, form, route of entry, host determinants and use of vaccines are discussed in Chapter 4.

FURTHER READING

Barrett J T 1974 Textbook of immunology, 2nd edn. Kimpton, London
Borek F 1972 Molecular size and shape of antigens. In: Borek F (ed) Immunogenicity. North Holland, Amsterdam, p 45
Boyd W C 1963 Fundamentals of immunology. Inter-science, London
Dumonde D C 1965 Tissue-specific antigens. Advances in Immunology 5:30
Gill T J 1972 The chemistry of antigens and its influence on immunogenicity. In: Borek F (ed) Immunogenicity. North Holland, Amsterdam, p 5

Heidelberger M 1956 Lectures in immunochemistry. Academic Press, New York
Kabat E A 1968 Structural concepts in immunology and immunochemistry. Holt, Rinehart & Winston, New York
Landsteiner K 1945 The specificity of serological reactions. Harvard University Press, Cambridge, Mass.
Sela M 1965 Immunological studies with synthetic polypeptides. Advances in Immunology 5:30
Sela M (ed) 1975 The antigens. Academic Press, New York

4

Acquired immunity

Objectives

On completion of this section the reader will able to:

1. Describe the two forms of adaptive immunity, humoral and cell-mediated.

2. Outline the main determinants in the genetic control of immunity.

3. Differentiate between active and passive immunity.

4. Starting with bone marrow stem cells, describe the development of the cells of the immune system.

5. Describe the filtration and trapping function of the lymphoid organs and draw a diagram of their general structure.

6. Briefly describe the evolution of the immune system.

7. Differentiate primary from secondary immune response; consider time of response, types of antibodies produced, longevity of the response.

8. List three determinants of acquired immunity.

9. Give examples of the three main types of adjuvants.

10. Draw a diagram of the IgG molecule; describe its possible evolution.

11. List in the form of a table the five classes of immunoglobulin and their characteristic properties.

12. Draw a diagram of the molecular structure of the IgG molecule and describe the functions of the individual domains and how diversity of the five regions is generated.

13. Define allotypes and idiotypes.

14. Describe two selective transport mechanisms for immunoglobulins.

15. List the cells concerned in the initiation of immunity and their characteristic surface markers and receptors.

16. Identify and outline the role of antigen presenting or inducer cells in the immune response.

17. Define immune tolerance.

18. Describe the role of T lymphocyte subclasses and how they are distinguished by differentiation antigens.

19. Outline the subcellular processes involved in immunoglobulin synthesis by B lymphocytes.

20. Define immunological memory.

21. Describe the differences between selective and directive theories of immunity and outline the clonal selection theory.

22. Describe the germline and somatic mutation hypothesis in the generation of antibody diversity.

23. Describe lymphocyte transformation.

24. List 10 cytokines (lymphokines and monokines) and describe their main role in immunity.

25. Briefly describe the role of the thymus in the immune response; what is thymic education?

26. Describe the main events in the cell-cooperative processes that lead to an immune response.

27. Describe the routes of lymphocyte recirculation and the advantages of the recirculation process.

28. Draw a diagram of the mouse and human MHC region and indicate the function of the different loci and on which cells they are present.

29. List the phagocytes of the immune system, describe their origin, regulation and function.

OVERVIEW

Microorganisms that overcome or circumvent the innate immune mechanisms come up against the body's second line of defence. This is the acquired or adaptive immune response and, as the description indicates, this form of immunity differs from innate immunity in that it does not pre-exist but is acquired by contact and adaptation to the inducing agent. All that pre-exists is a population of cells that are capable of recognizing, responding and remembering following their exposure to a foreign agent such as the antigens of a microorganism. The mechanisms by which cells of the immune system recognize, respond and remember their contact with antigen has been the main subject of study of immunologists during the last 20 years.

THE RESPONSE

Forms of response

1. This falls into two categories: a) a response that triggers certain cells of the immune system to manufacture globulin proteins that are secreted into the tissue fluids and blood and that are capable of binding to and neutralizing foreign antigens. This is the humoral immune response in which immunoglobulins (antibodies) are produced that have the ability to recognize and bind specifically to the antigen that induced their formation and not to other antigens; b) a response that requires the generation of certain types of lymphoid cells that themselves have the ability by means of surface receptors to recognize foreign materials such as microorganisms, or infected cells expressing the antigens of their infecting microorganism, and to attack and destroy them. This is called the cell-mediated immune response.

2. An acquired immune state may be induced in two main ways: a) by overt clinical infection or sometimes by subclinical (inapparent) infections — including gut flora, and by artificial immunization. This form of immunization is called active immunization; b) by transfer, either naturally via the placenta or in milk, or artificially by transfer of antibody made in another individual, or sometimes by lymphoid cells. This form of immunization is called passive immunization.

3. The first exposure of an individual to a foreign antigen results in the development of an immune response that takes a week or two to provide detectable levels of antibody or cell-mediated immunity and this is called a primary immune response. In contrast, a second exposure to the same antigen after primary immunity has developed leads to a very rapid and steeply rising level of immunity that persists at a plateau for weeks or months. Figure 4.11 (p. 88) shows the characteristics of the primary and secondary responses.

Features of the response

1. It is important to realize that the normal acquired immune response involves a combination of both forms of immunity and that they can interact with one another so that certain cells of the lymphoid system along with immunoglobulins can act together to destroy infected cells or microorganisms.

2. The immune response is a physiological reaction to the introduction into the body of foreign material, irrespective of whether it is harmful or not and this feature is used experimentally to work out the mechanisms of immunity using bland foreign materials such as foreign red blood cells or serum proteins.

3. In contrast to innate immunity the acquired response does not vary substantially between species but does vary to an extent between individuals within a species. This variation is under genetic control and takes two forms: a) control of the general capacity to produce an antibody response — first demonstrated by selectively breeding mice and guinea pigs on the basis of their ability to produce a good or poor immune response to several antigens, thus high and low responding groups were bred; b) control of the ability to respond to a particular antigen, usually a synthetic polypeptide. The genes controlling the ability to produce an immune response are sometimes called the immune response genes (Ir genes) and in the mouse are in the I region of chromosome 17 and in man in the DR region of chromosome 6. The activity of these genes has effects on the susceptibility of individuals to certain infectious diseases and will be discussed later.

4. An important feature of acquired immunity is that the immune system, after first exposure to a foreign antigen, develops a memory called immunological memory so that a recall reaction (sometimes called an anamnestic response) can develop quickly to a second exposure to the same antigen. This clearly has important consequences for protection against environmental infectious agents and sometimes persists for the lifetime of an individual (as in many viral infections). Lack of persistence of protection appears to be due not to loss of specific immunological memory but due to the fact that the infective agent may have changed its antigenic structure, as in the case of certain parasites, or that a new strain appears in the environment.

5. High doses of antigen tend to induce antibody of low average affinity whilst low doses induce high affinity antibody. This is because the lymphoid cells that have receptors that 'capture' the antigen vary in their ability to bind the antigen. Cells that bind strongly compete for the antigen with cells that bind the antigen weakly thus with low doses of antigen the stronger binding cells have an advantage. The antibody made by the stronger binding cells is itself better able to bind antigen and is thus of a higher affinity.

6. High doses of antigen are able to 'paralyse' the lymphoid cells so that they are unable to make specific antibody to the antigen. This is called immunological tolerance, the mechanisms of induction of which are complex and is brought about by certain infectious agents that shed large quantities of their surface antigens or exert direct effects on the function of cells of the immune system and will be dealt with in relation to specific infections later in the text.

7. The response is internally regulated both by feedback regulation due to antibodies and lymphoid cells, but also by immunoregulatory 'hormone-like' factors called cytokines produced by particular cells within the immune system (see p. 110).

8. Various hormones have been known for some time to influence the immune response by effects on the lymphoid tissues, for example, thyroid hormone and growth hormones enhance the response and glucocorticoids decrease it. Interactions between the neuroendocrine and immune systems in immunoregulatory processes are beginning to be understood, with pituitary peptides such as endorphins and corticotrophin having immunosuppressive effects. Brain macroglia (astrocytes, oligodendrocytes, ependymal cells) provide metabolic support and regulate the function of neurones. Macroglia respond to and synthesise several soluble factors that are either immunologically active or resemble lymphokines. Natural Killer (NK) cell activity (p. 64) has been found to be reduced in medical students stressed by examinations and recently divorced women have been shown, in a study in the US, to have reduced numbers of NK cells and other leucocytes together with increased herpes virus infections. These observations are seen as likely to lead to a better understanding of stress-related depression of immune reactivity and possibly of new strategies for prophylaxis and treatment of certain types of human disease. It is uncertain at present if the changes in immune reactivity noted after stress necessarily imply immune compromise.

Effector mechanisms

As indicated above there are two forms of acquired immunity — humoral or antibody-mediated and cellular or cell-mediated. To understand the details of the mechanisms of these types of immunity it is necessary to have a knowledge of the types of molecules and cells involved and these will be described later in this chapter.

In this introductory section it is sufficient to point out that in humoral immunity the molecules involved are immunoglobulins of which five classes have been described — immunoglobulins G, M, A, E and D. These are normally written as IgG, IgM, IgA, IgE and IgD. They are produced by a class of lymphocytes called B lymphocytes (and their differentiated form, plasma cells). These molecules show two main features:

1. The ability to combine with antigen by means of a complementary binding site the shape of which is determined by the sequence of amino acids in the binding site. The sequence of amino acids thus varies according to the antigenic specificity of the particular immunoglobulin. The elucidation of the genetic control of this variability has been an important subject of study for immunologists over the last few years.

2. The ability to take part in other biological activities, such as binding to receptors on phagocytes (referred to earlier), to activate the classical complement pathway, to allow transfer through membranes such as the placenta and to control the catabolism of the molecule.

Immunoglobulins act as effector molecules utilizing the above two features by combining with an infective agent by means of the complementary binding sites in the immunoglobulin molecule and then using one or more of the biological activities. This results in clumping of the infective agent, referred to as agglutination, or simply immobilizing the infective agent by linking different particles of the agent so that it is no longer free to move and grow in the tissues. Combination of the immunoglobulin with the infective particle can lead to its attachment to a phagocytic cell (and sometimes other cells) by the process of opsonization with subsequent phagocytosis and destruction of the infective agent. By activation of the complement system the infective agent is exposed to the lytic components of the complement cascade. The chemotactic and other components induce an inflammatory response leading to the attraction of leucocytes to the site of infection and to vascular changes so that immunoglobulins and cells can gain access to the site. Immunoglobulins have a further important role in neutralizing toxic products of microorganisms.

Cell mediated immunity is more complex and only incompletely understood. There are two main forms of cell mediated immunity that usually work together in eliminating infective agents.

1. Immunity dependent on macrophages, involving uptake and destruction of microorganisms usually but not always involving

immunoglobulins that bring about the attachment of the microorganism to the surface of the phagocyte. This form of immunity is regulated by cytokines produced by certain lymphocytes sometimes referred to a lymphokines (see p. 110). Macrophage mediated immunity is important particularly in infections involving intracellular infective agents such as viruses and intracellular bacteria or parasites.

2. Immunity dependent on a particular class of lymphocytes referred to as cytotoxic T lymphocytes. These cells recognize the antigens of microorganisms such as viruses on the surface of an infected cell bind to the surface of the cell and lyse the cell. Other ill-defined lymphocytes known as killer cells (K cells) can also destroy infected cells. There are two types, natural killer cells (NK cells) (p. 64) that act independently of immunoglobulins and kill infected cells directly and K cells that depend upon the initial attachment of immunoglobulin to the infected target cell. The K cells have receptors for a portion of the immunoglobulin molecule and bind in this way to the target cell. Phagocytes such as macrophages, neutrophils and eosinophils can also act as killer cells by a similar mechanism.

Further details of these forms of immunity will be described in the following sections.

The immune response — its origins in evolution

Organized lymphoid tissues are **absent in invertebrates** and the most primitive of the vertebrates, the hagfish. This system develops late in phylogeny and the first traces appear in the lamprey. Both these primitive vertebrates are, however, able to show a limited degree of adaptive immunity. Their serum contains a primitive form of immunoglobulin that appears to be related to IgM (see below), which has since become considerably diversified. The amphibians are the most primitive animals to show IgG, and all species higher in the evolutionary scale than birds have IgM, IgG and IgA.

The precursors of the early immunoglobulins are likely to have arisen in the prevertebrate era although as yet there is no direct evidence for this. It has been suggested that they may have arisen from receptors on the surface of phagocytes which enable the cells to distinguish foreign material from self. It seems possible that such receptors could have the molecular properties of the combining site of an antibody molecule (see below).

The **complement system** appeared some time later in evolution and is developed in the jawed vertebrate, the paddle fish. With increasing structural complexity of animal species the immune reaction has become more diversified and effective. However, once components of the immune system appear in evolution they are maintained with a remarkable constancy both at the molecular and functional level.

In the human, lymphoid tissue appears first in the thymus at about eight weeks' gestation. Peyer's patches are distinguishable by the fifth month and immunoglobulin secreting cells appear in the spleen and lymph nodes at about 20 weeks. From this period onwards both IgM and IgG globulins (p. 95) are synthesized by the fetus with IgM predominating. At birth the infant has a blood concentration of IgG comparable to, or sometimes higher than, that of maternal serum, having received IgG but not IgM via the placenta from the mother (p. 104). The rate of synthesis of IgM in the infant increases rapidly within the first few days of life but does not reach adult levels until about a year. This compares with the much slower rise in IgG and IgA globulins which do not reach adult levels until between the sixth and seventh years of life. Cell-mediated immune reactions can be stimulated at birth but these reactions (e.g. homograft rejection) may not be as powerful as in the adult, although the evidence for this is rather scanty.

Invertebrate immunity

For many years it had been generally assumed that the adaptive immune response was a characteristic of the vertebrates and that invertebrates lacked the ability to mount an immune response. The recent recognition of a limited ability in the most primitive of the vertebrates, the hagfish, to exhibit cell-mediated immunity, suggests that the origins of immune response may well have been rather earlier. Immunologists are now exploring the possibility that invertebrates can produce at least some form of adaptive immune response.

Specific recognition by certain primitive marine organisms (coelenterates) of the cells of unrelated species is a well-documented phenomenon and can be seen in colonial hydroids, gorgonians and reef-building corals. **Rejection of grafts** shows convincing specificity, but no immunological memory leading to accelerated rejection on second exposure has been demonstrated.

Invertebrates have a well developed **non-specific** cellular defence

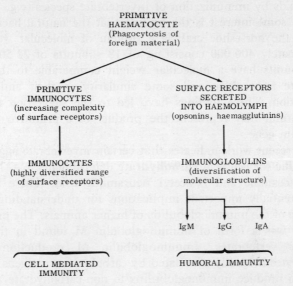

Fig. 4.1 Schematic view of proposed stages in evolutionary development of adaptive immune response

mechanism to cope with foreign materials that enter its tissues. The process is mediated by blood cells called **haemocytes** which phagocytose the foreign particle and localise it in a fibrous nodule. This process is quite distinct from the cell-mediated immune response of vertebrates as it does not result in the formation of a descendant family or clone of cells with a specificity limited to the inducing agent (Fig. 4.1). Evidence has, however, been obtained in work with annelids and echinoderms showing that they are capable of rejecting grafts from unrelated members of the same species. On repeated grafting **accelerated rejection** takes place indicating the development of what could be a secondary immune response. It seems clear that the mechanism underlying this rejection process is quite distinct from the non-specific haemocyte response to any foreign substance and may well turn out on further study to be a form of specific adaptive immune response.

The tissue fluids of invertebrates have been known for many years to contain a variety of **agglutinins** for vertberate eythrocytes. These haemagglutinins can be shown to act as **opsonins** (p. 103) facilitating phagocytosis. Many attempts have been made unsuccessfully to increase the quantity of these haemagglutinins in the tissue fluids by immunization of invertebrate species (e.g. in crayfish). Of some interest is the finding that the natural haemagglutinin of the horseshoe crab is a protein of molecular weight of approximately 400 000 consisting of 18 subunits of 22 500 each. The subunits have a molecular weight comparable to that of a vertebrate light chain and some similarity in their amino acid composition. These findings have led to the suggestion that the haeagglutinin may represent the product of a primitive form of light chain gene.

Some recent work indicates that certain invertebrate agglutinins are **specific** for cell wall **carbohydrate** determinants, e.g. N-acetyl D galactosamine and N-acetyl neuraminic acid. These findings have potentially important implications for understanding of the evolution of the immunoglobulins of higher animals. The precursor of these was a form of immunoglobulin M found in the most primitive vertebrates. Immunoglobulin M production by B lymphocytes is readily stimulated by carbohydrate antigens and the ability to produce immunoglobulins to non-carbohydrate antigens is probably a much more recently evolved and much more complicated process that requires co-operation between different cells of the lymphoid population.

Cell types resembling vertebrate lymphocytes have been observed in the tissue fluid of annelids but there seems to be considerable doubt that such cells are in fact the precursors of vertebrate lymphoid cells. Lymphocytes, macrophages and eosinophils do seem to be present in later phyla, the protochordates.

The finding of late complement components in invertebrates suggests that the alternate pathway (p. 27) may be phylogenetically more ancient than the classical complement system.

In conclusion it appears that immunological phenomena such as **recognition** and **phagocytosis** are found in the earliest eukaryotic cells. Recognition is responsible for maintenance of **specific partnerships** in metazoa, for exclusion of potentially harmful **microorganisms** and perhaps also for removal of altered or dead tissue constituents. **Cellular immune mechanisms,** such as rejection of unrelated tissue cells (initially without immunological memory), is a feature of all eukaryotic animals and precedes the development of humoral immunity. The emergence of organised lymphoid tissues occurred in the early vertebrate era and immune mechanisms became increasingly efficient with the development of cooperative relationships between the different cellular elements.

TISSUES AND CELLS OF THE IMMUNE SYSTEM

Primary lymphoid tissue

Bone marrow and fetal liver

The cells responsible for making the cellular components of the blood, a process called haemopoiesis, originate in the yolk sac of the embryo. These undifferentiated cells are found later in the fetal liver and later in the bone marrow. In the fully developed animal the bone marrow provides the haemopoietic stem cells from which arise the red cells, platelets, and leucocytes of the blood and tissues (Fig. 4.2). These stem cells can be shown to be pluripotent, as by chromosome marker techniques, each of the cell types that develop from the stem cell can be shown to have the same chromosome marker and appear to be derived from identical stem cells.

The first stage of differentiation involving synthesis of DNA by the stem cell under the influence of various glycoproteins derived from mature leucocytes leads to the proliferation of a cell type called a progenitor cell. It differs from the stem cell in that it is responsive to hormone-like factors that lead to further differentiation. The progenitor cells, under the influence of chemotactic factors, seed the different lymphoid organs where the later stages of differentiation take place. These are called haemopoiesis-inducing microenvironments (HIMs). Certain epithelial cells in these microenvironments produce hormone-like factors which are thought to act on the progenitor cells to induce a particular pathway of differentiation. For example, differentiation towards

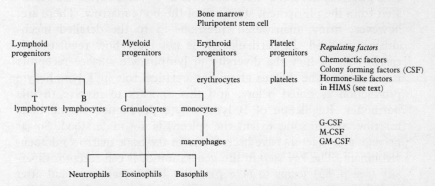

Fig. 4.2 Simplified scheme of haemopoiesis and regulation. CSF are a family of growth factors that regulate the survival, proliferation and differentiation of hemopoietic progenitor cells as well as the functional activity of mature cells.

erythrocytes in the microenvironment of the spleen under the influence of a factor called erythropoietin. Differentiation can occur towards certain lymphocyte types, e.g. thymic lymphocytes, in the thymus by a hormone called thymosin.

The process of differentiation is a continuous one because of the rapid turnover of blood cells. For example in man 1.6×10^9 neutrophils/kg of body weight are produced each day. There is great flexibility in the process so that even greater numbers of cells can be produced when required. The stimuli that lead to the production of these cells are very complex and not yet fully understood. They appear to involve what are called colony stimulating factors acting on the bone marrow stem cells. These factors are produced by blood leucocytes (including activated T lymphocytes p. 108), certain fetal tissues, and the placenta. The process can be modified to increased or decreased production by bacterial products such as endotoxin and various polysaccharide materials. Bone marrow damage by X-rays or cytotoxic drugs also leads to production of stem cell stimulating factors. The role of the colony stimulating factors in vivo has yet to be fully defined as have the environmental influences that enhance and suppress their production. The system has obvious physiological importance in the control of blood cell production including its ability to respond to inflammatory stimuli.

Lymphopoiesis

It is generally accepted that both B and T lymphocytes are generated from the pluripotent stem cell of the bone marrow. There are, however, many unanswered questions as to the detailed mechanisms involved. In particular, it is not clear how regulation is carried out or how the diversity of lymphocyte surface receptors is generated. The thymus gland has a critical role in T lymphocyte production as noted below, and this appears to involve thymic hormones. Regulation of B lymphocyte production in the bone marrow, and to some extent the spleen, is not understood. So far no regulatory factors have been found in the bone marrow microenvironment. The key step in the generation of B cell receptor diversity (see p. 85) seems to take place by DNA rearrangement after B and T cell subclasses have been formed but preceding synthesis of messenger RNA, and, therefore, before immunoglobulin is produced. It is thought that the stem cells resemble germ line cells and are not restricted with respect to the specificity of receptors that their progeny can produce.

The thymus

Development and structure

The thymus in mammals arises from the endoderm of the third and fourth branchial clefts and is the tissue in which lymphocytes can first be recognized. The thymus gland increases in size until puberty and then slowly atrophies although it is still readily recognizable in the adult. The thymus is a bilobed structure with an outer cortex and an inner medulla. The immature cells are in the cortex and pass into the medulla as they mature. The organ is divided into lobules with a network of epithelial cells superimposed on which are bone marrow derived interdigitating cells (see below). Unlike the spleen and lymph nodes there are no germinal centres and no plasma cells. Thus under normal physiological conditions the thymus cells do not make antibody. Plasma cells will appear only if antigen is injected directly into the organ. Hassall's corpuscles are a feature peculiar to the medulla of the thymus and consist of groups of reticular epithelial cells sometimes flattened and concentrically arranged around a central core of nuclear debris.

Cell turnover and humoral factors

The thymus can be shown, by tritiated thymidine incorporation studies, to be actively engaged in lymphopoiesis, there being a higher proportion of primitive actively dividing lymphoid cells than in any other lymphoid tissue such as the spleen or lymph nodes, and with a correspondingly high mitotic rate. Evidence suggests that the stimulus for thymocytes to divide arises in some way from the epithelial cells. The primitive cells in the thymus are slowly replaced during life by cells derived from the bone marrow that migrate via the bloodstream into the thymus. A small proportion of these cells leave the thymus and find their way to the peripheral lymphoid tissues; these are the **longlived lymphocytes** with a life of months in rodents and possibly years in man.

Maturation of T cells during the period they spend in the thymus has been shown to take place. The changes associated with this can be detected by means of **membrane antigens** on the T lympho-cytes. Identification of these antigens has been enormously helped by the advent of monoclonal antibodies (page 79). The main murine antigen markers are known as Thy (theta), TL and Ly anti-gens. The TL antigen is present on the lymphocytes that enter the thymus but is lost on maturation in the gland. The amount of Thy antigen is also much reduced during this period and the Ly anti-gens develop and are expressed on mature T lymphocytes. Various functional characteristics have been found to be associated with different Ly antigens and T lymphocytes carrying such antigens can thus be divided into **subpopulations**. The functional activities that can be defined on the basis of Ly markers are 'helper cell activity' (see cell co-operation, p. 71), cytolysis of allogeneic lymphocytes or tumour cells, i.e. 'cytotoxic T cells' and 'suppressor cell' activity involved in controlling B lymphocytes. Suppressor T cells in the mouse are characterized by surface markers (differen-tiation antigens) and are susceptible to thymectomy, X-irradiation, and cyclophosphamide. Suppressor cells express differentiation antigens, the Ly-2 and Ly-3 antigens as well as antigen coded by the I-J subregion (see p. 114). Helper T cells express Ly-1 antigen. About 60% of Ly-1 cells express an additional antigen, the Qa antigen, coded by a locus close to the H-2D end of the MHC complex in the mouse (Fig. 4.19). The Ly-1 Qa+ cells appear to control the generation of suppressor cells, probably by means of affects on a third subpopulation of lymphocytes expressing Ly-1, 2 and 3 antigens that themselves exert feedback inhibition of the Ly-2 suppressor cells. Human T cells express T1, T3 and T11 anti-gens on the majority of the cells and T4, T1 and T8 on subpo-pulations. Human helper T cells express T4 antigens and suppressor and cytotoxic cells express the T8 antigen. Table 4.1 shows the surface markers on mature murine and human T cells.

The regulatory circuits are very complex as are the experiments designed to elucidate their details. In simple terms, the Ly-1 cells can be thought of as the central lymphocyte population, rather like C3 in the complement system. These cells act to screen the surface of other cells, particularly macrophages, for foreign materials associ-ated with MHC molecules. When such foreign material is 'seen' by the Ly-1 cells, they induce a variety of effector cells to make a specific immune response and at the same time act on resting T cells causing them to emit various stimulatory and inhibitory stimuli. For a more detailed description of these complex regulatory

Table 4.1 Surface markers on mature human and mouse T cells

T Cell surface markers		Role
Human	Mouse	
T4 (CD4, Leu 3)	L3T4	Used by Th cells in T cell receptor recognition of MHC class 2 and antigen
T8 (CD8, Leu 2)	Ly2, 3	Used by Tc cells in T cell receptor recognition of MHC class 1 and antigen also present on Ts cells
T3		On all T cells, may be responsible for delivering activation signal to cell
	Thy-1	On all T cells, function unknown
T1		On most T cells (? Th, Tdh subsets)
T11		On all T cells, function unknown
HLA-DR	Ia	On all mitogen activated T cells
TAC		Interleukin-2 receptor

mechanisms, the reader is referred to the references under Further Reading.

One of the main functions of thymic differentiation is to produce a population of cells that can discriminate between self antigens and foreign antigens such as those expressed on microorganisms or the cells of unrelated individuals. How this is achieved is not yet resolved but one view widely held by immunologists is that T cells are educated within the thymus to recognize a particular group of antigens known as major histocompatibility (MHC) antigens

Table 4.2 Roles of T4 (CD4) helper T lymphocytes

Antigen recognition function in association with MHC class 2 antigens	Ability to respond to both soluble and cell-associated antigens
Helper function	Induce B cells to secrete immunoglobulins and precytotoxic T cells to become cytotoxic effector cells [T8 (CD8)]
Mitogenic function	Secrete leucocyte mitogenic factor that induces proliferation of T cells, B cells, null cells and macrophages
Regulation of suppression	Interact with T8 (CD8) cells to induce suppressor activity of responses to antigens, mitogens and mixed leucocyte reactions

(p. 113). The proposal is that one of the cell types in the thymus — the interdigitating cells — that are rich in MHC class 2 antigens present these to T cells so that they are then educated only to recognize foreign antigens if they are associated with the self MHC antigen. This idea comes from evidence that T helper cells can only recognize foreign antigen on inducer cells (such as macrophages) when the antigen is associated with class 2 MHC antigen (see p. 72 and Table 4.2).

The T4 receptor contains a variable domain (showing a 32% homology in amino acid sequences to the imunoglobulin variable domain), a joining region and a membrane spanning region. Both the T4 and T8 receptors share sequence and structural homology with immunoglobulin variable domains and are members of the **immunoglobulin supergene** family.

Secondary lymphoid tissues

The lymphoid tissues which are predominantly engaged in the immune response are the **lymph nodes, spleen** and **bone marrow**. Whilst the lung and to a lesser extent the liver can both take part in the immune response, their contribution is much less than that of the other tissues. The large overall contribution of the bone marrow is a reflection of the mass of this tissue throughout the skeleton. However, weight for weight the spleen and lymph nodes by far exceed the capacity for antibody production of the bone marrow. For this reason much effort has been expended in attempting to unravel the way in which the specialized lymphoid organs, the spleen and lymph nodes take up foreign antigens and initiate the immune process.

The role of the thymus gland is described above and co-operation between different cell populations in the early events preceding antibody synthesis will be described later in this chapter (p. 71).

The spleen, lymph nodes, bone marrow and other lymphatic tissues that engage in antibody production are **vascular filtration systems**. They depend on a three dimensional network of reticular cells and reticular fibres. In these filters, **antigen** is **trapped** and **cells** become lodged from the circulating blood and lymph and can **interact, differentiate** and **proliferate** in the organ. Collections of non-encapsulated lymphoid cells are found in various organs, especially associated with mucous membranes of the respiratory and gastrointestinal tract, e.g. tonsils and Peyer's patches. These

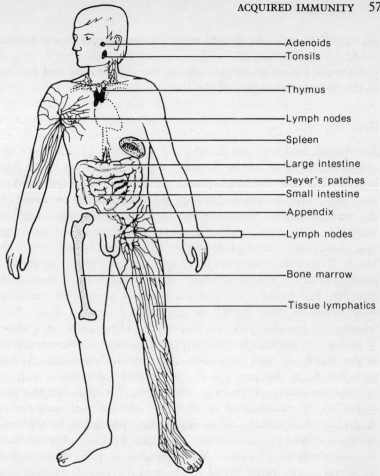

Adenoids
Tonsils
Thymus
Lymph nodes
Spleen
Large intestine
Peyer's patches
Small intestine
Appendix
Lymph nodes
Bone marrow
Tissue lymphatics

Fig. 4.3 Tissues and organs of the immune system. Human lymphoid system: lymphatic vessels collect interstitial fluid from extremities and carry lymphocytes and foreign materials to draining lymph nodes to initiate an immune response. Lymphatic vessels also leave lymph nodes and carry recirculating lymphocytes to neck veins to enter bloodstream. Lymphocytes leave blood via capillaries and via specialised blood vessels in the lymph nodes and spleen and recirculate. This allows recruitment of lymphocytes at sites of inflammation, replenishment of lymphoid organs if existing lymphocytes are destroyed by, for example, X-rays or infectious agents, and enables lymphocytes to have access to antigens anywhere in the tissues. Diagram also shows the bone marrow of a long bone from where the stem cells derive that develop into cells that populate the lymphoid organs (lymph nodes and spleen). Some of these stem cells, before entering these organs, pass via thymus gland and become thymus-derived or T lymphocytes. The respiratory and gastrointestinal tract have collections of lymphoid tissue — tonsils and adenoids of the oropharynx and Peyers patches and appendix of the intestine. The lymphoid tissues are filtering systems to remove foreign antigens from the bloodstream and lymph and where immune responses usually occur. (Reproduced from Blackwell C C, Weir D M 1981 Principles of infection and immunity in patient care. Churchill Livingstone, Edinburgh, p 61)

aggregates of cells are termed mucosal associated lymphoid tissue (MALT) (p. 61)

Figure 4.3 gives an overall view of the distribution and location of the tissues and organs of the immune system.

Gross structure

The **lymph nodes** of the human are structures of the shape and approximate size of a bean. In smaller animals they are of the same general structure but correspondingly smaller. The lymph flows from the limbs and organs through the lymph nodes on its way to the main lymphatic vessels of the neck and their union with the veins. The afferent lymphatics enter the capsule of the node (Fig. 4.4C) and the lymph leaves via the efferent lymphatics of the hilum. Trabeculae extend radially into the node from the capsule, passing from the marginal lymph sinus through the cortex to the medulla. The tissue of the gland consists of a reticular meshwork with dendritic cells spread on the surface and in which large numbers of **lymphocytes** are embedded. These cells are grouped in nodules or **follicles** in the cortex and form interconnected cords in the medullary area sometimes called medullary cords. Around each nodule in the cortex is a condensation of reticular cells. A reticular network provides a scaffolding for the lymphocytes, makes up the sinuses and supports the blood vessels and nerves. A nodule that enlarges after antigenic stimulation is termed a **germinal centre** and includes macrophages with cytoplasmic extensions or dendritic processes. **Macrophages** are present throughout the gland, many being found in the medullary area. **Plasma cells** and their precursors are also found, particularly at the cortico-medullary junction. Arteries enter the node at the hilum and their capillaries end up in post-capillary venules with a tall lining endothelium. Between and through these endothelial cells blood lymphocytes pass into the node.

The **spleen** (Fig. 4.5), like the lymph nodes, is enclosed by a capsule and divided by trabeculae into communicating compartments. The organ plays an important role in destruction of **red cells** and their production; as well as producing **platelets, granulocytes** and **lymphocytes**. Its major immunological role is to act as a filter for the bloodstream. The tissue consists of (a) the **white pulp** — around the branches of the splenic artery which are surrounded by periarterial lymphatic sheaths and lymphatic nodules or malpighian bodies, and (b) the **red pulp** — splenic

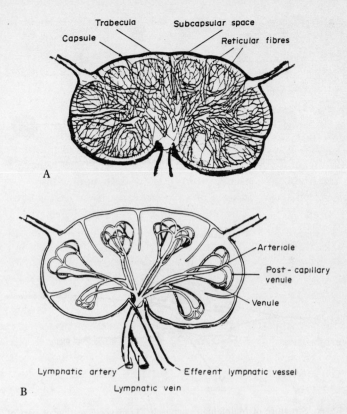

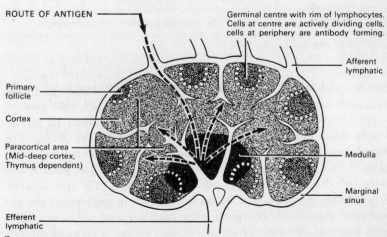

Fig. 4.4 A Network of reticular fibres on which other cells are embedded. **B.** Blood supply and postcapillary venules. **C.** General structure and route of antigen.

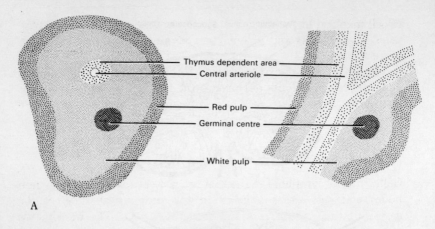

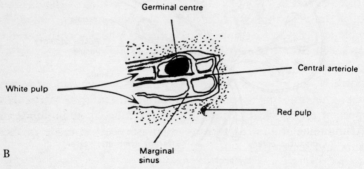

Fig. 4.5 A. Structure of Malpighian corpuscle. Transverse section of part of spleen showing area of white pulp related to central arteriole and considered to be thymus-dependent. **B.** Detail of the way the central arteriole divides to become the marginal sinus that allows the passage of lymphocytes into the white pulp where germinal centres form.

sinuses and splenic cords, the latter making up bands of tissue, reticulum cells, erythrocytes, lymphocytes and granulocytes — lying between the sinuses which are themselves lined by 'sinus-lining cells' held together by a network of reticular fibres. The blood leaves the white pulp via capillaries in the marginal sinus (Fig. 4.5B) and enters the red pulp passing into the sinuses and is collected up into venules and veins leaving by the splenic vein. The precise details of the blood circulation in the spleen are not yet fully elucidated, but particulate material and cells can clearly pass through the walls of splenic vessels or be discharged directly into the splenic tissue. It can thus be seen that the lymph nodes and spleen can be regarded as a complex organization of three types

of cell involved in the initiation of the immune reaction — lymphocytes, plasma cells and phagocytic cells of the mononuclear phagocyte system.

This account of the structure and histological detail of the spleen
and lymph nodes must not obsure the fact that many of the cells
in these organs are part of a mobile population circulating between
the blood and lymphoid tissues (p. 67).

Mucosal associated lymphoid tissue (MALT)

Collections of lymphoid tissue that are not encapsulated like lymph
nodes and spleen are situated in the submucosal areas of the
gastrointestinal, respiratory and urogenital tracts. The best known
of these aggregates of cells are the Peyer's patches of the gastrointestinal tract and the tonsils of the respiratory tract, where the
lymphoid cells are organized into distinct nodules with germinal
centres. Elsewhere the cells are not present in organized structures
and appear as diffuse collections of lymphoid cells in the lamina
propria of the intestinal wall, lining the bronchi and urogenital
tract. The mucosal associated lymphoid tissues are particularly
important for providing protection to the mucous membranes and
IgA immunoglobulin (as well as other isotypes) is made in these
tissues and secreted as secretory IgA (see p. 99).

Immune responses to food constituents

In infants and young children, antibodies to milk proteins can
frequently be detected. Experimental work in adult rabbits shows
that after feeding a protein such as bovine albumin all animals
made antibodies to the albumin. In humans, antibodies to bovine
albumin are found more frequently (75%) in children under 16
years than in older age groups (8%), indicating that there is a
substantial fall with increasing age. In patients with gastrointestinal
diseases such as ulcerative colitis, coeliac disease and idiopathic
steatorrhoea, raised levels of antibodies have been found to wheat
and milk protein fractions. It is not clear, however, if these antibodies are a primary cause of the gastrointestinal disease or
secondary to damage to the intestinal wall that has allowed food
antigens to enter the mucosa. High concentrations of circulating
antibodies to dietary proteins have been found to be associated with
forms of type 1 (anaphylactic) and type 3 (toxic complex) hypersensitivity (p. 232). Such individuals develop hypersensitivity

reactions following the oral or systemic administration of the dietary protein. It has been suggested that a mechanism involving T suppressor cells exists to limit the systemic response to antigens that enter by the gut. It is assumed that such suppression does not extend to local immune responses by the MALT that would be required to deal with intestinal pathogens. It has been proposed that a subpopulation of T cells called 'contrasuppressor cells' are present in the mucosal lymphoid tissues and are responsible for overcoming the effects of the T suppressor cells.

The situation with respect to cell mediated immune reactions in the gut is less clear. Chemicals such as 2.4 dinitrobenzene (DCNB) that are known to induce cell mediated responses when applied to the skin will, if given orally, either induce or abrogate pre-existing responses depending on the dose administered. Guinea pigs that have been sensitized to DCNB by applying it to the skin will develop mucosal lesions if the chemical is subsequently applied to the gut mucosa. It has been suggested that individuals who develop cell mediated immunity to antigens by skin contact may develop skin lesions following ingestion of the antigen via the gut. A large variety of chemicals are believed to be involved in such reactions, such as penicillin (traces of which may be found in cows milk), para-amino benzoic acid and other benzoate derivatives present in cosmetics, soaps, foodstuffs and soft drinks.

Skin associated lymphoid tissue (SALT)

The skin is the largest organ of the human body and has an important role in innate (p. 16) and acquired immunity. Lymphocytes are found widely distributed in the skin along with a family of skin dendritic antigen presenting cells (Langerhans cells, interdigitating cells and veiled cells). All the dendritic cells express class 2 MHC antigens and Langerhans and veiled cells (found in the draining lymph) also have Fc and C3 receptors. There are quite a large number of mast cells in the skin in addition to neutrophils. Mast cells appear to play a role in the regulation of the skin vasculature.

B cells and the bursa of Fabricius

The cells of the immune system concerned with producing circulating antibodies reside mainly in the corticomedullary junction and medullary cords of lymph nodes and the red pulp of the spleen.

The first evidence that B lymphocytes might be influenced by a non-thymic lymphoid organ came from phylogenetic studies in neonatal chickens which failed to develop normal immunological capacity after removal of the gut-associated lymphoid organ known as the **bursa of Fabricius**. Thymectomized chickens, as would be expected from the discussion above, fail to develop cell-mediated immune processes whilst capable of a humoral immune response. In striking contrast, bursectomized chickens fail to make immunoglobulins and have no plasma-cells or germinal centres in the lymphoid organs. Their cell-mediated mechanisms are, on the other hand, intact. Evidence is now emerging which suggests that there is a traffic of bursal lymphocytes to germinal centres in the spleen and lymph nodes comparable to that described in the thymus for bone marrow lymphocytes.

In mammalian species the bone marrow is the specific microenvironment where B cells differentiate from stem cells. Some 80% of the marrow small lymphocytes are of the B cell lineage. In the fetal liver and bone marrow the precursor cells cluster in the vicinity of macrophages and stromal cells. These cells seem essential for B cell development but the mechanisms are unknown. B lymphocytes develop without contact with antigen and move from the peripheral areas of the bone marrow to the centre. The immature rapidly dividing B cell precursors have μ heavy chains, characteristic of IgM (p. 99), but no light chains in their cytoplasm. There is a particular gene family in the chromosome of the B cell line for each of the two types of light chain, $\varkappa$ and κ, and a third for the various types of heavy chain. The three loci are unlinked and in the mouse are found in chromosome 6 and 12. The B lympho cyte family or clone that develops from a single stem cell is able to switch the expression of one type of heavy chain to another without changing the part of the molecule containing the amino acid sequences that bind antigen, the variable region (p. 96). The control of immunoglobulin class switching appears to involve T cell derived lymphokines. BCGF (p. 110) enhances production of antigen-specific IgM responses, whereas BCDF (p. 110) controls the appearance of IgG_1 antibodies. The earliest form of B cell (pre-B cell) is detectable in the fetal liver and bone marrow. It can synthesize IgM but this is found only in the cytoplasm; it appears later in the membrane, 16 to 17 days in mice and 9 days in man. The μ chain of the molecule as it appears in the membrane of the B cell is slightly different chemically from the secreted form of IgM. This seems to depend on there being two forms of μ mRNA derived from a single gene. The membrane form of the μ chain is 21 amino acids longer than the sacreted form and contains uncharged hydrophobic amino acids that are thought to anchor the μ chain in the membrane.

The diversity of amino acid sequences found in the part of the molecule that combines with antigen (variable region) is thought to be controlled by somatic mutation which is discussed more fully on page 85.

The immature B cells leave the bone marrow and migrate to the secondary lymphoid tissues. At the same time surface IgM increases in density. During this period the B cells can become tolerant. It has been recently proposed that the cells may be more susceptible to tolerance induction during the G_1 phase of the cell cycle. Before reaching lymphoid follicles B cells meet T cells and interdigitating cells. These cells are thought to present antigen and activate the B cells that then migrate to the lymphoid follicles and at the same time lose their IgD. Without meeting antigen virgin B cells are short lived. Most of the proliferating B cells in the follicles die and are phagocytosed by tingible-body macrophages. Surviving B cells are surrounded by follicular dendritic cells (found only in follicles) that appear to ensure their survival. The follicular dendritic cells have Fc and C3b receptors and retain antigen in form of immune complexes. Various receptors become detectable on B cells: Fc, Ia and C3 receptors.

Null cells

Amongst the cells of the immune system are a population of lymphocyte-like cells that express Fc receptors and contain large granules in their cytoplasm. Their origin and lineage is uncertain but they share some monocyte and T cell characteristics expressing most of the markers that have been associated with T cells in mice and humans as well as certain markers restricted to macrophages. This cell population is sometimes referred to a 'null cells' and includes natural killer cells (NK cells) along with a smaller number of myeloid stem cells and immature T or B cells. NK cells are believed by some immunologists to be prethymic T cells. The main function associated with NK cells is the non-specific killing of tumour cells and virally infected cells. They also appear to have a role in regulation of lymphoid and other haemopoietic cell populations. NK cells can kill autologous, allogenic and xenogenic cells (p. 194) and do not require recognition of antigens in association with MHC products in contrast to cytotoxic T cells. It has been recently proposed that NK cell activity should be referred to as non-MHC — restricted cytotoxicity and that the cells should be termed N Lymphocytes. Interleukin-2 activated NK cells have been associated with a phenomenon termed lymphokine activated killer cell activity. In most experimental models NK cells have been found to be mainly involved in the prevention of tumour metastases. The cells may have originally evolved as regulators of haemopoietic stem cells and later developed into a host defence mechanism directed against intracellular parasites and tumours (see also p. 111).

Phagocytes

Main phagocytes in immunity — neutrophils and monocytes/macrophages

Phagocytic cells of both the polymorphonuclear granulocyte series, the neutrophil and the monocyte/macrophage series, play a very important role in immunity by removing, by the process of phago-cytosis, microorganisms or inert particles that may enter the blood stream or tissues (Fig. 4.6). They also are the source of many pharmacologically active mediators of the inflammatory response and the macrophage plays a crucial role as one of the main inducer cells of acquired immunity. The macrophage forms a link between innate and acquired immunity. Both types of cell have powerful microbicidal activities using oxygen-dependent and independent mechanisms. They contain enzymes that catalyse the conversion of oxygen atoms to superoxide and the potent oxidizing agents hypochlorite and hydroxyl radicals. At the same time as destroying microorganisms, these highly reactive compounds can injure the cells of the host and have recently been shown to have mutagenic effects. Neutrophils that make up over 90% of the circulating granulocytes and 60% of the total leucocytes in the blood (with large reserves in the bone marrow), by means of proteolytic enzymes, solubilize and remove cellular debris at the site of an inflammatory response. The macrophage (2.7×10^5 per ml of blood in humans) is the source of mediators that play an important role in regulating the immune response as well as being involved in microbicidal and tumoricidal activities, lipid metabolism and regulation of granulocyte and erythrocyte pools by colony stimulating factors.

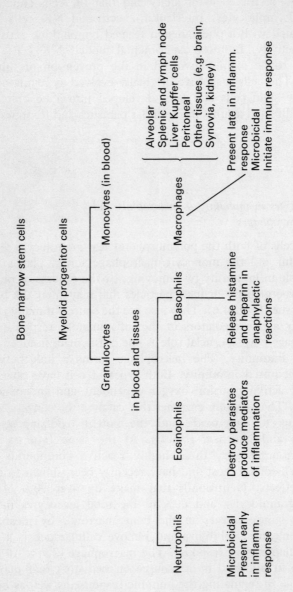

Fig. 4.6 Origin, differentiation and main functions in immunity of phagocytes.

Other granulocytes — eosinophils, mast cells and basophils

The role of eosinophils (2.5% of the blood leucocytes in healthy humans) has been controversial for a number of years, with their main function perceived as a modifier of allergic reactions by destroying mast cell products such as histamine and slow-reacting substance of anaphylaxis (SRS-A). This view is now changing in view of evidence that eosinophils produce a mediator of the inflammatory response, leukotriene C (that increases capillary permeability and contracts smooth muscle), as well as a factor that activates platelets (PAF). Furthermore eosinophils are known to make oxygen radicals (with microbicidal and cytocidal activity) and to destroy parasites and tumour cells and they are regulated by interleukin 4 (p. 110). Basophils and mast cells (0.2% of the blood leucocytes) may originate from the same progenitors but show morphological and biochemical differences that may be the result of environmental factors at their site of localization. Their granules contain histamine and heparin and other mediators such as slow reacting substance of anaphylaxis (SRS-A) and eosinophil chemotactic factor (ECF). These mediators are released from the granules of the cell when antibody on their surface (IgE, p. 225) interacts with antigen. Their main role appears to be in allergic reactions (p. 226). Figure 4.6 summarizes the origin and main functions of these cell types.

Recirculation of lymphocytes

In a previous section (p. 51) consideration was given to the traffic of lymphocytes from the bone marrow via the thymus to the lymph nodes. This journey, during which the cells are maturing and proliferating, probably takes a period of weeks. Another form of lymphocytic traffic also exists, involving a non-dividing population of small lymphocytes with a potential life-span of many months and derived mainly from the thymus. This journey is measured in hours rather than days (Fig. 4.7). This traffic takes the form of a **recirculation** of small lymphocytes between the blood and lymphoid tissue, and thus each small lymphocyte may be exchanged between these two compartments very many times during its lifetime. One of the main advantages to the individual of such a recirculation process is that, for example, during the course of a natural infection the continual traffic of lymphocytes would enable very many different lymphocytes to have **access to the antigen** with the result that there would be a good chance that

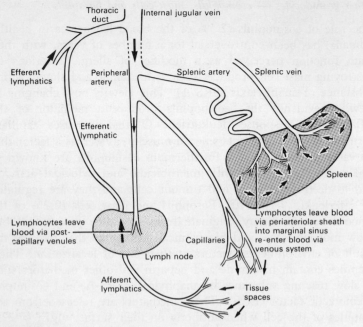

Fig. 4.7 Schematic view of main pathways of lymphocyte circulation

a lymphocyte carrying antibody receptor for the particular antigen would come across it and initiate an immune reaction. Another possible role of this recirculation process is that it can be used to **replenish** the lymphoid tissue of, for example, the spleen which might have been depleted by X-irradiation, trauma or infection.

There is convincing evidence that lymphoid tissues can **recruit** lymphocytes from the recirculating pool. If a rat spleen is irradiated immediately after an intravenous injection of sheep red cells the antibody response is only slightly delayed. However, if whole-body irradiation is given after the initial splenic irradiation there is complete suppression of the anti-sheep cell response. It thus seems likely that without whole-body irradiation the irradiateed spleen is able to recruit a fresh supply of lymphocytes from the circulating pool.

Another situation in which recirculation of lymphocytes could be helpful in the induction of an immune response is when the local concentration of antigen might be sufficient to induce tolerance rather than immunity in a static cell population. The passage of lymphocytes through an area where antigen had been localized and concentrated on the dendritic processes of macrophages might facilitate the induction of immunity.

The routes of lymphocyte recirculation

There are three main areas where the migration or transfer of lymphocytes from the blood takes place: the **lymph nodes** and Peyer's patches, the **spleen** and the peripheral **blood vessels**. Most is known about the mechanism of transfer in the lymph nodes where studies using the electron microscope show that small lymphocytes actually penetrate and traverse the cytoplasm of the cuboidal endothelial cells of the postcapillary venules. These **postcapillary venules** are confined on the deep and mid zones of the lymph node cortex and are unusual in that their endothelial cells are hypertrophied and cuboidal in appearance in comparison with the flattened endothelium of normal postcapillary venules found elsewhere. From the lymph node cortex the lymphocytes pass through the node to the medullary sinuses and then to the efferent lymphatics.

The precise routes of lymphocyte migration in the peripheral blood circulation are not clear, but the migration seems to be on a much smaller scale than in lymphoid tissues and almost certainly takes place across capillary walls. The flow can be increased if a local granuloma is formed in response to some foreign agent; then the migration from blood to lymph can be as great as in the lymph nodes themselves.

In the spleen, postcapillary venules have not been described and it appears that small lymphocytes enter the periarteriolar sheath from the blood, passing between the cells rather than through them as in the postcapillary venules. The cells later re-enter the blood within the spleen rather than leave via the lymphatics.

THE CELLS CONCERNED IN THE IMMUNE RESPONSE

Antigen localization and contact with macrophages and lymphocytes

A simplified picture of the cellular mechanisms leading to antibody formation is that antibodies of different specificities are made by different families of **clones** of cells, each family being genetically programmed to make antibody of only **one specificity**. There is evidence to show that the cells carry at least part of the molecule of their particular antibody exposed on the cell membrane as a receptor for antigen. Thus when an antigen is injected into the body and comes in contact with lymphoid cells it combines with those exposed antibody receptors which are best able to fit the determinant groups of the antigen molecule.

The way this is brought about can be seen when isotope-labelled antigen is injected into an animal. It is first rapidly localized in the sinus-lining macrophages in the marginal zone around the malpighian bodies in the spleen or the medullary macrophages of the lymph nodes (Fig. 4.4C), depending on the route of injection (p. 89). After this localization, plasma cell precursors (probably small lymphocytes) at the corticomedullary junction of the lymph nodes are triggered to proliferate and differentiate into antibody-producing cells; after partial degradation in the macrophage, antigenic fragments are passed on to the lymphocytes (see p. 75). It is also possible for some antigens to react directly with the lymphocytes themselves (see below). This stimulation and proliferation leads to the development of lymphoid follicles, which are localised collections of active lymphoid cells taking part in the primary immune response.

Subsequent contact with antigen now results in a rather different pattern of localization influenced by the presence of secreted antibody to the antigen; antigen, whilst still taken up by medullary macrophages, is also localized on the surface of **dendritic macrophages** (macrophages with cytoplasmic extensions) which interdigitate with each other and with the lymphoid cells of the lymphoid follicles or malpighian bodies. This localization seems to depend on antibody at the surface of the macrophage. B lymphocytes themselves may also come directly in contact with antigen. They can be shown to have portions of the immunoglobulin molecule on their surface (see below) because they can readily be stimulated to respond by transformation, to contact with antibodies directed at various parts of the immunoglobulin molecule. The specificity of these surface immunoglobulins is determined by the **genetic constitution** of the particular lymphocyte. Nossal in Australia was able to isolate single antibody-producing cells in a 'microdroplet' and show that such cells taken from an animal immunized with salmonella produced only one type of antibody. It has been inferred from this that the cell receptor and the secreted antibody are of the same specificity and it has been found that receptors can only be seen clearly on the antibody secreting cell population (i.e. the B cells).

Immunoglobulin heavy chains are present as a component of the immunoglobulin receptor on B cells; they are μ chains as found in IgM and the molecule appears to be an IgM subunit (similar in MW to IgG and called IgMs). B lymphocytes prior to antigenic stimulation are believed to synthesize around 250 to 5000 subunits of IgM per hour per cell. The molecules are shed from the surface membrane into the extracellular fluid.

The B cell membrane possesses **receptors** for the Fc fragment of the immunoglobulin molecule and a receptor for the activated complement component C3. The major role of the receptors (CR1 and CR2) that can bind several of the split components of C3 is believed to be the binding of antigen-antibody complexes that develop within germinal centres of the lymphoid tissues. This appears to act as a growth promoting stimulus to the B cells to synthesize DNA and secrete immunoglobulins. One of the receptors (CR2) that seems to be restricted to B cells acts as the receptor for the Epstein-Barr virus (p. 141) that acts as a polyclonal activator for human B cells. The detailed mechanisms underlying these proposals are as yet far from being resolved and await a much clearer understanding of the gene complexes for the various receptors and their products as represented in the cell membrane.

Microscopic examination of lymphocytes exposed to antigen has shown that antigen tends to bind preferentially to certain areas of the lymphocyte membrane rather than uniformly over the cell surface. The surface immunoglobulin receptors seem to be able to **coalesce** at points around the cell membrane, suggesting that they have a degree of mobility. This finding is consistent with current views on the structure of cell membranes indicating that they are made up of a lipid bilayer containing protein molecules that can move around, coalesce and separate when for example the pH of the surrounding medium is changed.

Properties of antigen, cell co-operation and activation of lymphocytes

Binding of antigen to the immunoglobulin receptors on a B lymphocyte, whilst a necessary prelude to activation of the cell for immunoglobulin synthesis, is not in itself sufficient to ensure B cell stimulation. For successful activation the antigen molecule must have additional properties, rather like the mitogenic properties of phytohaemagglutin (see p. 106), which provide a 'signal' to activate the cell.

Certain antigens, e.g. bacterial lipopolysaccharides, have this property and can stimulate B cells unaided. Other antigens, e.g. serum proteins, although able to bind to the B cell, are unable to deliver the activating 'signal'. These latter antigens require the assistance of T lymphocytes to **co-operate** with the B lymphocyte and provide the necessary stimulus for activation.

The observations that led to these conclusions allowed the identification of two categories of antigen: (1) those that bind and activate B lymphocytes without the assistance of T lymphocytes, referred to as **T-independent antigens**, and (2) those that can bind to B lymphocytes but require the co-operation of T lymphocytes for B cell activation, referred to as **T-dependent antigens**.

T cell recognition

Despite the fact that considerable detail is known of the structure of the alpha and beta chains of the T cell receptor, it is still not clear how this receptor recognizes antigen in the context of polymorphic class 2 MHC molecules found in a species. The V regions of the alpha and beta chains together form the antigen binding domain. The V beta genes of the mouse are the most thoroughly studied and like immunoglobulin genes (with which they share many homologous regions) are divided into separate V, J and D segments that are assembled by recombination during T cell development to form a V beta gene associated with either of two constant genes. The V beta gene repertoire is much smaller than that of the immunoglobulin heavy or light chain genes and it seems likely that beta chain somatic diversification depends on a greater contribution from J and D gene segments than in immunoglobulins. This at least partially compensates for the limited number of V beta gene segments and allows an extensive repertoire of antigen recognizing structures in the T cell receptor. It has been proposed that T cell receptors may bind to antigen with a lower affinity than immunoglobulin and this also would be expected to increase their binding repertoire.

As previously noted, T cells recognize antigen in association with MHC antigens. Helper T cells usually recognize antigen in association with class 2 MHC antigens and cytotoxic T cells in association with class 1 MHC antigens. These cells carry different T cell differentiation antigens T4 in the case of human T helper cells and T8 in T cytotoxic cells. The possibility that these molecules are the recognition units for class 1 and class 2 MHC antigens respectively is suggested by the fact that monoclonal antibodies against the T4 or T8 determinants will inhibit MHC class restricted activities of these cells. A further surface antigen, T3, is found on all mature T cells and may be a 'framework' or constant segment of the T cell receptor perhaps responsible for transmitting an 'activation' signal to the cell when the receptor binds antigen. The T cell binds antigen by receptors that recognise determinants on the protein molecule that carries within it smaller (haptenic) determinant groups with which B cells can interact (but not respond to without T cell cooperation). This effect is called the **carrier effect** and was originally shown using haptenic groups such as dinitrophenol (DNP) attached to a protein carrier like bovine gamma globulin (BGG) or ovalbumin (OA). T cells appear to recognize the carrier and B cells the hapten. An animal immunized to DNP-BGG would not respond to a subsequent challenge with DNP-OA, indicating the need for T cells to recognize the carrier before B cells could respond to the hapten.

Table 4.3 summarizes the main characteristic of T and B lymphocytes. The linear amino acid sequences recognised by T cells are exposed in large molecules that are degraded (processed; see p. 75) by inducer cells. In contrast B cells recognise superficial non-linear determinants.

Table 4.3 Characteristics of T and B lymphocytes

	Percentage of cells (mice)	
	T lymphocytes	B lymphocytes
Location		
Peripheral blood lymphocytes	60–85%	25–35%
Lymph node cells	60–75%	25–35%
Splenic lymphocytes	25–45%	60–60%
Bone marrow cells	1–5%	35–45%
Thymus cells	> 95%	negligible
Thoracic duct cells	80–90%	10–20%
Markers		
Thy 1 antigen	present	absent
TL	present	absent
H-2 antigens	present	present
Ly antigen	present	present
	(Ly, 1, 2, 3)	(Ly 5)
Immunoglobulin		
IgG or IgA or IgM		
or IgD or IgE	absent	present
Fc and C3 receptors	absent	present
	(usually)	

The role of macrophages in antibody production

Macrophages and other inducer cells (Langerhans' cells of the skin and dendritic cells in the lymphoid tissues) play an important role in the **initiation of the immune response** by T and B lymphocytes (Table 4.4). It has been known for some years that macrophages are required in order to obtain an immune response to sheep red blood cells by mouse spleen cells in vitro, and these findings have since been confirmed with a number of antigens and in different species. The source of the macrophages was found to be important, and whilst those from the spleen or peritoneal cavity were effective, macrophages from the lung (alveolar macrophages) and liver (Kuppfer cells) were not able to cooperate with lymphocytes in the initiation of an immune response. The latter cells do, however, possess many features — functional and morphological — of macrophages, including the ability to adhere to glass, to phago-cytose particles and to be cytotoxic for antibody coated cells.

Immune responses induced in vitro in spleen cell suspensions suggest that the macrophage appears to be necessary for an immune response to occur to T-dependent antigens (see above) and its pres-ence has been shown to be necessary for the triggering of B lymphocytes by at least some T-independent antigens.

Macrophages may also function by **concentrating antigen** in 'critical sites', such as the follicles and medulla of the lymph nodes, thereby optimizing the chances of contact with lymphocytes.

Table 4.4 Cells concerned with initiation of immune response

Cell	Essential functions
Macrophages, Langerhans' cells, dendritic cells	Remove and catabolize excess antigen Localize and retain antigen at 'critical sites' and present antigen to lymphocytes Regulate activities of lymphocytes by soluble factors Bind antigen-antibody complexes by Fc and C3 receptors
T lymphocytes	Act as 'helper' cells for certain antigens (T-dependent) Regulate activities of macrophages and B lymphocytes and recruit other T lymhocytes by soluble factors
B lymphocytes	Immunoglobulin production Binding of antigen by Ig receptors and responding to T-independent antigens. Fc and C3 receptors binding antigen-antibody complexes and possible role in activating the B lymphocytes and regulating their activity

Some antigen may be retained at the surface of macrophages where it serves as a **depot of antigen** for the maintenance of the immune response. It it also possible that some antigen retained within the macrophage will function in this way although antigen can also be **catabolised** within the macrophage and later eliminated from the body as breakdown products. Macrophages have receptors for the Fc component of immunoglobulin and for C3b (p. 25). These will enable complexes of antibody and antigen to adhere to the macrophage membrane and be subsequently internalized.

ESSENTIAL STEPS IN THE GENERATION OF AN IMMUNE RESPONSE

The response depends on four cell types and the various cytokines that they produce as regulators of the response. Antigen first comes into contact with a group of cells called inducer cells or sometimes antigen presenting cells (APC). The main feature of an inducer cells is the presence of class 2 MHC antigens in its membrane. As noted previously (p. 72), antigen is only recognized as foreign by T helper cells if it is associated with class 2 antigens. Class 2 antigens are in general limited to cells of the immune system but stimuli like gamma interferon can bring about its expression in fibroblasts and endothelial cells so that they might act as inducer cells. The main inducer cells are macrophages, dendritic cells in the lymphoid tissues, Langerhans' cells in the skin (that can carry antigen to the lymph nodes) and B lymphocytes. One of the essential functions of inducer cells is to take up antigen and 'process' it to a suitable form for re-expression of the cell surface in association with the class 2 antigen. It is uncertain at present if antigen 'processing' is required for all types of antigen as there is evidence that under certain circumstances presentation can occur without processing. A requirement for processing is indicated by the finding that fixed (killed) APC can present peptides to Tk cells whereas they generally cannot present the native protein. The other feature associated with inducer cells is their ability to produce interleukin-1 with its wide ranging effects (see p. 110). The activity crucial to its role in the induction of immunity is its effect on helper T lymphocytes that initiates the cascade of T cell lymphokines (p. 108).

The next stage in the process is the recognition of the class two associated antigen on the inducer cell by the T helper cells by means of its T cell receptor (p. 72). This is a heterodimer consisting of an alpha and beta chain coded for on different chromosomes (14 and 6 respectively in the mouse and 14 and 7 in man). The various lymphokines produced by the helper T cell, including B cell growth and differentiation factors, lead to both humoral and cell mediated immunity with the proliferation and clonal expansion of B cells, plasma cells, cytotoxic T cells (Tc), T cells involved in delayed hypersensitivity reactions (Tdh cells) based on their ability to produce various lymphokines and, finally, T suppressor cells (Ts) that regulate the immune response. Recruitment of fresh supplies of both lymphocytes and phagocytes from the bone marrow is brought about by cytokines called colony-stimulating factors such as interleukin 3. A recently described, interleukin (IL-4) appears to act as a B cell growth factor for IgE production as well as inducing eosinophil proliferation. It is not yet clear if synthesis of other immunoglobulin isotypes is controlled in the same way.

Immune tolerance

Another possible result of the interaction of certain types of antigen e.g. soluble protein antigens, with the surface of lymphocytes is that the cell is prevented in some way from transforming for antibody production and is thus functionally eliminated from further participation in the immune response. This phenomenon is known as **immune tolerance** and is specific for the inducing antigen; the term is used by immunologists to indicate a state in which the individual is unable to response to a specific antigen or hapten. The phenomenon was recognised in 1924 by Glenny and Hopkins. Owen in 1945 observed that dizygotic cattle twins parabiosed in utero by placental fusion were permanent chimeras with respect to their red cells. Immune tolerance was first studied experimentally by Medawar and his colleagues in mice injected neonatally with cells from another strain of mice (i.e. containing transplantation antigens) (p. 194). The injected mice were later able to accept grafts from the strain of mice which had donated the original injected cells.

It has since been found that tolerance to a large variety of antigens can be readily induced when the antigens are injected neonatally. Tolerance can also be induced in the adult provided more antigen is given to take into account the maturity of the lymphoid system, the larger size of the lymphoid organs and more cells to paralyse. A notable advance was made in this field when Mitchison, using serum protein antigens, showed that there was another form of tolerance inducible by very small doses of antigen. This was termed **low zone tolerance** in contrast to the high zone tolerance previously described. Doses between these two levels were found to immunise. Other workers have confirmed these findings with different types of antigen.

Tolerance induced in either the T cell or B cell populations of lymphocytes results (as would be predicted from what is known of co-operation between the two cell populations) in tolerance of the whole animal to the antigen used to induce tolerance. This was established by transferring either tolerant T cells or tolerant B cells to a recipient mouse that had been irradiated and injected with normal cells of one or other population (i.e. T or B cells). Tolerant T cells would not co-operate with normal B cells to produce an immune response to human gammaglobulin and tolerant B cells would not co-operate with normal T cells to produce a response. The T cell population appeared to retain their tolerance for rather longer than the B cells (approximately 150 days compared to 50 days).

Suppressor T cells play an important role in tolerance induction by recognising the idiotypic determinants (p. 99) of the surface immunoglobulins of B cells and could be responsible for maintaining self-tolerance by suppressing those B cells expressing anti-self immunoglobulin receptors.

Immunoglobulin synthesis

After the initial changes of transformation of lymphocytes have been set in motion, the actual **synthesis** of large amounts of immunoglobulin takes place. Two types of cells have been shown to be engaged in this process: (1) cells of the **plasmocytic** series and (2) cells of the **lymphocytic** series (small, medium and large lymphocytes). Of these two types the plasma cell line makes the largest contribution to immunoglobulin production and when single cells from immunized animals are examined in microdrops it can be shown that two-thirds of the **antibody-producing cells** are of this type (Fig. 4.8). An important characteristic of any cell making immunoglobulin is the presence of a **rough endoplasmic reticulum** (formed by the attachment of protein-synthesising polyribosomes to the convoluted endoplasmic reticulum membrane). The lymphocytes contain less of this than do plasma cells. It has been shown by a number of techniques that the immunoglobulin is localized in the spaces of the endoplasmic reticulum where it sometimes forms distinct aggregates termed Russell bodies.

In the spleen the cells engaged in antibody production tend to

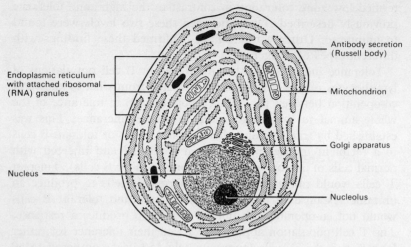

Antibody secretion
(Russell body)

Endoplasmic reticulum
with attached ribosomal
(RNA) granules

Mitochondrion

Golgi apparatus

Nucleus

Nucleolus

Fig. 4.8 Plasma cell

be found in the **red pulp**, and in the lymph glands in the **cortex**.

Individual immunoglobulin-producing cells appear to be able to synthesize the whole molecule, both heavy and light polypeptide chains (p. 94). It has also been found that the individual cells make only one class of immunoglobulin and that the light chains are restricted to only one of the two types (K and L, p. 97). It is very unusual to find an immunoglobulin secreting cell synthesizing more than one class of immunoglobulin, although B cells in the early stages of an immune response can be shown to be secreting IgM antibody. They later switch to the synthesis of IgG antibody and thus at any one time produce only one class of immunoglobulin. Recent evidence indicates that the same cell can switch back to IgM production during a secondary response. The IgG that is produced is of the same specificity as the earlier IgM and almost certainly involves continued synthesis of the same light chain and the same variable region of the heavy chain; only the constant region is altered. The genetic mechanisms may be a translocation event whereby the variable region gene becomes dissociated from the μ constant region gene and associates with the γ constant region gene. This IgM-IgC switch seems very likely to depend upon the influence of T cells on the B-cell population.

The actual synthesis of immunoglobulin (after DNA has directed the synthesis of the appropriate mRNA) is carried out on the ribosomes of the producing cell, tRNAs sequentially adding amino acids to the growing polypeptide chain. Different ribosomes synthesise heavy and light chains, and assembly (by disulphide bond formation) takes place after the chains have been released into the cisternae of the endoplasmic reticulum. Polymerization of immunoglobulin molecules to form IgM involves the addition of J chains and carbohydrate groups just prior to its release from the cell.

Monoclonal antibodies

A very important advance in the rapidly expanding field of biotechnology comes from the development by Milstein and Kohler in Cambridge of 'immortal' cell lines capable of producing antibody of any required specificity, indefinitely, in cell culture conditions.

In conventional immunization procedures injection of purified antigen leads to the production of an antiserum containing antibodies with a wide range of specificities for different determinants on the antigen molecule. It is virtually impossible to separate the different antibodies to obtain those of a particular specificity. The technique used to produce monoclonal antibodies does not require the preparation of purified antigen for injection and enables the selection of a cell producing antibody of a single specificity that is then grown in bulk to produce large amounts of the specific antibody.

The principle behind the method is the fusing of cells from an immunized animal with cells of a cultured myeloma cell line. Polyethylene glycol is the agent used to fuse the two types of cell. The myeloma cells are selected for their ability to grow in 8-azaguanine because they lack the enzyme hypoxanthine guanine phosphoribosyl transferase. This enzyme is required for rapid growth in tissue culture medium containing hypoxanthine, aminopterin and thymidine (HAT medium).

After fusion, the cells are grown in HAT medium in a number of wells for 10–14 days. The supernatants of each well are then tested for antibody activity. Clones that secrete the required antibodies, usually only a small proportion of the cultures, are selected and grown in bulk. This can be done either in culture or as tumours in the peritoneal cavity of mice; the antibodies are secreted into the tissue culture fluid or the peritoneal fluid of the mice. The technique is outlined in Figure 4.9 and Table 4.5.

The potential value of the technique is vast and will enable the

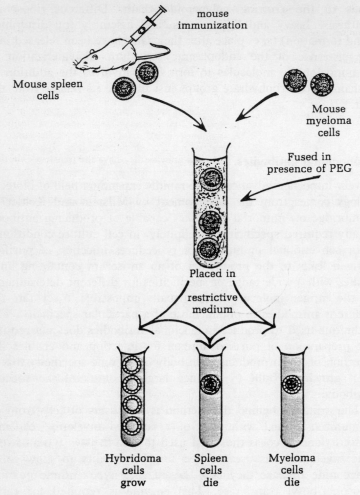

mouse
immunization

Mouse spleen
cells

Mouse
myeloma
cells

Fused in
presence of PEG

Placed in

restrictive
medium

Hybridoma
cells
grow

Spleen
cells
die

Myeloma
cells
die

Fig. 4.9 Production of monoclonal antibodies.

identification of differentiation antigens on cells, cell receptors, tumour antigens, histocompatibility antigens, microorganisms and their products or tissue cells. New applications are appearing continually and radioimmunoassay techniques, tissue typing and serotyping of microorganisms will be revolutionised within the next few years. The regulation of the immune response by such antibodies is not inconceivable and the passive use of monoclonal antibodies to treat infections or tumours is within the bounds of possibility. The use of antibody to D antigen of the rhesus system

Table 4.5 Steps in preparation of monoclonal antibody

Immunization	Mouse (or rat) immunized with antigen — primary — then booster immunization
Fusion	Spleen cells taken from immunized mouse and fused with a myeloma cell (a mutant not producing antibody) using polyethylene glycol
Selection of hybridoma	Myeloma cells used lack an enzyme hypoxanthine phosphoribosyl transferase so cannot grow in a medium containing hypoxanthine, aminopterin and thymidine (HAT medium). Spleen cells cannot grow as not a continuous cell line. Hybridoma cells can grow as they have the transferase derived from the spleen cells and the capacity of the myeloma to grow in continuous culture
Screening	Clones are screened for antibody production (may represent about 10% of the cells)
Propagation	Positive clones are propagated from single cell preparations and should produce 10–100 μg/ml of specific antibody. Can be grown in mouse peritoneal cavity and ascitic fluid containing antibody collected
Storage	Antibody freeze dried or hybridoma cells stored at $-70°C$ as stock cultures

(see p. 187) to prevent haemolytic disease of the newborn will be of immediate value and anti-idiotypic (p. 99) autoantibody potentially could suppress autoantibody formation.

The extension of the technique to cell-mediated immunity is now under way using activated T lymphocytes fused with lymphoma cells. Such hybridomas offer the possibility of enhancing suppressor or helper cell activity to particular antigens and could have wide applications in the future.

THE CELLULAR PROCESSES INVOLVED IN IMMUNITY

Learning and memory

The outstanding feature underlying these mechanisms is that the immune response is a **learning process** at the cellular level.

After initial contact with an antigen the cells of the immune system retain a memory which can be evoked on subsequent contact with the antigen, and furthermore, like other learning processes, the immune system becomes increasingly skilled with continued experience of a particular antigen. The antibody which is synthesised becomes increasingly more effective in binding with antigens, as those cells which are best able to produce a 'good fitting' (avid) antibody molecule are selected from the population of antibody-forming cells. At the same time increasing numbers of committed cells are added to the immune system on repeated contact with antigen and the magnitude of the response is increased (p. 88). This increase in quantity and **avidity** of antibody can lead for example to increased efficiency in neturalizing an infective agent or its toxic products so that a well-immunized animal would be able to withstand a dose of the agent which might be lethal to a poorly immunised animal.

The immunological memory can exist for the lifetime of an individual and implies that memory T and B cells are long-lived. Some of these cells are likely to be non-dividing and others divide at a low frequency. The intermitotic intervals can extend from a few months in rodents to at least 10 years in man.

Theories of immunity

Two main theories have evolved which account for the development of an immune response and are referred to as **directive** and **selective** theories.

Directive theory

The **directive** theory was formulated by Haurowitz, Mudd and Alexander in the early 1930s and later modified by Pauling. The antigen is visualized as a mould or template which can enter any immunoglobulin-producing cell and cause the pattern of amino acids laid down to be modified so that it will fit the template, resulting in the synthesis of a molecule with a spatial configuration complementary to that of the antigen molecule. To account for the continued production of antibody it is assumed that the antigen, or part of it, remains in the cell to direct future antibody production. Alternatively, it is proposed that the antigen modifies the genetic information in the DNA of the cell so that it and its daughter cells continue to produce the specific immunoglobulin.

Selective theory

In contrast, the **selective** theory proposes that antigen selects, from the population of cells capable of making antibody, only those few cells that already have the inherent ability to make an immunoglobulin specific for the antigen. The antigen serves simply as a trigger on reacting with antibody receptor sites at the lymphocyte cell membrane. The **clonal selection theory** of Burnet is the best known of the selective theories and was formulated and modified over the years to take account of the hitherto unexplained phenomenon of recognition by the normal individual of tissue antigens as part of self and distinguishing these from foreign non-self antigens. Such an explanation became necessary with the description of human diseases where self-recognition breaks down and self antigen is treated as if it were foreign antigen — so-called autoimmune disease (p. 246). The theory proposes that the cells of the antibody-forming system have arisen by random mutation resulting in the emergence of small numbers of cells or clones of cells differentiated so as to be capable of producing one or a very small number of specific antibodies. Contact by such differentiated cells with self or foreign antigenic material during fetal life before the cells have reached maturity, would lead to suppression rather than stimulation of antibody formation against the particular antigen concerned — **immune tolerance**. That this could occur was illustrated by Medawar and his colleagues. Mice could be induced to accept potentially incompatible skin grafts by pretreatment during neonatal life with the appropriate 'transplantation antigen'. These studies were the forerunner of much further work in this field and it has now been shown that tolerance can also be induced even in adult animals if antigen is given in suitable doses and in an appropriate manner. However, it is more difficult to do this in the adult, the immature immune system of the neonatal animal being more susceptible. X-irradiation of an adult is frequently used as an aid in tolerance induction.

Burnet has since suggested that the initial contact with self antigens leading to the elimination of 'self-reactive clones' or 'forbidden clones', may take place in the thymus, this organ acting as a **censor** of the lymphoid cells. This idea is supported by the very rapid turn-over of lymphocytes in that organ and by the emergence of self-reactive antibody-producing cells in the absence of the thymus (see p. 55). The view is held by some immunologists that the ageing process may in part be due to a failure in these proposed controlling mechanisms, i.e. a gradual loss of efficiency of the censorship role of the thymus associated with its atrophy later in life.

The immune response to an antigen and the consequences of repeated stimulation can readily be explained in terms of the selective theory.

Antigen introduced into an animal comes in contact with lymphocytes carrying receptors corresponding to the antigenic determinants of the antigen molecule (p. 31). Some receptors (high affinity receptors) will fit the determinant well whilst others (low affinity receptors) will not fit so well. The dose of antigen given will have an affect on whether more antigen is bound by high or low affinity receptors — the less antigen given, the greater the chance that cells with high affinity receptors will bind antigen. With increasing doses of antigen more will be available to combine with the lymphocytes with the weaker lower affinity receptors. The consequence of this is that large doses of antigen will generate antibody of low average affinity and small doses will generate high affinity antibody. On subsequent administration of antigen, antibodies of progressively **higher affinity** will be produced. This is because after the first dose of antigen its concentration will gradually fall in the tissues as it is gradually catabolized and eliminated, resulting in less antigen being available for the lymphocytes with low affinity receptors. In these circumstances, lymphocytes with high receptors will preferentially bind the small amounts of antigen remaining and will consequently be stimulated to produce high affinity antibody. This 'selection' of lymphocytes will be reflected in the **affinity** of the antibody stimulated by subsequent doses of antigen given to the immunised animal.

Implications and variations of theories

The theory outlined above suggests that early contact with self antigens leads to the individual developing an immune system which is suppressed or tolerant towards self antigens. The unblocking of a cell inherently capable of producing antibody against self antigen would explain **autoantibody** formation (p. 249). It is for this aspect of immunity in particular that the clonal selection theory provides a more plausible explanation than the directive theory which requires that all antibody-forming cells are blocked by every self antigen rather than only those cells capable of responding specifically to each antigen concerned. The other main characteristics of antibody formation — the specificity of antibody for antigen and differences between the primary and secondary responses — can be explained equally well by either theory; the

clonal selection theory is however the most complete attempt so far
to take into account all the known facts of antibody production.

A number of variations of Burnet's original selective hypothesis
have been proposed in the last new years but all maintain the
assumption that the cell is already programmed to produce a
specific antibody. It has been postulated, for example, that each
potentially immunologically competent cell carries chromosomal
DNA genes for a large variety of different types of antibody and
is thus capable of responding to many antigens (sometimes referred
to as the 'germ line theory'). An alternative proposal is that all
antibody-producing cells may initially make identical immunoglobulins. During the lifetime of the individual variability of amino acid
sequence appears due to crossing over during mitosis of the nucleotides responsible for coding and **variable** amino acid sequences of
the Fab portion of the molecule. There is a clear survival value in
such a variation-producing mechanism resulting in the production
of immunoglobulins capable of reacting with a wide range of
environmental antigens. Similarly there is survival value in the
maintenance of those parts of the gene carrying the nucleotide
sequences for the **constant** parts of the immunoglobulin molecule
which maintain is structural integrity.

Molecular genetics of immunoglobulin synthesis

Recent advances in recombinant DNA technology and structural
analysis of proteins have provided much information on the hierarch-
ical organization of the domains within the immunoglobulin
molecule and the way that combinatorial diversity has been created.

The genes for the kappa and lambda light chains and the heavy
chains are carried on different chromosomes (2, 22 and 14 in man)
and are divided into coding exons and non-coding (silent) introns
like the genes for other macromolecules. Most detail is known
about the mouse kappa and lambda genes. The kappa genes are
on chromosome 6 and consist of three sets of genes for the Variable
(V), Joining (J) and Constant (C) regions. The lambda gene on
chromosome 10 consists of two pairs of V genes and three pairs of
J and C genes. The heavy chain gene on chromosome 12 in the
mouse is made up of four gene segments V, D, J and C in a cluster
of between 100 and 200 different segments each of about 295 base
pairs.

Variability in amino acid sequence for antibodies of different
specificity is created by rearrangements of the different gene

segments noted above that code for the variable region of the molecule, i.e. V and J segments for the light chains and V, D and J segments for the heavy chains. The random rearrangements that arise generate enormous diversity in the immunoglobulin population so that between 10^6 and 10^7 different specificities appear. In addition to this somatic mutation that occurs during differentiation of a clone of B cells, another source of diversity also makes a contribution. A lack of precision has been found in the DNA splicing machinery that fuses V, D and J segments so that the site of the junction between the different regions varies by several base pairs.

Estimates of the mutation rate indicates that one change in the variable region occurs for 3–30 cell divisions in the B cells and this is much higher than that found normally in eukaryotic cells. The effect of the combinatorial changes results in a population of cells that carry a very wide range of specificities for antigen so that the resulting antibody is 'fine tuned' to match the inducing antigen.

THE IMMUNE RESPONSE

Immunoglobulin production — the humoral antibody response

The antibody response resulting from exposure to antigenic substances has certain well-defined characteristics. After first meeting the antigen there is an interval of about two weeks before antibody can be found in the blood, and during this initial period there is intense activity in the antibody-forming tissues. This can be shown by studies with isotope-labelled precursors of cell components, for example tritiated thymidine, to show DNA synthesis or carbon-14 labelled amino acids in protein synthesis. Following antigenic stimulation there is a rapid increase in cell proliferation and synthesis of protein in the cells of the lymphoid organs indicated by the incorporation of the labelled materials. If the lymphoid cell population of a rat is depleted by placing a cannula in the thoracic duct and draining off the lymph, then no such cell proliferation takes place and there is no antibody response. In contrast in a normal animal immunized, for instance with sheep red blood cells, lymphocytes taken from the spleen or lymph nodes can be shown to have synthesized anti-sheep cell antibodies. If sheep red cells are mixed with the spleen or lymph gland cells the red cells aggregate around individual lymphocytes giving a rosette appearance when examined microscopically (Fig. 4.10).

IMMUNO-CYTO-ADHERENCE
Rosette technique

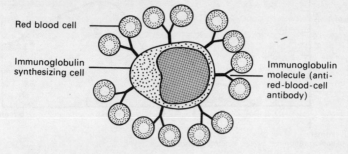

Red blood cell

Immunoglobulin
synthesizing cell

Immunoglobulin
molecule (anti-
red-blood-cell
antibody)

LOCALISED HAEMOLYSIS IN GEL
Jerne Plaque technique

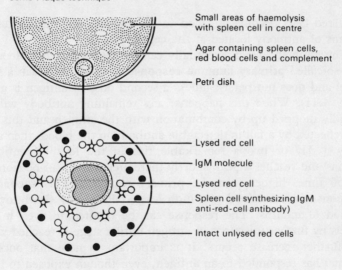

Small areas of haemolysis
with spleen cell in centre

Agar containing spleen cells,
red blood cells and complement

Petri dish

Lysed red cell

IgM molecule

Lysed red cell

Spleen cell synthesizing IgM
anti-red-cell antibody)

Intact unlysed red cells

Fig. 4.10 Two methods for demonstrating antibody formation by single cells. In the immuno-cyto-adherence test spleen cells from an animal immunized with, for example, sheep red blood cells, are mixed with the red cell antigen and after a period of incubation 'rosettes' are formed as shown. The red cells often completely surround the antibody-producing spleen cells. In the Jerne plaque technique, the spleen cells from the sheep-cell immunized animal are mixed with the red cell antigen in soft agar and when complement (guinea-pig serum) is layered on the surface, lysis of the red cells occurs. This happens because the antibody produced by the spleen cell has diffused into the surrounding agar and coated the red cells. This enables the complement system to be activated with the resulting lysis of the red cell (see p. 27 for the description of complement lysis)

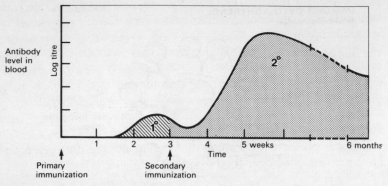

Antibody level in blood — Log titre

1   2   3   4   5 weeks   6 months
Time

↑ Primary immunization   ↑ Secondary immunization

1°   2°

Fig. 4.11 The antibody response

The red cells become attached to the surface of lymphocytes by means of antibody located at the cell membrane.

The antibody which eventually can be detected in the blood — the so-called **primary immune response** — does not reach a high level and does not persist unless a second dose of antigen is given (Fig. 4.11). When this happens, any remaining antibody will be rapidly mopped up by combination with the antigen and this will be reflected by a fall in detectable antibody in the blood; then after only a day or two a remarkable rise in the level of antibody begins and reaches a peak shortly thereafter which can be from 10 to 50 times higher than the primary response. This **secondary response** is maintained at a high level, falling only slowly over a period of months. The response can be boosted to even higher levels by further injections of antigen until a stage is reached when no further increase occurs. It is important to note that once an animal has responded to an antigen, even though exposed to it on only one occasion, the animal retains a **memory** of the antigen so that even after an interval of months or years it is able to react by means of a secondary response with a rapid mobilization of antibody-forming cells. Hence vaccination against an infective agent such as smallpox or poliomyelitis virus provides many years of useful protection against infection, even though soon after vaccination the level of antibodies falls to a low level, since the memory has been retained.

To obtain a maximum response, the **interval** between the primary and secondary injections should not be too short and an interval of less than 10 days is likely to reduce the level of the secondary response; subsequent injections should be spaced out to weeks, then to months (p. 165). This allows time for the increase in numbers of antibody-forming cells which can be stimulated by subsequent injections. The lymphocytes engaged in the initiation of humoral antibody production are derived from the bone marrow and are referred to as **B cells**. This cell differentiates into the main antibody synthesising cell — the **plasma cell**. The characteristics of this cell population were discussed earlier in this chapter.

Some of the host determinants of acquired immunity have already been mentioned. The nature of the antigen, the form in which it is presented, the route of injection and the dose given also have marked effects on the response.

Determinants of acquired immunity

Form, dose and route of entry of antigen

The determinants of antigenic specificity have been discussed above (p. 31), as have the affect of molecular weight and the need for foreignness of the antigenic material. It is, however, possible to enhance the natural ability of an antigen to induce an immune response by altering it or mixing it with another substance (called an adjuvant). A procedure of much practical value is to alter the **physical state** of the antigen by adsorbing it on to mineral gels such as aluminium hydroxide or phosphate. These alum-precipitated antigens are widely used as immunizing agents for humans. Such particulate forms of antigens seem to be able to initiate antibody production much more effectively than the same antigens in non-particulate form. This effect is not fully understood but may be due to a direct effect of the particulate material on the lymphocyte cell membrane leading to more effective transformation of the cell for antibody formation than can be brought about by antigen in solution.

An additional factor which may be important for some types of antigen is that particulate material is more readily phagocytosed by macrophages. These cells have been shown in certain situations to make a contribution by serving as a store of antigen for later release and stimulation of lymphocytes. It has been suggested that macrophages may also improve the antigenicity of weak antigens by altering them in some way before passing them on to lymphocytes. It is conceivable also that by removing antigen from the circulation they protect the lymphocytes from the effects of excess antigen which would be likely to paralyse the lymphocytes rather than initiate antibody production (see also 74). For a protein antigen a dose of a few hundred microgrammes is required to stimulate the production of detectable circulating antibody. The increase in antibody response is small in proportion to the increase in dose of antigen given and is approximately proportional to the square root of the increase in antigen administered until an upper limit is reached. An increase above this level can, as indicated above, result in specific paralysis of the antibody-forming tissues. This form of inhibition, sometimes referred to as **immunological tolerance**, is specific only for the antigen which brought it about. The lymphoid tissues remain normally responsive to other antigens.

Other methods have been developed to enhance the antibody response, although at present they are used mainly in experimental work. The most important of these consists of the preparation of a **water-in-oil emulsion** (Fig. 4.12): an aqueous solution of antigen is emulsified in a light mineral soil so that tiny drops of antigen solution are dispersed throughout the oil. The emulsion forms a depot of antigen in the subcutaneous tissues from which small quantities of antigen are continually released, sometimes for a year or more. An influenza vaccine in this form has been used successfully in man. New possibilities have been opened up by the development in Edinburgh of a multiple form of emulsion, in which the aqueous solution is first dispersed in oil and the oil is finally dispersed in a water phase. These emulsions are stable and much less viscous and less difficult to inject that the water-in-oil type. An even better response is achieved if killed tubercle bacilli are included in the emulsion; a wax constituent of the bacterial wall is responsible for this effect. The bacterial product appears to

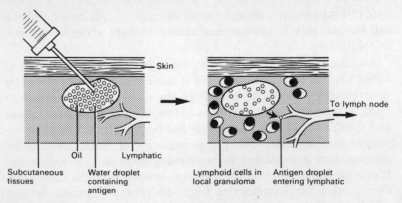

| Subcutaneous tissues | Water droplet containing antigen | Oil | Lymphatic | Lymphoid cells in local granuloma | Antigen droplet entering lymphatic | Skin | To lymph node |

Fig. 4.12 Water in oil adjuvant (depot forming adjuvant)

Table 4.6 Adjuvants

Type	Example	Main effects
Depot or repository		
Aluminium and calcium compounds	Aluminium phosphate	Slow release of antigen and local granuloma
Water in oil emulsions of antigen	Freund's incomplete	Slow release of antigen, emulsion droplets carry antigen to lymph nodes, local granuloma
Bacterial		
Mycobacteria	BCG (sometimes in water-in-oil emulsion — Freund's complete)	Stimulation of macrophage activity, increases numbers of antibody-producing cells
Anaerobic coryneforms	*Corynebacterium parvum*	Stimulation of macrophage activity, augmentation of certain classes of immunoglobulin e.g. IgM. Immunostimulation for antibody responses and immunosuppression of cell-mediated immune responsiveness.
Bordetella	*B. pertussis*	Activation of macrophages, lymphocytosis (shift of lymphocytes from T and B cell areas of lymphoid tissues)
Bacterial polysaccharides	various Gram-negative organisms	Activation of lymphocytes
Chemical		
Lysolecithin analogues	C_{18} ether hydroxy lysolecithin	Activation of macrophages
Lysozome labilizers	Vitamin A, beryllium salts silica	Activation of macrophages
Polyanions	Double, stranded, natural and synthetic polyribonucleic acids	Increase numbers of memory cells, activation of T lymphocytes and macrophages (interferon production)
Fungal polysaccharides	Lentinan (a glucose polymer)	Not known (possible stimulation of T lymphocytes)
Imidazole derivative	Levamisole	Not known

stimulate the cells involved in the immune response. Such emulsions are of course only suitable for experimental work and are often termed **Freund's** adjuvants after their originator.

The advantages of these **adjuvant** methods of immunization are that both the primary and secondary immune response are achieved by only one injection of antigen and that the peak level of antibody is maintained over a long period by the small quantities of antigen released from the depot.

Table 4.6 gives a list of examples of the three main types of adjuvant that are used: **depot** or **repository, bacterial** and **chemical**. The main effects of these adjuvants on the immune system (where known) are shown in the table. In the last few years adjuvants have been widely employed in tumour immunotherapy, both in experimental animals and man, and this is discussed further on page 217).

If an antigen is given intravenously most of the antibody is produced by the spleen, and some in the lung and bone marrow; on the other hand, if given subcutaneously or intradermally, the antigen travels via lymphatics to the local lymph nodes where antibody production is initiated. When antigen is given with adjuvants, there is a local accumulation of inflammatory cells, and antibody production occurs in the resulting granulomatous tissue as well as in the draining lymph nodes.

THE IMMUNOGLOBULINS

Enormous advances have been made in the last decade in knowledge of the chemical structure of immunoglobulins and the relationship of the **structure** to the **biological activities** of the molecule. These have enabled immunologists to agree internationally on a nomenclature which distinguishes a number of different classes of immunoglobulin on structural rather than functional characteristics. It was the practice to refer to an antibody as an agglutinin, a neutralizing or a precipitating antibody, when it was not realized that each of these activities could be exhibited by a chemically heterogeneous population of molecules and could be shared by the same molecule. Other classifications were dependent on the behaviour of the molecules in electrophoresis, which did little more than split the population up into still heterogeneous groups of proteins differing in their overall charge and molecular size.

Methods have been developed in America for the fragmentation of the immunoglobulin molecule by chemical cleavage in Edelman's laboratory, and by pepsin digestion by Nisonoff. Porter in Britain was the first to achieve cleavage with retention of biological activity of the fragments using papain digestion. These studies gave

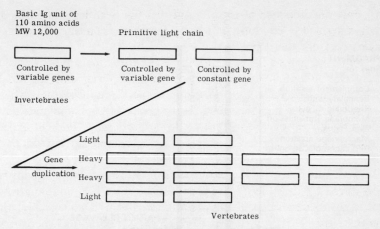

Fig. 4.13 Possible evolution of the immunoglobulin molecule

impetus to the work which now has enabled immunologists to distinguish five main classes of immunoglobulin each based on a similar polypeptide chain structure consisting of two pairs of 'heavy' and 'light' chains joined by disulphide bonds sometimes occurring as multiples of this basic unit.

It is considered that the molecule is based on a **12-unit structure**, each unit or domain consisting of a polypeptide chain with 110 amino acids of mol.wt 12 000 Daltons. Each light chain of mol.wt 25 000 Daltons consists of two of the basic units and each heavy chain four basic units. Heterogeneity of immunoglobulin structure occurs within this general framework with some of the basic units being affected more than others. Figure 4.13 shows a tentative view of how the molecule may have evolved from the basic unit, perhaps arising as a receptor on a phagocytic cell. The ancestral molecules, consisting of a single domain that immunoglobulin may have evolved from, are β2 microglobulin and Thy-1. These molecules form part of the array of substances found on the surface of various tissue cells. β2 microglobulin is a component of certain histocompatibility glycoprotein antigens and these are known to be involved in recognition of similarities and differences between cells. The evolutionary advantage provided by antibody-like molecules has ensured their maintenance and diversification over hundreds of millions of years. A picture of the immunoglobulin molecule has been built up and is represented in Figure 4.14. The general arrangement has been confirmed by electron microscopy.

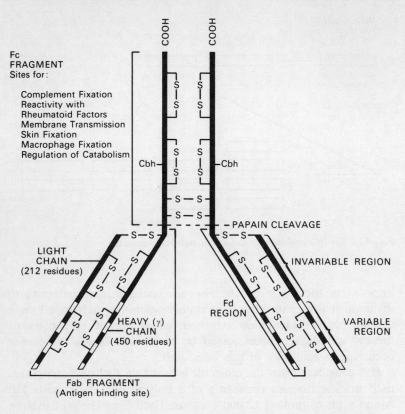

Fig. 4.14 Diagrammatic view of structural arrangements of polypeptide chains of immunoglobulin molecule. The chains are held together by three disulphide bonds. Pepsin splits the molecule, leaving an Fc fragment (crystallizable) and Fd parts of the heavy chains with attached light chains — the whole making Fab (or antigen binding) fragments. The N terminal ends of the light and heavy chains have variable sequences of amino acids as shown by the broken line. There are also a number of intra-chain disulphide bonds which influence the shape of individual chains. The carbohydrate (Cbh) groups may be concerned with the catabolism of the molecule

On the basis of marked **antigenic differences** in the **heavy chains** it has been possible to define **five classes** of human immunoglobulin, using the technique of immunoelectrophoresis. These are referred to as IgG, IgM, IgA, IgE and IgD (Table 4.7 and Fig. 4.15). IgM seems to have been the first immunoglobulin molecule to evolve. IgG and IgA probably evolved from the IgM by loss of single basic unit (domain) from the heavy chains (see below).

Table 4.7 Immunoglobulin classes

Immunoglobulin class	Molecular characteristic	Approximate serum concentration (mg/100 ml)	Molecular weight (Daltons)	Half life (days)	Heavy chain	Biological activities
IgG	Monomer	1100	150 000	21	gamma	Toxin neutralization Agglutination Opsonins Bacteriolytic (with complement) Ag/Ab complexes can mediate tissue injury IgG is late antibody
IgM	Monomeric on B cells Pentamer in serum with J chain	100	900 000	5	mu	IgM is early antibody and antigen receptor on B lymphocytes
IgA	Monomer and dimer with J chain and secretory piece	250	150 000–350 000	6	alpha	Surface protection Toxin neutralization
IgD	Monomer	3	180 000	3	delta	Antigen receptor on B lymphocytes
IgE	Monomer	0.1	190 000	2	epsilon	Antibody involved in allergic type l hypersensitivity reactions Immunity in worm infections

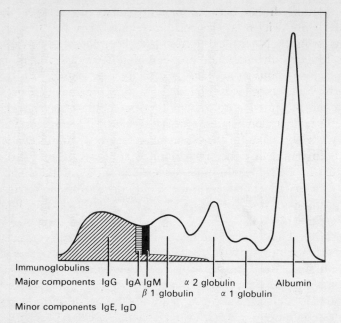

Immunoglobulins

Major components IgG IgA IgM   α 2 globulin   Albumin

β 1 globulin   α 1 globulin

Minor components IgE, IgD

Fig. 4.15 Electrophoretogram obtained by u.v. scanning of paper electrophoresis strip and showing diagrammatically the main components of human serum and the immunoglobulin classes

Immunoglobulin G or IgG

This is the major immunoglobulin component of serum making up 75% of the total and having a molecular weight of 160 000 Daltons in the human. The molecule has two antigen-binding sites as shown in Figure 14.14 on what are termed the **Fab** portions of the molecule and involving part of both the heavy and light chains. The amino acid sequences have been worked out in whole or in part for a number of light and heavy chains in various species, using myeloma proteins which are present as a homogeneous population in the serum of individuals with plasma cell tumours in sufficient quantity to enable studies of this type to be made.

The light chains can be shown to consist of two parts joined together. One has a **constant** sequence of amino acids at the C terminal end of the chain, common to the light chains of the species under study. The other part is at the N terminal end in which **variation** occurs in the sequence of the 107 amino acids. The variable portion differs between one myeloma and another, being similar only within a particular myeloma. Up to 50% of the positions in the N terminal portion have been found to be variable. This leads to an enormous number of different permutations of sequence and thus in antibody specificity. An animal may have a repertoire of a thousand different V_L and V_H regions that between them can account for up to a million potential antibody specificities. The other domains, one in light chains and three or four in heavy chains, make up the constant or C region. Similar variation has been found in rather more limited studies of the N terminal end of the **heavy chain**. The variable portions of the light and heavy chains are contained in the Fab portion of the molecule and it is in this **variable portion** of the chain that the **antigen-binding** site is present.

As larger numbers of immunoglobulins have been sequenced, it has become apparent that the amino acid variability tends to be concentrated in three so-called **hypervariable** regions. The remaining amino acid sequences of the variable regions, when one immunoglobulin is compared with another, fall into V region subclasses (four for K chain V regions and five for L chain).

The discovery of V region subclasses demonstrates that V region sequences have been more **strictly conserved** during evolution than those of the constant regions. No species-specific amino acid residues have so far been found in the variable portion and this suggests that during embryogenesis a single gene controls the development of the entire range of variability in the light chains. This gene probably arose early in evolution and the survival value associated with diversification of the antigen-binding site has ensured its maintenance since then.

The **light chains** are of two distinct types known as K or L (κ or λ) chains. In any one individual, both K and L chains are produced but they are not found together in the same immunoglobulin molecule. K and L chains are present in a ratio of about 2:1 in any one individual. Two intrachain disulphide bonds (Fig. 4.14) occur in almost exactly the same position in both K and L chains and both chains have cysteine as the terminal amino acid at the carboxyl end. This serves for the attachment to the heavy chains. These facts suggest a **common genetic origin** of K and L chains which, although they have **diverged** during evolution, have retained many common structural characteristics.

The **heavy chains** are specific for each class; in the human IgG molecule the heavy chain or γ chain exists in four different forms,

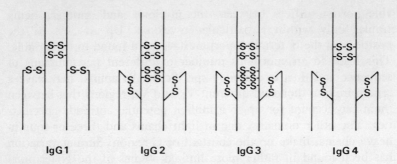

Fig. 4.16 IgG subclasses showing variable arrangements of the disulphide bonds

IgG1, IgG2, IgG3 and IgG4, which can be distinguished by specific antisera able to detect differences in the Fc fragment of the heavy chains. Sixty-five per cent of the IgG molecules in human serum are of the IgG1 subclass, 23% of the IgG2 and 8% and 4% IgG3 and 4. Differences have been found in the numbers and position of the disulphide bonds in the different IgG subclasses and these are shown diagrammatically in Figure 4.16. Disulphide bonds are essential to the normal 3-dimensional structure of immunoglobulin molecules and differences in their location may be reflected in different biological activities.

The separate immunoglobulin chains consist of repeating homologous units called **domains**; two for light chains, four to five for heavy chains (μ and ε heavy chains have five). A so-called **'hinge'** region occurs on heavy chains of all classes except IgM. It is inserted between the Fd and Fc portions and contains the inter-heavy-chain disulphide bridges. The domain at the amino terminal end of each H and L chain is the variable or V region referred to above and is the part which recognizes and binds foreign antigens.

The domains show many **homologies** in their amino acid sequences and were probably derived from an ancestral gene coding for the length of one domain. This gene was presumably doubled then redoubled and, within each resulting gene, crossing-over and mutation has since led to the differences that can now be detected in their products. The further back in evolution that divergence between the genes took place the fewer the similarities. The generation of subclasses is relatively recent in evolution and there is therefore a high degree of homology.

Individuals can be subdivided on the basis of certain characteristics of their immunoglobulin molecules. These are comparable to the blood groups but instead of involving antigenic differences in the surface antigens of red cells, they depend on antigenic differences in the light and heavy chains of the immunoglobulin molecule. These genetically determined subgroups are known as **allotypes**. Three main groups, Gm, Km and Am, have been found and each can be subdivided. The antigenic determinants of the Gm groups are carried in the γ chains of the IgG molecule only. In contrast the Km factors are present in the K light chains of each of the immunoglobulin classes. Am allotypes have been found in the IgA2 subclass.

The variable portions of the heavy and light chains of the Fab fragment have also been shown to carry antigenic determinants. These depend on the amino acid sequences in the variable portion that determine the specificity of the antibody. Thus Fab fragments of different specificity have different antigenic determinants. These are called **idiotypic** determinants and are characteristic of the particular clone of cells producing a specific antibody and have proved of considerable value to immunologists as a way of following the activity of a particular clone of cells by identifying the idiotypic marker. Isotypes also exist and are due to antigenic determinants on all molecules of a certain class or subsclass of heavy chains or of certain light chains.

IgM, IgA and IgD

Like IgG globulin each of these classes of immunoglobulin in man has been found to contain K and L light chains. The heavy chains, on the other hand, are unique for each of these types of immunoglobulin, IgM containing μ chains. The μ chains have five subunits or domains (one variable and four constant) compared with four subunits in γ and α heavy chains. IgM in membrane-bound form on B cells has an additional hydrophobic portion that traverses the B cell membrane with a short positively charged sequence of amino acids in the cytoplasm of the cell. Thus the μ chain of secreted IgM has 21 fewer residues than the membrane-bound form. The extra residues of the latter anchor the molecule in the B cell membrane. Membrane immunoglobulins do not form polymers of the basic 4-chain unit. Secreted immunoglobulins are released from the cell by reverse pinocytosis. IgE (see p. 226), like IgM, also has an extra domain in its ε heavy chains. IgA have α chains and IgD δ chains and it is these differences which enable them to be distinguished one from another. There are two subclasses of IgA (IgA1 and

IgA2). IgA2 is unusual in that the light chains are linked to each other by disulphide bonds instead of to the heavy chains (they are linked covalently to the heavy chains in this subclass). IgA1 accounts for 90% of the total serum IgA in contrast to secretions, where IgA2 makes up as much as 60% of the total. IgM globulin, with a molecular weight of about 900 000 Daltons, can be split by reduction of disulphide bonds into five subunits. These subunits have a molecular weight of 180 000 Daltons and like IgG have two heavy and two light chains.

Until recently most studies on the number of antigen-binding sites of IgM antibody showed that the molecule had only 5 binding sites despite the fact that theoretically 10 were present. Both human and rabbit IgM however have now been shown to have the 10 sites and it is believed that the 2 binding sites on each are unable to combine with antigen with similar efficiency thus making it difficult to demonstrate all 10 sites. Polymeric forms of IgA and the IgM molecule have been shown to have a small polypeptide called the J chain.

This polypepide has a molecular weight of about 15 000 Daltons and differs in structure from all known immunoglobulin polypeptide chains. It is rich in cysteine residues and appears to exist in a molar ratio of one J chain per polymer regardless of how many immunoglobulin subunits make up the polymer. The J chain makes up about 1% of the IgM molecule by weight and in the IgA molecule about 3%.

The role of the J chain is not entirely clear but the fact that it is added at the final polymerisation stage just before the molecule is secreted at the cell membrane of the synthesizing cell suggests that it may be required in the secretion process. It is noteworthy that IgM subunits are not found free in the serum, although polymers of IgM without J chain are found in certain pathological conditions. The role of the J chain in the IgA molecule may be to activate the transport molecules that carry IgA through the mucous membranes and may perhaps be responsible for the ability of the IgA molecule to bind the secretory piece (see p. 105). The molecular structure of some of these immunoglobulins is shown in Figures 4.17 and 4.18.

Structure and function of immunoglobulins

Knowledge gained from the structural studies discussed above has

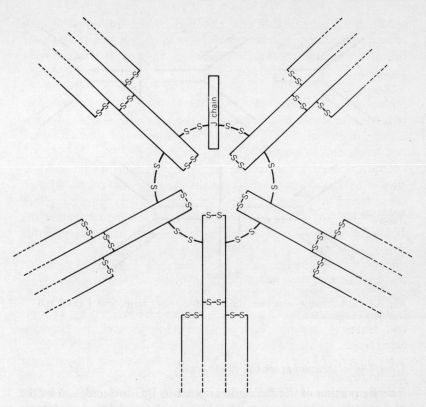

Fig. 4.17 IgM structure showing five subunits and multiple combining sites

helped towards an understanding of the biological activities of the immunoglobulin molecule and it is now possible to pinpoint areas of the molecule responsible for different activities. The areas of the light and heavy chains (Fab portion) containing the variable sequences are the site of that part of the molecule with the capacity to combine with antigen. The heavy chain component (Fd portion) seems in some studies to contain as much as 85% of the antigen-binding ability although this is not always so. The light chain component, although usually inactive alone, seems to act together with the heavy chain to form a stable antigen-binding site. The flexibility and independent movement of the Fab portion of IgG enables the molecule to bind to single particles containing repeating epitopes irrespective of how they are arranged.

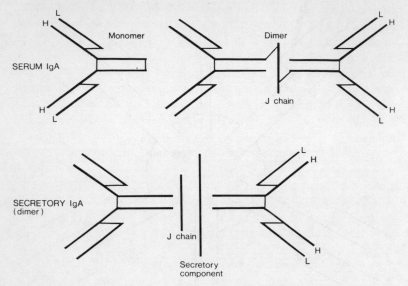

Fig. 4.18 IgA showing monomer, dimer and secretory form, with J chain and secretory component.

Complement activation and agglutination

The Fc portion of the molecule appears in IgG molecules to be the major component responsible for activating the complement system, although this does not occur unless two or more molecules of IgG are brought into close apposition. It is not certain exactly what changes in molecular configuration or other effects take place when the molecules come close together but isolated Fc fragments do not activate complement and will do so only if aggregated first. The flexibility of the molecule in the 'hinge' region appears to be important in enabling C1q of the complement system (p. 25) to bind to the Cγ2 domain of IgG. This flexibility in contrast is absent from the hinge region of the IgM molecule and the binding of C1q to its Cμ3 and/or 4 domain is believed to be dependent on as yet undefined interactions between domains when the Fab regions bind to antigen. The subclasses of IgG (Fig. 4.16) vary in their ability to bind complement components. IgG3 appears to bind C1q seven times more effectively than IgG1 and IgG4 does not bind complement at all.

It has been calculated that a single IgM molecule attached to a red cell by its multiple combining sites can bring about lysis whereas 1000 IgG molecules are required for the same effect. Humphrey and Dourmashkin, who came to these conclusions, assumed that as two IgG molecules must come together for complement activation, a large number of IgG molecules would be required for this to occur as the antigenic determinants are spread evenly over the surface of the red cell. Agglutination is brought about by the linking of particulate antigens such as red cells or bacteria by the two Fab fragments of the immunoglobulin molecule.

As might be expected from knowledge of the structure of the IgM molecule, its five combining sites make it a very efficient agglutinating antibody molecule and rabbit IgM antibacterial antibody is known to be 22 times as active as IgG antibody (mol/mol) in bringing about bacterial agglutination. Because of its large molecular size IgM is largely confined to the bloodstream and probably plays an important role in protection. Deficiency of IgM is often associated with susceptibility to septicaemia. IgG antibodies on the other hand are more effective than IgM antibodies at neutralising diphtheria toxin, lysozyme or viruses such as poliovirus. Whilst some of this activity was present in isolated Fab fragments, the evidence from virus neutralization indicates that the Fc fragment may assist the Fab fragments in neutralization of virus infectivity. The molecular basis for such effects has yet to be elucidated.

Tissue fixation and opsonization

The ability of immunoglobulin to attach to tissue cells appears to be a well-marked feature of the IgE class of immunoglobulin responsible in humans for various forms of hypersensitivity reaction (p. 226) and may be dependent on the activity of the Fc portion of the molecule. This is suggested by studies of the ability of immunoglobulin fragments to adhere to guinea-pig skin and produce a particular form of hypersensitivity reaction that is known as passive cutaneous anaphylaxis. Immunoglobulin antibody specific for particulate antigens such as bacteria plays a valuable role by coating the surface and making the antigen more susceptible to phagocytosis. These are known as opsonizing antibodies and IgM antibodies perform this role particularly efficiently. In the rabbit it has been shown that IgM anti-salmonella antibodies are some 500 to 1000 times more effective than IgG antibodies as opsonizing agents.

How opsonization is brought about is not clear; it is possible that antibody may alter the surface properties, such as the surface charge of a particulate antigen, and thus perhaps reduce electrostatic repulsion between phagocyte and antigen. It also can be shown that the $C_\gamma 3$ of the Fc fragments of the antibody have an affinity for the Fc receptor of the macrophage and thus link the particulate antigen (attached by means of the antibody combining sites) to the macrophage (attached by the Fc fragment). Antibody with the ability to attach to macrophages by means of the Fc fragment has been described in the guinea-pig and is known as cytophilic antibody. Antigen-antibody complexes appear to be localized in the lymphoid follicles of lymph glands due to the activity of the Fc portion of the immunoglobulin molecule.

The presence of immunoglobulin molecules as receptors for antigen on the surface of lymphocytes has been confirmed by a variety of techniques. B lymphocytes can clearly be shown to have light chains and heavy (μ) chains on their surface.

Recent work indicates that IgD is present on the majority of B lymphocytes in the cord blood of human infants and in a lesser proportion of adult B lymphocytes. The molecule does not cross the placenta and is absent from cord serum. The significance of these observations is not yet clear. A similar immunoglobulin has been found in the mouse and occurs together with other classes of immunoglobulin on a substantial proportion of B cells in the spleen, lymph nodes and Peyer's patches. Immature B cells (uncommitted) appear to have μ (IgM) heavy chains and later to develop δ (IgD) chains in addition (see also p. 63). At a later stage in differentiation δ and γ (IgG) chains are formed without μ chains. Human IgD has a heavy chain consisting of four domains with an Fc region that is highly resistant to proteolysis. An unusual structural feature is a long hinge region that might be important in the cross-linking of membrane associated IgD (sIgD) by antigen. It has been proposed that IgD on B lymphocytes may be involved in processing of antigen. The immunoglobulin appears to be able to induce a T cell population with receptors for IgD that can enhance antibody responses.

Selective transport

The newborn animal, emerging from an environment where it has been sheltered from antigenic stimuli, is protected by maternal immunoglobulins transmitted from the mother. These antibodies often reach a level higher than in the mother and persist longer in the circulation of the young animal than they would do in the adult. This transferred **passive immunity** tides the infant over the period until its own immunological system begins to mature.

In humans, IgG globulins can pass through the placenta and reach the fetal circulation; this is not a simple filtration process, but is due to selective transfer of the molecules involving a part of the Fc fragment of IgG heavy chains. This property is a feature only of the γ heavy chains of IgG and has not been found in the μ and α chains of IgM and IgA. This mechanism seems to be limited to **primates** whilst in **ruminants** maternal immunoglobulins from the colostrum reach the fetus through the intestinal epithelium.

Another selective transport mechanism is found with IgA globulins which are selectively secreted into saliva and respiratory and intestinal **mucuous secretions** as well as into the **colostrum**. The site of synthesis of IgA is in submucosal plasma cells of the **lamina propria** of the gastrointestinal tract and in the salivary glands and mammary glands. In the lamina propria of human gastrointestinal tract the IgA-producing cells outnumber the IgG cells by about 20:1 in contrast to lymph nodes and spleen where the ratio is 1:3 (IgA:IgG). The IgA found in mucous secretions is manufactured as a dimer with a J chain component and has an attached **secretory** or transport component not found except in small amounts in serum IgA. The secretory component is synthesized by epithelial cells and is added to the molecule during its passage into the mucous secretions from the lamina propria, underlying the mucous membrane of the gut and respiratory tract. The secretory component has a molecular weight of 70 000 Daltons, the J chain 15 000 Daltons and the secretory IgA is an 11S molecule of molecular weight 400 000 Daltons. The IgM present in secretions has also been found to have secretory component bound to it, whilst any IgG or IgE found in secretions does not. About 4% of the plasma cells of the respiratory and gastrointestinal mucosa are making IgE and, like IgA-producing cells, contribute to serum IgE levels.

In contrast to other immunoglobulins, salivary and colostral IgA, probably because of the attached secretory piece, appear to be relatively resistant to digestion by proteolytic enzymes. This would clearly be an advantage in allowing this immunoglobulin to remain active and able to perform a protective role in the intestinal tract. It has been suggested recently that the main function of the secretory component is to anchor the dimeric form of IgA to the mucous surface to prevent it being swept away by the secretions. Much effort is being expended by laboratory workers in studying the role of IgA as a protective mechanism at the mucous surface and the possible future use of vaccines designed to stimulate this form of antibody response may be of considerable value.

An interesting suggestion has been made, supported by some experimental evidence, that IgA in the mucous secretions may inhibit the binding of potentially pathogenic microorganisms to the mucous membranes and thus prevent infection. IgA may play a role by combining with food constituents that could act as allergens and prevent their passage through the gut wall. This idea is supported by the finding that infants with reduced serum IgA levels soon after birth seem more likely to develop allergic states at about 1 year of age. See page 136 for further discussion of IgA activity.

THE CELL-MEDIATED ACQUIRED IMMUNE RESPONSE

In the immunologically mature individual, contact with an antigen leads not only to the production of circulating antibody, but also to the development of a separate cell-mediated form of response. In both types initial contact with the antigen is necessary and the response is specific for the antigen. Cell-mediated immunity occurs particularly in infections by agents which enter the cells such as viruses, tubercle bacilli and *Brucella* species (p. 124). It can also develop after skin contact with certain simple chemical substances (p. 237). The sequence of steps leading to this form of immunity is essentially no different from that leading to the antibody response but the response is initiated in different areas of the spleen and lymph nodes (white pulp around the central arterioles of the spleen and the paracortical areas of the lymph nodes); these areas are under the control of the thymus gland (p. 53).

A characteristic of these thymus-dependent lymphocytes is that they can be stimulated to differentiate and divide by plant extracts known as phytohaemagglutinins (PHA) and by certain extracts of microorganisms such as streptolysin S from streptococci. These substances, sometimes referred to as mitogens, appear to act on the small lymphocytes of all vertebrates so far examined and induce enlargement of the cells, increased synthesis of RNA followed later by DNA synthesis. The plant extracts are specific for sugar determinants present in the lymphocyte cell membrane, and interaction

Table 4.8 Main steps in lymphocyte transformation

1. Reaction of inducer at plasma membrane — PHA or antigen
2. Increased synthesis of RNA in 30 min to 2 hours
3. Morphological changes — enlargement of the cell, changes in nucleus,
   (transformation)   increases in lysosome granules and endocytosis
                                  (commences at about 20 hours)
4. Increase in thymidine incorporation into DNA about 36 hours for PHA and
   40 hours for antigens. Mitosis

leads to 'triggering' of the activity of the cell. This involves biochemical changes that are now beginning to be understood and include transport of ions (e.g. Ca^{2+}), amino acids and nucleotides through the cell membrane leading to purine synthesis and finally cell division. This process is known as **lymphocyte transformation** and can be brought about in sensitized lymphocytes on subsequent exposure to the sensitizing antigen (see Table 4.8). Transformation is readily measured in vitro by culturing the cells in the presence of labelled precursors of nucleic acids, e.g. ^{14}C thymidine for DNA synthesis or ^{14}C uridine for RNA synthesis. The test can be used to detect sensitisation to an antigen and the non-specific plant mitogens are used as a test of the competence of the cell-mediated immune system. Lymphocytes from an individual with, for example, an immune deficiency state (Ch. 9) with thymic aplasia and consequent defective cell-mediated immunity would be unable to transform in the presence of PHA. Transformation of lymphocytes to PHA is reduced in certain virus infections (p. 149).

Mechanisms of cell-mediated immunity

Lymphocyte activation products

Cell-mediated immunity dependent on these activated lymphocytes is usually recognized by means of a skin test (e.g. intradermal injection) with the antigen that, in an individual who has developed a cell-mediated immune response, results in an inflammatory reaction at the injection site. When examined histologically it can be seen that the tissues at the injection site have been infiltrated by mononuclear cells, mainly lymphocytes and a few macrophages. There is considerable experimental evidence that the majority of the infiltrating cells are not the activated (or sensitized) lymphocytes that have previously been sensitized to antigen but uncommitted cells attracted by soluble products of the sensitized lymphocytes.

Cytokines

Cells of the lymphoid system secrete a number of mediators called cytokines that play important roles in the regulation of the immune system. **Cytokines** produced by macrophages are termed monokines and by lymphocytes **lymphokines** and those specifically involved in interactions between leucocytes are called **interleukins**. Lymphokines were the first to be discovered and are produced mainly by T lymphocytes although B lymphocytes can also make a contribution. Numerous activities are associated with lymphokines but have not all been identified with a particular molecular species. Lymphokines affecting the function of phagocytes were the first to be described and include a factor that inhibits the migration of macrophages (MIF) thus retaining them at the site of an inflammatory response. Once retained they are activated by gamma interferon from lymphocytes an activity that used to be ascribed to macrophage activating factor (MAF) before it was found largely to be due to interferon. Macrophage activation is a very complex but crucial process in cellular immunity involving membrane changes such as receptor expression and increase in microbicidal factors both oxygen dependent and independent as well as lysosomal enzymes. Another important lymphokine is one with chemotactic activity for macrophages and there is a separate one for neutrophils that bring such cells to the site of an inflammatory response. Yet another activity called colony stimulating activity stimulates the bone marrow to replenish the levels of circulating phagocytes. Lymphokines affecting other cells include interleukin-2 one of the most important lymphokines as it triggers the production of a number of other lymphokines including factors that stimulate B lymphocytes to grow and differentiate, B cell growth and differentiation factors (BCGF and BCGF) as well as the chemotactic, colony-stimulating factors and interferons (alpha, beta and gamma) (Table 4.9). A better understanding of these lymphokines is emerging with the cloning of T cells (produced, for example, by fusing T cells to form a hybridoma with T cell lymphoma cells). Interferons, interleukin-2 and tumour necrosis factor are now available in purified form as a result of cloning techniques and can thus be studied in isolation rather than as one of a mixture of activities in the supernatants of cultured lymphocytes. The more recently described interleukins-3 and 4 are described as having effects on mast cell and eosinophil proliferation respectively. IL-3 appears to be a colony-stimulating factor and IL-4 has effects on B cell growth leading to IgE production.

Table 4.9 Sources of interferons

α interferons	1] Leucocytes + virus 2] Lymphoblastoid cell lines + virus 3] Bacteria or yeasts by recombinant DNA technology (each produces a different subtype approx 20 amino acids differ in each subtype)
β interferons	1] Fibroblast + virus or chemicals 2] Bacteria by recombinant DNA technology
γ interferons	1] Leucocytes + antigen or mitogen 2] Bacteria by recombinant DNA technology

Recent evidence suggests that IL-4 is a B cell growth factor regulating B cell activation, proliferation and antibody formation. It seems likely that there may be as many as 4 cytokines regulating T cells and 5 regulating B cells and that an Interleukin–IL-5 may be responsible for induction of IL-2 receptors on T cells.

Monokines produced by macrophages include interferons and interleukin-1 as well as a variety of mediators such as prostaglandins, complement factors, microbicidal and tumoricidal factors and factors with effects on tissue organization (elastase, collagenase, hyaluronidase angiogenesis factor). Interleukin-1 is particularly important in the regulation of the immune response as it is responsible for stimulating T helper cells (T4/CD4 cells) to produce interleukin-2. There are two forms of interleukin-1 the alpha and beta forms with extracellular activity being due to a 17 KDa molecule cleaved from a precursor molecule. The alpha form appears to be able to be cleaved more effectively than the beta form to the active molecule. Interleukin-1 has a multitude of inflammatory effects both on cells of the immune system and other cells. It acts as a pyrogen by effecting the temperature control centre of the brain and initiates the production of acute phase proteins by the liver (e.g. C reactive protein). As noted above, it initiates the cascade of reactions that follow interleukin-2 production by T helper cells and recent evidence has implicated interleukin-1 in activating phospholipase enzymes (PLA2) that can hydrolyse membrane phospholipids. Interleukin-1 is produced by a variety of cell types as well as macrophages, in particular those cells that like macrophages act as inducer cells for the immune response (dendritic cells, Langerhans' cells and B cells) as well as other cells (epithelial cells, fibroblasts and neutrophils), usually after stimulation by the membrane triggering agent, bacterial endotoxin. Interleukin-1 production is associated with the expression of class

Table 4.10 Lymphokines and monokines

Factor	Source	Functions
Mitogenic factor Blastogenic factor Lymphocyte transformation factor	lymphocytes	Recruitment of additional lymphocytes. Initiating lymphocyte proliferation to enhance response
Chemotactic factors	lymphocytes	Part of inflammatory response to attract macrophages and neutrophils to site of immune response
Interferons	lymphocytes and macrophages	Provides protection against viral replication; activates macrophages and natural killer cells
Interleukin-1	macrophages (dendritic cells, PMN, lymphocytes, glial cells, kidney mesangial cells, skin cells)	Imunopotentiation — stimulates T-helper cells (increases IL-2 receptors) and thymocytes to proliferate and produce mature T-cells that release their own growth promoting factors; stimulates liver cells to produce 'acute phase proteins' and induces fever. Chemotactic to PMN awnd Lymphocytes, Local cytotoxic effects
Interleukin-2	lymphocytes	Promotes proliferation of T-helper and cytotoxic cells
Interleukin-3 and 4	lymphocytes	Proliferation of bone marrow precursor cells
B cell growth and differentiation factors (BCGF/BCDF)	lymphocytes	Promotes (along with other factors) B cell differentiation towards antibody production
Tumour necrosis factor (TNF) Lymphotoxin (LT)	lymphocytes	cytostatic for some tumours, tumour necrosis in vivo, induces monocyte cytotoxicity. Activates PMN, Fibroblast growth factor, induction of β and γ interferon, fever induction, cartilage matrix resorption, induction of IL-1, oynovia) collagenase and PGE_2.
Macrophage inhibition factor Macrophage aggregation factor	lymphocytes	Retains macrophages at site of inflammatory response
Macrophage activating factor	lymphocytes	Triggers microbicidal and tumoricidal activity in macrophages

TNF is indistinguishable functionally from lymphotoxin. They are 32% homologous in structure, compete for the same receptor and cause fragmentation of the DNA of the target cell. The genes for TNF (α and β) map between the class III region and the mouse H-2 D locus (Fig. 4.19).

2 MHC antigens on the cell and thus with the ability of the cell to present antigen to T helper cells for the induction of immunity.

Table 4.10 lists a variety of lymphokines and cytokines that are involved in the regulation of cells of the immune system. Their other main functions being in recruitment, retention and activation of the cells in an inflammatory response.

Effects of interferons

Interferons have a wide variety of effects including stimulation of cytotoxic, natural killer and B cells. They are involved in recovery from virus infections. They inhibit some enzyme functions such as ornithine decarboxylase and increase others such as protein kinase. Changes are induced in the cell membrane such as increased expression of MHC antigens and sometimes increases in net negative charge.

In commercial production a lymphoblastoid cell line selected for its ability to produce large amounts of alpha interferon is grown in large volumes with the addition of sodium butyrate to increase yield. Sendai virus is used to induce the cells to produce interferon that is then purified by precipiatation, solvent extraction and chromatography. See page 218 for discussion of its use in clinical practice.

An association has been noted between virus infections of the upper respiratory tract and exacerbation of type 1 hypersensitivity. The effect may be due to interferon production that enhances release of histamine from basophils. Other suggested causes are virus induced suppression of T suppressor cell activity leading to enhanced IgE production or mucosal damage by virus allowing access of allergen in a susceptible individual.

Cytotoxic cells. Understanding of the mechanism of killing of cytotoxic T cells (Tc) and natural killer cells (NK) (p. 64) has been helped by cloning techniques. There is now good evidence that cytolytic lymphocyte clones contain in their granules cytotoxic protein molecules termed 'perforins' that are activated by Ca^{++} to induce transmembrane pores on the target cell. Cell death results in the same way as with late complement components by loss of cellular content through the pores. Cloned NK cells have been shown to contain granule associated highly negatively charged proteoglycans that are believed to be responsible for target cell lysis.

In vivo role of cell-mediated immunity

Cell-mediated immune responses are involved in protection against various infective agents (p. 139). They may also serve an important physiological role in the normal individual bringing about the elimination of spontaneously arising neoplastic cells which might represent a potential threat to the individual. In support of the existence of such an **immunological surveillance** mechanism (Ch. 8), it has been found that the incidence of tumours is highest at the two extremes of life when the immunological mechanisms are at their least efficient. The cell-mediated immune system is under the influence of the thymus and the cells are referred to as thymus-dependent or T cells. After thymectomy in mice the incidence of tumours induced by chemical carcinogens and viruses has been found to be significantly higher than in sham-thymectomised controls. The thymus has been found to be absent in certain rare immune deficiency states of children (p. 241). In such conditions there is a deficiency of lymphocytes from the areas of spleen and lymph nodes under thymic control. Cell-mediated immune reactions are absent and there is an inability to deal with virus infections. This type of cell-mediated immune mechanism would be likely to have arise **early in evolution** with the development of multicellular organisms and would have additional survival value in that it would also be effective against exogenous parasites.

Cell co-operation and the genetic control of the immune response

The mechanisms by which immunocompetent cells co-operate together to produce an immune response have begun to be resolved with the use of advances in molecular genetics and cell cloning techniques. The identification of a variety of interleukins that act as mediators regulating interactions between leucocytes has been one of the most important advances. Much knowledge has been gained on the genes controlling the ability of the immunocompetent cells to respond to antigens that are genetically very closely related to those genes controlling certain important cell surface antigens. These antigens are those involved in rejection of grafts and on transfer of a graft of tissue to an unrelated (allogeneic) recipient are recognised as foreign. An immune response is initiated and the graft is rejected (see p. 200).

The cell surface antigens are known as **histocompatibility** antigens and the group of genes that determines the expression of these antigens as the **major histocompatibility complex** (MHC). In the mouse these genes are present in chromosome number 17 and 6 in humans.

The glycoprotein gene products are expressed on the surface of various cells and three classes of MHC gene products have been identified that are important in immunity.

Class 1 antigens determine graft rejection and also associate with viral antigens enabling the infected cell to be recognized by cytotoxic T cells. Class 2 antigens act as receptors for the presentation of antigen to helper T cells. These antigens are sometimes referred to as immune response or IR gene products. Class 3 antigens are involved in the production of components of the complement system (p. 25).

Class 1 antigens are expressed on most nucleated cells (this enables tissue cells infected with a virus to be recognized by cytotoxic T cells). Class 2 antigens are more restricted and are found on macrophages dendritic cells in the lymph nodes and spleen. Langerhans' cells in the skin. B lymphocytes, activated T lymphocytes, vascular endothelium and some epithelial cells. Gamma interferon can promote and increase the expression of class 2 antigens on various cells types.

Figure 4.19 shows the arrangement of the genes in the MHC of mouse and man. The class 1 and 2 antigens are glycoproteins made up of two chains with an extracellular, a hydrophobic transmembrane and a cytoplasmic segment. Class 1 antigens consist of a highly polymorphic heavy chain of 45 kDa and a non-poly-

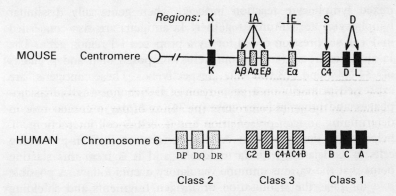

Fig. 4.19 Simplified view of the major histocompatibility gene complex.

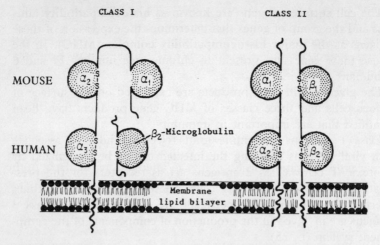

Fig. 4.20 Simplified digram of the structure of class 1 and class 2 MHC gene products.

morphic, non-glycosylated light chain of 12 kDa (beta 2 microglobulin) and class 2 antigens of an alpha and a beta chain of 34 and 28 kDa respectively. Figure 4.20 illustrates the structure of these antigens.

The I region in the mouse and the D region in man contains genes which function as lymphocyte activating determinants and code for membrane — associated antigens, the Ia antigens. Figure 4.19 shows the subgroups so far determined within the I region. Various roles have been found for the different I regions in the immune response. Antisera against I region associated antigens block certain functions of the immune system, for example, the mixed lymphocyte reaction induced when genetically dissimilar lymphocytes are cultured together. Ia antigens are also concerned in T cell suppression coded for by a proposed I-J region gene. The Ia antigens are surface glycoproteins composed of α and β chains of 34 000 and 28 000 kDa respectively. These antigens are expressed primarily on a proportion of B lymphocytes and macrophages and other inducer cells (p. 74) and play a crucial role in determining antigen presentation and T cell-B cell interactions. T helper cells detect antigen on the surfaces of antigen-presenting cells in association with Ia molecules and it is from this starting point that the various immune regulatory events follow. A possible role for Ia is the stabilisation of antigen fragments and shielding them from proteolytic digestion.

The first clues that the MHC genes were involved in cell cooperation came from studies on collaboration between thymocytes and
bone marrow cells in the immune response to sheep red blood cells.
It was found that allogeneic thymocytes and bone marrow cells
collaborate poorly and that the most efficient response was
produced when the cells were from syngeneic donors. Genetic
analysis revealed that concordance in the I region of the mouse
MHC genes was necessary for efficient collaboration. The same
conclusions have more recently been drawn from studies of collaboration between macrophages and lymphocytes. These studies have
important implications in immunity to infection, particularly in the
case of virus infections, and are discussed more fully in Chapter
5. Thus, in conclusion, activation of T lymphocytes usually
requires the simultaneous association of the T cell receptor with
antigen and MHC class two products on the inducer/antigen
presenting cell or, in the case of cytotoxic T lymphocytes, with
MHC class one and antigen. Other non-polymorphic T cell surface
molecules are also involved in the cell co-operative process although
their precise roles are not clear. These include human T4 (CD 4),
murine L3T4, human T8 (CD 8), murine Lyt2 and LFA-1 that
take part in the formation of a stable T cell receptor-antigen-MHC
complex.

Table 4.11 provides a summary of the pathways leading to the
different forms of immune response.

Table 4.11 Summary of stages in antibody and cell-mediated immune response

Main pathway
Dendritic cells and macrophages → ingestion → digestion and re-expression on
surface. Interleukin-1 production

Minor pathway
B-lymphocytes → antigen bound to Ig receptors on those cells expressing Ig
specific for the antigen — which can in special circumstances,
trigger B-cells directly

1. Antigen recognized on macrophages or B-lymphocytes in association with
MHC class 2 molecules by T-helper lymphocytes. This triggers interleukin-
2 production by T helper cells
2. Interleukin-1 from macrophages increases the number of receptors on T
helper cells for interleukin-2
3. Mitosis, production of B cell growth factors and clonal expression resulting in
generation of effector T- and B-lymphocytes:
(a) Cytotoxic T cell — T_c
(b) Delayed hypersensitivity T-cell — T_{dh} that produce lymphokines
(c) Suppressor T-cells — T_s regulate immune response
(d) B-lymphocytes differentiate into plasma cells to produce immunoglobulins

FURTHER READING

Adams D 1982 Molecules, membranes and macrophage activation. Immunology Today 3:285

Honjo T 1983 Immunoglobulin genes. Annual Review of Immunology 1:499

Howard M, Paul W E 1983 Regulation of B cell growth and differentiation by soluble factors. Annual Review of Immunology 1:307

Immunology Today, published monthly by Elsevier/North Holland Biomedical Press. Contains invaluable reviews and articles on current developments

Inglis J 1982 B lymphocytes today. Elsevier Biomedical Press, Amsterdam

Inglis J 1983 T lymphocytes today: Elsevier Biomedical Press, Amsterdam

Kaufman J F, Anffray C, Korman A J, Shackelford D A, Strominger J L 1984 The class II molecules of the human, murine major histocompatibility complex. Cell 38:1

Lachman L B, Maizel A L 1983 Human immunoregulatory molecules. Interleukin 1, and interleukin 2 and B cell growth factor. Contemporary and Topical Molecular Immunology 9:147

McConnell I, Munro A, Waldmann H 1981 The immune system, 2nd edn. Blackwell Scientific Publications, Oxford

Moller G 1982 Interleukins and lymphocyte activation. Immunology Review 63

Robertson M 1984 T cell antigen receptor. Nature 312:16

Roitt I M 1984 Essential immunology. Blackwell Scientific Publications, Oxford

Roitt I M, Brostoff J, Male D K 1985 Immunology. Churchill Livingstone, Edinburgh.

Stites D P, Stobo J D, Fudenberg H H, Wells J V (eds) 1984 Basic and clinical immunology 5th edn. Lange Medical Publications, Los Altos.

Tonegawa S 1983 Somatic generation of antibody diversity. Nature 302:573

Tonegawa S 1900 Molecules of the immune system. Scientific American 253:104

Turner M W 1983 Immunoglobulins. In: Holborow E J, Reeves W G (eds) Immunology in medicine, 2nd edn. Grune and Stratton, London

Unanue E R 1984 Antigen-presenting function of macrophages. Annual Review of Immunology 2:395

Williamson A R, Turner M W 1985 Essential immunogenetics. Blackwell Scientific Publications, Oxford

Immunology in Action

5

Infection, immunity and protection

Objectives

On completion of this section the reader will be able to:

1. Differentiate infection from disease.
2. Define the compromised host syndrome and give three examples.
3. List two common commensal organisms present on skin, in throat, nasopharynx, oropharynx, small intestine, large intestine, and female genital tract.
4. List two ways in which the normal flora of the body prevents colonization and infection by pathogenic organisms and list two conditions by which this ecological balance can be disturbed.
5. Give four examples of the mechanisms by which microorganisms can escape the immune response and establish themselves in the host's tissues.
6. List three factors that contribute to 'non-specific' immunity to microorganisms.
7. Describe the role of immunological memory in the mechanisms of immunity to bacterial and viral infections.
8. Define antigenic drift.
9. Give three examples of bacteria and viruses that interfere with the development of acquired immunity.
10. List two factors associated with difficulty in development of an immune response to protozoa and helminths.
11. Describe with the aid of a diagram the various consequences following stimulation of the T lymphocyte response to a microorganism.
12. List three bacterial and three viral vaccines; describe their use in prophylaxis, and list any contraindications for their use.
13. Describe how recombinant DNA techniques are being used to develop new vaccines.
14. Outline the contribution immune complexes make to bacterial and viral pathogenesis.

In the normal healthy individual, despite popular belief, the relationship between microorganisms and ourselves is usually a harmless one. Saprophytic or commensal microorganisms grow and reproduce without apparent damage to either host or microbe. As Lewis Thomas points out in his essay on 'Germs' (*The Lives of a Cell*, Bantam Books), 'we have always been a relatively minor interest of the vast microbial world' and human disease is not 'the work of an organized, modernized kind of demonology, in which bacteria are the most visible and centrally placed adversaries. . . . Most bacteria are totally preoccupied with browsing, altering the configurations of organic molecules so that they become usable for the energy needs of other forms of life'. The normal flora of humans is shown in Figures 5.1 to 5.3 and gives examples of bacteria, fungi and protozoa which are commensals. Parasitic microorganisms can very often be considered to be foolish commensals that do not recognise a good situation.

Modern medical science has managed to eliminate many of the classical infectious diseases, but has also helped to create new ones which result from interference with normal host defence mechanisms — consequent upon medical and surgical procedures such as chemotherapy, catherization, immunosuppression and X-irradiation. Infections that develop in this way are known as iatrogenic (physician-induced) diseases in which host defence mechanisms have been **compromised** in some way (Table 5.1).

It is important to differentiate infection from disease. A host may be infected with a particular microorganism and be unaware of the presence of the microorganism. If the microbe reproduces itself to such an extent that toxic products or sheer numbers of organisms begin to harm the host then a disease process has developed. It is well known that certain viruses cause latent infections (e.g. Herpes simplex) and only cause disease (e.g. cold sores) under circumstances when the host defences are impaired. Other examples are the carriage of potentially pathogenic bacteria in the nose, throat or bowel, e.g. pneumococci, streptococci or salmonellae. This is known as the carrier state and is a source of infection to other individuals.

Evasion

Once a microorganism becomes established in the tissues, having escaped the innate defence mechanisms described in Chapter 2, the microorganism can often make use of a number of evasion

NOSE & NASAL PHARYNX

Staphylococci
Diphtheroids
<u>Neisseria</u> sp
<u>Haemophilus</u> sp

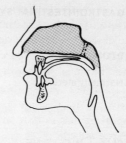

OROPHARYNX

Staphylococci
<u>Streptococcus</u> sp
<u>Neisseria</u> sp
<u>Haemophilus</u> sp

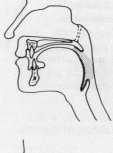

MOUTH

Staphylococci
Streptococci
<u>Actinomyces</u> sp
<u>Haemophilus</u> sp
Yeasts
Enteric bacteria
Anaerobic bacteria
Spirochaetes

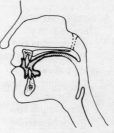

SKIN

Staphylococci
Streptococci
<u>Corynebacterium</u>
<u>Propionibacterium</u>
Yeasts
Diphtheroids
Enteric bacteria (rare)

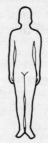

Fig. 5.1 Normal flora of the skin, mouth, nose and nasopharynx, and the oropharynx. (Reproduced from Blackwell C C, Weir D M 1981 Principles of infection and immunity in patient care. Churchill Livingstone, Edinburgh, p. 53)

GASTROINTESTINAL SYSTEM

STOMACH

Normally sterile

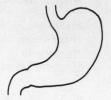

SMALL INTESTINE

Lactobacilli
Enterococci
Diphtheroids
Yeasts (<u>Candida</u>) } Small numbers
Enteric bacteria
Anaerobic gram
negative bacilli

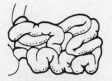

LARGE INTESTINE

Anaerobic bacteria
   gram negative
     <u>Bacteroides</u> spp
     <u>Fusobacterium</u> spp
   gram positive
     <u>Eubacterium</u> spp
     Lactobacilli
     <u>Clostridium</u> spp
     <u>Bifidobacterium</u>
     Streptococci

Facultative and aerobic organisms
   Staphylococci
   Enterococci
   Enteric bacteria
   <u>Proteus</u> spp
   <u>Pseudomonas</u> spp
   Yeasts (<u>Candida</u>)

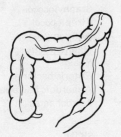

Fig. 5.2 Normal flora of the gastrointestinal system. (Reproduced from Blackwell & Weir 1981, p. 54)

strategies that protect it from the immune reactions of the host, including interference with phagocytic activity and antibody function.

GENITOURINARY TRACT

KIDNEYS AND BLADDER

Normally sterile

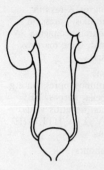

VAGINA AND CERVIX
Anaerobic bacteria
  Lactobacilli
  Streptococci
  Bacteroides spp
  Clostridium spp
  Bifidobacterium
  Eubacterium

Aerobic bacteria
  Diphtheroids
  Staphylococci
  Enterococci
  Strep. pyogenes (group B)
  Enteric bacteria

Yeasts
  Candida
Protozoa
  Trichomonas vaginalis
  (10-15% normal women)

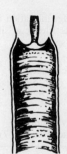

Fig. 5.3 Normal flora of the genitourinary tract. (Reproduced from Blackwell & Weir 1981, p. 55)

For example, the pneumococcus secretes large quantities of capsular polysaccharide that repels phagocytes and mops up antibody as it is produced, thus allowing the pneumococcus itself to proliferate unhindered. Trypanosomes appear to change their surface antigenic make-up from one generation to the next, so that the antibody made in response to the antigens of the original organism is inactive against the second generation of organisms.

Table 5.1 The compromised host

Predisposing factor	Effect on immune system	Type of infection
Drug or X-rays in immunosuppression Allograft recipients (renal, bone marrow, heart)	Diminished cell-mediated and humoral immunity	Lung infections, bacteraemia, fungal infections, urinary tract infections
Virus immunosuppression e.g. rubella, herpes, EB virus, hepatitis virus HIV (LAV/HTLV III) virus	Replication of virus in lymphoid cells with resulting impaired function	Secondary bacterial infections (also fungal and protozoal in AIDS)
Tumours	Replacement of cells of immune system	Bacteraemia, pneumonia, urinary tract infections
Malnutrition	Lymphoid hypoplasia Decrease in circulating lymphocytes Decreased phagocytic ability	Measles, tuberculosis, respiratory infections, gastrointestinal infections
Smoking, inhalation of dust particles (e.g. silica, fungal spores)	Inflammatory lung changes, immune complex deposition to fungal spores	Chronic respiratory infections, allergic responses
Chronic endocrine disease (e.g. diabetes)	Decreased phagocytic activity	Staph. infections Tuberculosis Respiratory infections, bacteraemia etc.
Primary immune deficiency (see Ch. 7)	Diminished cell-mediated and/or humoral immunity	

Many microorganisms, particularly tubercle bacilli, brucellae and many viruses, disappear inside tissue cells before sufficient antibody is produced to act against them. In the last few years it has been found that leprosy bacilli, which are similar in many ways to tubercle bacilli, have the ability to grow in the thymus-dependent areas of the lymphoid tissues. This affects the development of a cell-mediated immune response against the invading organisms and allows its unhindered proliferation. The same appears to be true for cutaneous leishmaniasis where instances have been described of a loss of cell-mediated immunity. In short, a particular microorganism is pathogenic because in some way it is able to circumvent, at least initially, the immune mechanisms of the host. Table 5.2 gives a list of microorganisms that have been shown to interfere with cell-mediated immune function. In a situ-

Table 5.2 Microorganisms affecting cell mediated immune function

Bacteria	Viruses	Fungi
M. tuberculosis	Influenza	*Coccidioides*
M.leprae	Viral hepatitis	*Cryptococcus*
T. pallidum	Herpes simplex	*Histoplasma*
Brucella abortus	Cytomegalovirus	*Candida*
Salmonella spp.	HIV (LAV/HTLV III)	
	Measles	
	Mumps	
	Rubella	
	Infectious mononucleosis	

ation where the host immune defence mechanisms are defective in some way (often called the compromised host), the distinction between pathogenic and non-pathogenic microorganisms becomes unimportant. All microorganisms that are human parasites have the capacity to produce disease in such a defective host. The breakdown of the normal host-parasite relationship then assumes central importance. Restoration of normal immune function is likely to be of more importance in the recovery of the patient than specific antimicrobial drug treatment.

Aggressins and impedins

These are a rather ill-defined group of bacterial products (Table 5.3), the presence of which is associated with virulence. If antibody to the aggressin is present the pathogenicity of the microorganism is likely to be reduced. They are usually enzymes and many have damaging effects on leucocyte function, for example leucocidins produced by many Gram-positive bacteria. *Staphylococcus aureus* produces at least three separate leucocidins acting on macrophages and polymorphonuclear leucocytes causing membrane disruption and degranulation. Injection of these substances into experimental animals can lead to leucopenia. The leucocidin diphosphopyridine nucleotidase acts within the phagocyte and destroys it. DNAases and nicotine adenine dinucleotidase have a similar effect. Other aggressins such as hyaluronidase act as spreading factors enabling dissemination of microorganisms through the tissues. Protein A from staphylococci combines with the Fc portion of the IgG immunoglobulin molecule (except IgG_3 subclass) and prevents complexes of antibody and antigen binding to the Fc receptor on phagocytes. This is an example of what is termed an **impedin** as are the IgA proteases produced by Neisseriae and certain streptococci (Table 5.3). Tables 5.4 and 5.5 show various ways microorganisms can evade immune mechanisms or interfere with induction of immunity.

Table 5.3 Some examples of bacterial aggressins and 'impedins'

Staphylococci	Coagulase
	Leucocidins
	Hyaluronidase
	Protein A
Streptococci	Haemolysins
	Hyaluronidase
	Fibrinolysin
	Leucocidins
Neisseria gonorrhoea	IgA proteases
N. meningitidis	
Strept. sanguis	
Ps. aeruginosa	Collagenase
	Elastase

Table 5.4 Evasion mechanisms

Microorganism	Product or characteristic	Effect
Staphylococci	Catalase	Protects from phagocyte H_2O_2
	Protein A	Binds antibody and interferes with opsonization
	Peptidoglycan	Inhibition of leucocyte migration
	Capsular material	Interference with opsonization
	Leucocidin	Cytotoxic and leucotoxic
	Haemolysin	Leucotoxic
	Coagulase	? inhibition of phagocytosis
Streptococci	Capsular polysaccharide	Inhibition of phagocytosis
	Streptolysins	Cytotoxic, inhibits chemotaxis, inhibition of macrophage migration ? inhibit lymphocyte proliferation
Gonococci and meningococci	IgA proteases	Digests and inactivates IgA
Trypanosomes, malaria parasites	Change membrane components in successive generations	Renders immune response to earlier generation ineffective
Intracellular organisms (tubercle bacilli, brucella, viruses)	Ability to survive within cells	Avoid destruction by antibody

Table 5.5 *Microorganisms that interfere with induction of acquired immunity*

Microorganism	Effect
Measles, rubella, herpes, hepatitis viruses Lymphadenopathy associated virus of AIDS (HIV)	Infection of cells of immune system and interference with induction of acquired immunity and expression of cell-mediated immunity
Malaria parasites	Depressed lymphocyte responsiveness to mitogens and some antigens
Leprosy bacilli	Alteration in T:B cell ratio with reduction in expression of complement receptors (? blocked by immune complexes)
	Non-specific impairment of cell-mediated immune response
Trichphyton fungi	Repeated exposure to tricophyton leads to relative allergy to the fungal antigens and reduced inflammatory response
Schistosomes	Incorporate host antigens and prevent recognition of their antigens
Influenza viruses	Suppress mitogenic responses of lymphocytes
	? Disables macrophages leading to secondary bacterial infection
Herpes simplex and cytomegalovirus	Induce Fc receptors on infected cell that bind and thus inactivate antiviral antibody

Epithelial attachment and infection

Bacteria

The attachment of a microorganism to an epithelial surface is a prerequisite for the development of an infectious process (excluding entry at sites of trauma). The mucosal surfaces of the respiratory, intestinal and genitourinary tracts are of primary importance as sites of attachment of microorganisms. Certain streptococci that are normal inhabitants of the mouth have been shown to adhere to epithelial cells of the cheek, whilst others preferentially attach to tooth surfaces. Specific attachment of various bacteria to different parts of the intestinal tract may account for the nature of the indigenous flora of the gut. It is suggested that the pathogenicity of *Salmonella typhi* and *Corynebacterium diphtheriae* depends on their ability to attach to the intestinal or pharyngeal mucosa respectively and *Neisseria gonorrhoeae* is believed to attach to epithelial cells of the genitourinary tract by means of its 'pili'. This organism at the same time appears to secrete an enzyme that breaks down

Table 5.6 Portals of entry of microorganisms

Portal of entry	Infection
Ingestion	Food poisoning, cholera, dysentery
Inhalation	Measles, cold, flu
Sexual contact	Gonorrhoea; syphilis; herpes virus, HIV
Iatrogenic	Heart valves, pacemakers, wound infections
Zoonoses	Malaria, salmonellosis, encephalitis, typhus
Self-infection	Urinary tract, eye infection, appendicitis
Accidental	Drug users, motor accidents

secretory IgA_1, whilst IgA_2 is not affected. The portal of entry of microorganisms in a number of infective states in shown in Table 5.6. Bacteria (Fig. 5.4) have an inner cell membrane and a peptidoglycan cell wall. Outside these basic structures there can be a variety of other components such as proteins, capsules, lipopolysaccharide or teichoic acids. There also may be organelles involved in motility (flagella) or adherence to the host's cells (fimbriae or

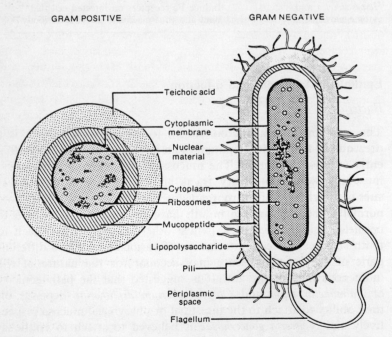

GRAM POSITIVE   GRAM NEGATIVE

Teichoic acid
Cytoplasmic membrane
Nuclear material
Cytoplasm
Ribosomes
Mucopeptide
Lipopolysaccharide
Pili
Periplasmic space
Flagellum

Fig. 5.4 Schematic representation of a Gram-positive bacterium and a Gram-negative bacterium.

pili). These are some of the components to which the immune system directs its responses. In general, peptidoglycan is attacked by lysosomal enzymes and the outer lipid layer of Gram-negative bacteria by cationic proteins and complement components. Flagella or fimbriae can be recognized and attacked by antibodies. The capsular material of some bacteria enables them to resist phago-cytosis or the shedding of excess capsule will mop up antibodies. Table 5.4 lists some of the ways in which products of microorganisms interfere with immune mechanisms.

Viruses (Fig. 5.5)

In virus infections the most common portals of entry are after inhalation into the upper respiratory tract (rhinoviruses), ingestion via the intestinal tract (enteroviruses), injection by insect vectors (togavirus) or contaminated needles (hepatitis B, HIV). Herpes simplex virus enters by direct contact with mucous membranes.

Once the virus has entered the tissues, cells must be available that carry receptor sites for the virus and that allow viral repli-cation. After the virus penetrates its target cells and replicates it may or may not cause disease at this site. Rhinoviruses, for example, after replication at the site of entry, cause localized disease. Virus may enter the blood or lymphatic system of nerve tissues and spread to other tissues or organs that may become secondary sites of infection, with associated damage to tissues and cells. Togavirus, transmitted to horses by mosquito vectors after local replication, spreads through the blood stream to the brain where further viral replication occurs. Herpes simplex is spread by way of nerve tissue. Herpes viruses are examples of viruses that become dormant and cause disease later, for example, if the immune system is compro-mised in some way. Abortive virus infection can occur when the infected cell is unable to support viral replication, but even in this situation disease can result.

Knowledge of the replication cycle of viruses is relevant to the understanding of viral immunity. After attachment and penetration of its target cell the virus is 'uncoated' by cellular enzymes that attack and partially remove viral capsid. Viral DNA then enters the host cell nucleus via the nuclear pores and is then transcribed by host cell DNA-dependent RNA polymerase. Viral messenger RNA (mRNA) is transported to the cytoplasm and translated into proteins by cellular ribosomes and tRNA molecules. Viral poly-

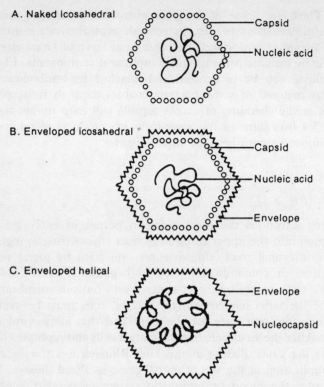

A. Naked icosahedral — Capsid — Nucleic acid

B. Enveloped icosahedral — Capsid — Nucleic acid — Envelope

C. Enveloped helical — Envelope — Nucleocapsid

Fig. 5.5 Schematic diagram of three examples of animal virus structure: the **capsid** is an outer symmetrical protein shell, when associated with the nucleic acid it is called the **nucleocapsid** (C). The capsid protects the nucleic acid, facilitates attachment to target cell, confers symmetry, usually icosahedral or helical (exceptions are poxviruses and hepatitis virus that are more complex) and confers antigenicity. Naked viruses (A) have no envelope. The envelope (B) consists of proteins, lipids and carbohydrates. Retroviruses are unique and have no envelope but two capsid shells (one as in A and one associated with nucleus, i.e. a nucleocapsid — C). Retroviruses have double-stranded RNA.

peptides then migrate either to the nucleus or to the cell membrane where they become the target of antibody or cell-mediated immunity (see p. 140). The site of virion assembly for all DNA viruses (except pox viruses) is the host cell nucleus. Virions are transported to the cell surface and released and this is sometimes associated with lysis of the cell.

Penetration and uncoating of RNA viruses is basically the same as for DNA viruses but replication does not usually involve the host cell nucleus. Replication of RNA viruses varies according to the type of RNA and involves the synthesis of RNA-dependent

RNA polymerase. This enzyme is either derived from the parental RNA or brought into the cell by the virions. Retroviruses, in contrast, carry the genetic information for induction of an RNA dependent DNA polymerase called 'reverse transcriptase' that catalyses the synthesis of double-stranded DNA complementary to the viral RNA. The DNA integrates into the host cell nucleus and is used as a template for the transcription of RNA that is then translated for viral protein production.

Most enveloped RNA viruses are released from the cell by budding through the cell membrane and it is at this stage that they are susceptible to antibody and cell-mediated immunity.

The viral coded antigens (either those inserted into the host cell membrane or associated with the virion) are the ones recognized by the immune system. Viruses can also induce host-coded antigens and, whilst these can serve as markers of virus infection, they are unimportant as far as immunity is concerned. Intracytoplasmic or intranuclear viral antigens are also not accessible to antibody or cell-mediated immune mechanisms. Some viruses spread from one cell to another cell in contact with it, without being released. In this case also the immune system is ineffective.

Infection, inflammation and immunity

The innate immune mechanisms that protect the individual (mechanical barriers, antibacterial substances and phagocytosis) have been discussed in Chapter 2 and this discussion is concerned with the protective responses that form a second line of defence. The microorganism, having successfully avoided the innate immune mechanisms, starts to proliferate in the tissues and its toxic products trigger an inflammatory response. The response is initiated by the release of vasoactive amines, principally histamine and SRS-A from mast cells. The resulting increase in vascular permeability leads to an exudation of serum proteins including components of complement, antibodies, blood clotting factors and phagocytic cells. Phagocytic cells are attracted to the site of inflammation by chemotactic factors generated by interaction of components of the complement system with antibody. C5a act as a chemotaxin. Anaphylatoxins generated at the same time increase vascular permeability and further encourage exudation of fluid and cells at the site of inflammation. See Chapter 2 (p. 21) for a more detailed discussion of the inflammatory response.

Many types of microorganisms (e.g. staphylococci, streptococci) are effectively dealt with by the polymorphs and the intensity and duration of the inflammatory process depends on the degree of success with which the microorganism initially established itself. This in turn depends on the extent of the injury, the amount of associated tissue damage and the number and type of microorganisms introduced. A localized abscess may arise at the site of infection.

Some capsulate microorganisms (e.g. pneumococci) are able to resist phagocytosis and are not dealt with effectively until large amounts of antibody are made. These mop up the released capsular polysaccharide and phagocytosis occurs. If bacteria are not eliminated at the site of entry and continue to proliferate, they may pass via the lymphatics to the regional lymph nodes causing their enlargement (lymphadenitis). Other microorganisms (e.g. diphtheria, tetanus, cholera) produce exotoxins and are called **toxigenic** organisms. In this situation they can produce their damaging effects without migrating from their site of entry. Immunity in this situation requires the development of specific **antitoxins** (see below).

The types of infection described above are usually referred to as **acute infections** and contrast with protracted or **chronic infection** which is usually induced by microorganisms that are adapted to live within the cells of the host. Included amongst these are mycobacterial infections (e.g. tuberculosis, leprosy) brucella infections and virus infections. In these infections cell-mediated immunity plays a predominant part in the final elimination of the microorganism.

IMMUNITY IN INFECTION

The immune system, as has been noted in Chapter 4, has evolved the capacity to respond and react to a large variety of foreign molecules whilst at the same time avoiding self-reactivity. The capacity of the individual to resist infection can be explained in terms of the clonal selection theory of acquired immunity with the production of a specific immune response. To understand the detailed cellular events and differences in responses to infection of individuals it is necessary to take into account more recently acquired knowledge of the role of the major histocompatibility complex (MHC) in determining the outcome of an immune response. The MHC is a highly polymorphic system of genes that control the expression of the cell surface molecules involved in immunity (see p. 112).

The existence of such a polymorphic system will inevitably result in individuals with different immunological potentials to respond to a given challenge. Whilst some individuals will be well prepared to resist an infectious agent others will be at risk. It will come as no surprise to find that certain infective states are linked with the MHC. For example, the association between viral hepatitis and the HLA-A8 antigen on lymphocytes (see p. 225). There are many examples of such associations in viral infections of mice.

The evolutionary advantage to a species of such as polymorphic set of determinants of immunity, with its attendant survival value and possibility of adaptation, is clearly an advantage in dealing with unforeseen challenges.

Association between certain infections and the blood group status of the individual has also been established. Individuals of blood group O are more susceptible than those of other blood groups to cholera. There is also an increased susceptibility if they do not secrete blood group substances into their tissue fluids and mucous secretions (i.e. are non-secretors). Carriers of streptococci tend to be non-secretors. In studies of a Chilean population it was found that people of blood group B had a 50% greater probability than non-B persons of contracting *E. coli* urinary tract infections. Blood group B individuals are more susceptible to gonococcal infections. Non-B persons and non-secretors are more susceptible to rheumatic fever and rheumatic heart disease. In the author's laboratory, blood group B and AB non-secretors have been found to be three times more susceptible to urinary tract infections and non-secretors were much more prevalent amongst cases of meningococcal meningitis is studies carried out with samples from Scotland, Iceland and northern Nigeria. We have also found increased numbers of non-secretors in insulin dependent (type 1) diabetes and ankylosing spondylitis, both of which may have an infectious basis.

Bacterial infection

Antibody-mediated immunity

Antitoxins. Many microorganisms owe their pathogenic abilities to the production of **exotoxins**. Amongst diseases dependent on this type of mechanism are diphtheria, cholera, tetanus, gas gangrene and botulism.

Diphtheria toxin, for example, is a polypeptide chain with a molecular weight of about 62 000 daltons. The intact molecule is not active but requires the reduction of one disulphide bridge and hydrolysis of the peptide chain to release an active fragment. This is believe to occur on the membrane of host cells resulting in the entry of the toxic fragment into the cell where it interferes with protein synthesis. The cholera toxin owes its effects to its ability to bind to a specific glycolipid of the intestinal cell wall. A toxin constituent then passes through the cell wall, enters the cytoplasm and irreversibly 'switches on' the adenyl cyclase (the cyclic AMP-making enzyme). The 'activated' cell then proceeds to secrete fluid into the intestinal lumen resulting in massive fluid loss from the tissues.

Antibodies either acquired by immunization or previous infection, or given passively as antiserum, are able to **neutralize** bacterial toxins (Fig. 5.6). To give protection, antibodies must either be present in sufficient quantity, as they would after administration of antiserum, or be produced faster than the toxin is produced by the microorganism. This would be likely to occur if the individual had previously been exposed to the organism or its products by natural infection or artificial immunization. In such a situation the infected individual would be able to mount a rapid

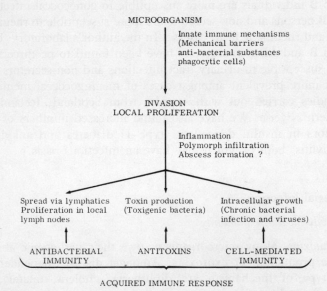

Fig. 5.6 Scheme showing the progress of infection and the immunological defence mechanisms

secondary immune response (p. 88). The previously exposed individual can be said to have an **immunological memory** of the toxin, having a population of cells ready and waiting to respond rapidly to the slightest whiff of the exotoxin. The infected individual with no 'immunological memory' may require to be given antibody prophylactically in order to tide him over the first stages of infection.

Bacterial toxins have been largely identified as enzymatic in nature and the antibody in some way is able to interfere with the ability of the enzyme to interact with its substrate. The antibody is not thought to interact with the active site of the enzyme but the nearer it reacts to this the more effective is its neutralizing power likely to be. The most probable explanation of the inhibitory effect of antibody is that is produces what is called 'steric hindrance', which simply means that it gets in the way and physically prevents the enzymes from coming in close apposition to its substrate (Fig. 5.7). This idea is supported by the finding that antibody is much more effective against enzymes which have high molecular weight substrates than it is against those with low molecular weight

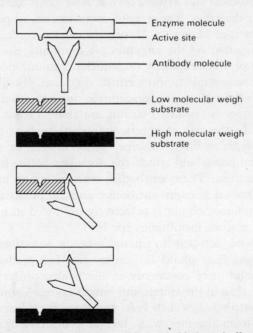

Fig. 5.7 Diagrammatic view of the possible 'steric hindrance' effect of antibody against an enzyme toxin. A low molecular weight substrate avoids the blocking effect of the antibody molecule. The closer the antibody is attached to the active site of the enzyme the more effective will be its blocking action

substrates. Figure 5.7 shows how such a low molecular weight substrate can still come in contact with the active site of the enzyme even in the presence of antibody.

Antibacterial immunity. In the case of a microorganism that does not secrete exotoxins, the protection afforded by antibodies depends on the direct effect of antibodies attached to the surface of the microorganism. This can have a number of effects, the most important of which is in encouraging phagocytosis by macrophages of the blood (monocytes) or the polymorphonuclear leucocytes. Phagocytic cells have receptors for a site on the Fc fragment of immunoglobulin G (particularly the human IgG 1 and IgG 3 subclasses) that is exposed after the immunoglobulin has combined with its antigen. There are also receptors for the C3b component of complement. This means that a bacterium coated with antibody and complement will adhere to a phagocytic cell and become susceptible to phagocytosis (see also p. 24). The phagocytic cell in many instances can then digest the microorganism by secreting into the phagocytic vacuole a variety of digestive enzymes carried in the intracellular lysosomes. However, some microorganisms such as the streptococci and *Mycobacterium tuberculosis* are able to resist intracellular digestion. The streptococcus carries, as part of its cell wall, a substance known as M protein, which confers the ability to resist digestion by the enzymes. If immunity exists to the M protein, by previous exposure or artificial immunization, the streptococcus is susceptible to intracellular digestion. Rough (avirulent) strains of salmonellae are susceptible to intracellular digestion whilst the smooth (virulent) strains are able to resist digestion in some way. In the case of enteric infections such as those due to *Salmonella typhi* or *Vibrio cholerae*, antibodies can be secreted into the intestinal lumen and attack the organism before it invades the intestinal mucosa. These antibodies secreted by an immune individual are known as copro-antibodies and are predominantly IgA. The IgA immunoglobulin is selectively produced in intestinal and respiratory mucous membranes (p. 105).

IgA can be detected in many mucous secretions in higher concentrations than found in serum, and IgA-producing plasma cells are found more commonly in the lamina propria of mucous membranes than in the spleen and lymph nodes. Various functions have been attributed to such IgA, and there is evidence that it acts as an anti-toxin together with IgG in protection against experimental cholera infection. Another suggested function of IgA is that by reacting with gut microorganisms it prevents their adherence to the gut wall. This is suggested by experiments in mice in which cholera organisms were prevented from adhering to the gut wall by the presence of IgA. A further function of IgA is suggested by work with IgA fractions of human colostrum, which bind to *E. coli* together with complement. The effect of this on the lipopolysaccharide of the bacterial cell wall is postulated to lead to the exposure of the underlying mucopeptide. This enables the enzyme lysozyme (p. 18) to digest the mucopeptide layer with resulting lysis of the bacterium. Gram-negative organisms such as *E. coli* are normally resistant to the effects of lysozyme (Fig. 5.8). It should be noted that these effects have been shown by *in vitro* assays and may not reflect what occurs in the intact animal. Other effects of antibody reacting with the surface of the microorganism are cell lysis, brought about by the activation of the complement system, and simple localization of the organism by agglutination or clumping.

It is even conceivable that antibody acts by coating growing bacteria so that their daughter cells, when formed, remain in a clump instead of dispersing. Attachment of bacteria to the host's red blood cells in the presence of antibody and complement is another way in which phagocytosis is encouraged. This phenomenon is known as **immune adherence**, the attachment to red cells takes place by means of C3b receptors in the red cell membrane.

Apart from the clumping effect on the bacteria, agglutination seems to have little effect on the viability or respiratory activity of the organisms, although it is conceivable that the bacteria at the centre of a large mass of clumped organisms would be limited in their metabolic activity simply by a lack of sufficient nutrient material. Recent work suggest that antibody can inhibit the uptake of iron by some bacteria and that its lack can inhibit their growth.

A protective role for IgE has been suggested by the discovery of

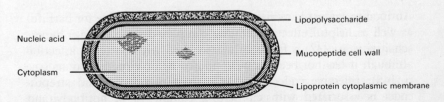

Nucleic acid

Cytoplasm

Lipopolysaccharide

Mucopeptide cell wall

Lipoprotein cytoplasmic membrane

Fig. 5.8 Gram negative bacillus showing lipopolysaccharide which protects mucopeptide cell wall from the effects of the mucolytic enzyme lysozyme. IgA + complement may attack the lipopolysaccharide and allow access of lysozyme to the cell wall

a similar distribution of this immunoglobulin to that found for IgA in the mucous secretions produced by local plasma cells. IgE is known to attach to the surface of mast cells and on combination with antigen, degranulation of the mast cell occurs with histamine release. These reactions in the allergic individual lead to hypersensitivity states (p. 226). If it occurs on a smaller scale in a localized area it might be helpful in bringing about an inflammatory response with consequent elimination of a microorganism (See also p. 161).

Humoral immunity in bacterial infections — summary

1. Antibody can neutralize bacterial toxins from, for example, diphtheria, cholera, tetanus and botulism organisms.
2. Antibody can attach to the surface of bacteria and:
   (a) act as an opsonin enabling phagocytosis, e.g. IgG and IgM
   (b) prevent the adherence of microorganisms to their target cell, e.g. IgA in the gut
   (c) activate the complement system leading to bacterial lysis
   (d) clump bacteria (agglutination) leading to phagocytosis
   (e) attach bacteria to host red blood cells or platelets by C3b receptors, so that the complex is phagocytosed (immune adherence)
   (f) inhibit the uptake of iron by bacteria by preventing bacteria from releasing their iron binding compounds
   (g) IgE attached to mast cells interacts with microbial surface to cause histamine release with inflammatory response and elimination of microorganism (if this occurs excessively, it can lead to hypersensitivity — Ch. 9)
   (h) inhibits motility and possibly the metabolic activity of bacteria.

Immune complexes in bacterial infections

Antibodies against bacterial antigens can be responsible for harmful as well as helpful effects. Immune complex disease (type 3 hypersensitivity, p. 232) is frequently associated with bacterial infection although it has not been as well studied as in virus infections (see p. 145). Infective endocarditis due to staphylococci and streptococci is associated with circulating complexes of antibody and bacterial antigens and, whilst helpful in diagnosis, can also lead to joint and kidney lesions as well as vasculitis and skin rashes. Other sequelae of acute streptococcal infection, such as rheumatic fever and poststreptococcal glomerulonephritis, are associated with deposition of immune complexes and release of inflammatory mediators (see p. 233). Other examples of bacterial infection where immune complexes may play a role in pathogenesis are leprosy, typhoid fever and gonorrhoea.

Acquired cellular immunity

Macrophage-dependent cellular immunity (see Fig. 5.9). The interrelations of antibody-mediated immune mechanisms and acquired cellular immunity are not yet clearly defined. It is known, however, that macrophages from animals immune to tubercle bacilli are more actively phagocytic than those taken from a normal animal. The cells spread out more than unstimulated macrophages when cultured in a glass chamber, and are more heavily endowed with mitochondria and lysosomes. The cellular immunity fades with time but can be recalled in an accelerated manner only by exposure to the original antigenic stimulus. Enhancement of cellular immunity has been reported with macrophages from brucella-infected animals; such cells restricted the intracellular growth of brucellae

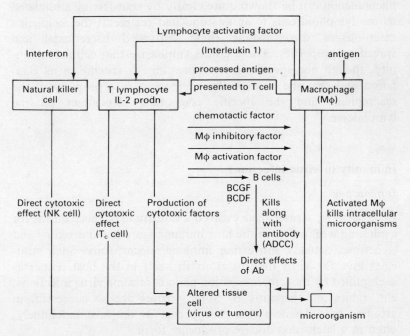

Fig. 5.9 T lymphocyte — macrophage relationships.

although the enhancement was dependent on the initial immunisation with a living virulent strain of the organism. The same phenomenon has been found after *Listeria monocytogenes* infection in mice in which macrophages isolated from the peritoneal cavity acquire an increased resistance to listeria and at the same time an increased intracellular resistance to tubercle bacilli and brucellae. This increased resistance is **non-specific** in the immunological sense in that the enhanced activity of the macrophage is directed not only at the species of organism responsible for the initial infection but also at other species.

The non-specific enhancement of macrophage activity, including their ability to kill microorganisms and spread themselves throughout the peritoneal cavity to mop up an infectious agent, appears to depend upon the transfer of lymphokines from lymphoid cells which have reacted immunologically to the initial injection of microorganisms. Thus the first part of the response depends on a specific immune reaction on the part of lymphoid cells to an agent such as *L. monocytogenes*; these cells proliferate and in turn activate the macrophages so that not only do they handle listeria more effectively but also other bacterial agents. This phenomenon can be shown quite clearly by transferring stimulated mouse lymphoid cells to an unstimulated recipient; the recipient's macrophages then assume these enhanced bactericidal and spreading properties. These points emphasize that cellular immunity, though non-specific in its expression, is specific in its elicitation and that the non-specific component is a property of the macrophage and the specific component dependent on the lymphocyte.

Immunity in virus infections

Introduction

Like bacteria, viruses have evolved a multitude of mechanisms for exploiting weaknesses in the host immune system and avoiding and sometimes actually subverting immune mechanisms. Such strategies give the virus time to establish itself in the host tissues as exemplified by the long incubation periods of some virus infections, e.g. rabies and hepatitis B. Some viruses are so successful in avoiding host defences that they persist in the host indefinitely, often in a latent non-disease producing form.

One of the most important strategies developed by viruses is to

Table 5.7 Examples of subvertive effects of viruses on immune function

Virus	Cells infected	Effects
HIV (HTLV III)	T lymphocytes, B lymphocytes, monocytes/macrophages, microglial brain cells	Cytopathogenicity loss of T4/CD4 (receptor for virus). Depletion and impaired functioning of infected cells
Lactic dehydrogenase virus (LDV) of mice	Macrophages bearing class 2 MHC (Ia) antigens	Depletion of Ia +ve cells with depressed antigen presenting function of macrophages
Semliki Forest virus	Cells bearing class 1 MHC antigens (sometimes class 1-ve cells also)	? Removal of class 1 antigens from cell surface and interference with Tc cell killing mechanism
Adenoviruses	Viral glycoproteins attach to class 1 MHC antigen	
Epstein Barr virus	B lymphocytes (via C3d receptor)	Polyclonal activation of B cells
Hepatitis B virus	Liver cells	Release of viral antigen, ? tolerance induction in B cells with failure to produce antibodies to viral surface antigen
Lymphocytic choriomeningitis virus (LCM) in mice	T lymphocytes	Clonal deletion of T cells with loss of response to virus

Other possible, but as yet unresolved, effects of viruses include production of immunomodulatory substances by viruses with effects on T helper and cytotoxic cells and on production of cytokines such as interleukins one and two. Some viruses can affect phagocyte function and immune complexes with viral antigen can have effects on the immune system (see text).

infect cells of the immune system itself (Table 5.7). The effect of this is often to disable the normal functioning of the cell type that has been infected. Many common human viruses infect cells of the immune system including rubella, mumps, measles, certain adenoviruses, most herpes viruses and sometimes hepatitis B virus. The most recent example of viral interference with the functioning of cells of the immune system are human immunodeficiency virus (HIV) infections. This is the name proposed by an international committee for the lymphadenopathy or HTLV III virus that is responsible for the acquired immunodeficiency syndrome AIDS (see below). Studies carried out in response to the emergence of this very serious disease have advanced knowledge to a substantial degree on the mechanisms and consequences of infection by this and a number of other viruses. The consequences of viral infections of cells of the immune system have been categorized as:

1. Infections that cause temporary immune deficiency to unrelated antigens (and sometimes to antigens of the infecting virus, as seen in mouse reovirus, herpes simplex and influenza infections). It is well known that patients who have suffered from virus infections such as influenza, rubella, measles and cytomegalovirus are susceptible to bacterial and other infections. This is sometimes associated with depressed immunoglobulin synthesis by lymphocytes and interference with the antimicrobial functions of phagocytes.

2. Permanent depression of immunity to unrelated antigens (and occasionally to antigens of the infecting virus). The acquired immunodeficiency syndrome is an example of such an effect where the patient becomes susceptible to otherwise harmless protozoa, bacteria, viruses and fungi (see below).

Antibody-mediated immunity

Virus infections, particularly those caused by enteroviruses, are frequent and severe when humoral immunity is impaired as in inherited immunodeficiency states. In Bruton type deficiencies (see p. 240) poliomyelitis may develop after vaccination; meningoencephalitis caused by echovirus and coxsackie virus, may also be seen. In a variety of mouse experimental models the administration of immunosuppressive drugs has shown that antibody is essential for recovery from a number of virus infections, including influenza and coxsackie viruses. Antibody appears to operate through opsonization followed by ingestion by macrophages or by neutralization of virus haemagglutinins.

In many situations viruses seem to be able to escape these protective mechanisms of the host and remain infective, even when complexed with antibody. Some viruses become latent, e.g. the herpes group, and are reactivated despite the presence of circulating antibody, passing from cell to cell without entering the bloodstream. Other escape mechanisms, such as that of the influenza virus, are discussed below.

Bloodstream or surface protection. In virus infections the efficiency of antibody depends largely on whether the virus passes through the bloodstream in order to reach its target organ. A well-known example of a virus which follows such a route is the **polio virus**; this crosses the intestinal wall, enters the bloodstream and passes to the spinal cord and brain where it proliferates. Small amounts of antibody in the blood can **neutralize** the virus before it reaches its target cells in the nervous system. A number of other viruses behave in the same way and pass through the bloodstream on their way to their target organ; examples are the viruses of measles, mumps, rubella and chickenpox. Disease caused by these viruses is characterised by a **prolonged** incubation period.

In comparison, in another group of virus diseases with a **short** incubation period such as influenza and the common cold, the viruses do not pass through the bloodstream, as their target organ is their site of entry to the body, namely the respiratory mucous membranes. In this type of infection, even a high blood level of antibody will be relatively ineffective against these viruses in comparison with its effect on the blood-borne viruses. For this antibody to act on such respiratory viruses it must pass through the mucous membranes into the respiratory secretion. Examination of the antibody content of mucous secretion has shown that in contrast to the blood there is very little IgG antibody and often no IgM and it thus appears that the mucous membranes are not very permeable to antibodies of these classes. However, it has been found that the predominant immunoglobulin in these secretions is IgA manufactured by plasma cells in the lamina propria of the mucous membranes. IgA present in nasal secretions has been shown to be responsible for most of the neutralizing activity against common cold viruses. One conclusion which can be drawn from this is that conventional immunization methods designed to produce high blood levels of antibody are unlikely to be effective against viruses which attack the mucous membranes, and some effort is being directed at developing methods for stimulating local antibody production of IgA type in the mucous membranes themselves. An example of this is the intranasal administration of a live attenuated influenza virus which has been used extensively in the United States and the Soviet Union and is now available in Britain.

It is generally believed that the best way to achieve protection against a viral disease is to use a live virus vaccine and it is clear that natural infections of humans by influenza virus confers more complete and long-lasting protection than does vaccination. There is evidence that cytotoxic T lymphocytes may be as important as immunoglobulins in this protection. Inactivated influenza vaccines and subunit vaccines result in antibody production but are much less efficient in inducing cytotoxic T lymphocytes in mice. The neutralizing antibodies generated in influenza infection are highly specific for the haemagglutinin of the infecting virus. In contrast, cytotoxic T lymphocytes appear not to discriminate between different type A influenza viruses. Thus for efficient long-term immunity live vaccines appear to be preferable to inactivated vaccines.

The high degree of immunity provided by the oral polio vaccine seems likely in part to be due to locally produced antibody in the gut neutralizing the virus even before it reaches the bloodstream. The presence of IgA antibody against polio virus has recently been demonstrated in the faeces, in duodenal fluid and in saliva. In contrast, after injection of inactivated virus vaccine no such antibodies could be found. The nasopharyngeal antibodies have been shown to persist for at least 300 days which is consistent with the long-term protection that the oral vaccine affords. It is of some interest that the levels of IgA antipolio antibody were found to be lower in children who had their tonsils and adenoids removed. Furthermore, primary vaccination in such children produced lower levels of these specific antibodies than in children who had not had their tonsils removed.

Persistence of virus and 'antigenic drift'. One of the major differences between viral and bacterial immunity is that the former is usually of much longer duration and in many instances lifelong, e.g. in measles and mumps. An explanation of this may be that some virus remains within tissue cells and is protected from immune rejection. Occasionally some virus material is released and thus maintains a persisting level of immunity. The possibility exists that such virus antigen will combine with antibody resulting in the formation of **toxic complexes** with ensuing hypersensitivity of type three (p. 232). The existence of such a phenomenon could have considerable importance in the pathogenesis of some viral diseases.

In those virus infections in which repeated attacks occur, e.g. influenza and the common cold, fresh infection is due to different strains of the virus which are relatively insusceptible to the antibodies induced by previous infection by other strains. Evidence for a persisting immunity to virus comes from studies in the Faroe islands where successive measles epidemics were separated by intervals of 65 and 31 years. Only those who had not been previously infected developed the disease. Persistence of antibody can also be shown after virus and other infections, for example in Eskimos, 40 years after polio virus infection.

Influenza epidemics have occurred at 2 to 3 year intervals over the last 40 years and type B virus outbreaks tend to alternate with type A epidemics. Type A virus is responsible for pandemic influenza infections. Type C influenza virus rarely, if ever, gives rise to epidemics and no variants have been reported since it was first isolated in 1950. The main viral antigen responsible for inducing immunity is the haemagglutinin (HA). It is sometimes called the 'V' antigen and is thought to be located on the spikes projecting from the viral envelope. Influenza viruses types A and B have different HA antigens and within these two types are a number of distinct families with HA antigens which differ markedly from one another. Antigenic differences between HA antigens form the basis for classification of the viruses into families of the same type. Neuraminidase is also a surface antigen of influenza viruses and is responsible for the ability of the viruses to attach to tissue cells including red blood cells. This allows its laboratory detection in a haemagglutination test (see p. 278). In type A infection, the families A, A_0, and A_2 have appeared successively, and each in turn has dominated the epidemic history of influenza for periods of 10 to 15 years and is then displaced by later antigenic variants. It is believed that this 'antigen drift' from one virus family to another is one of progressive mutation, and that immunity against earlier strains becomes obsolete once further antigenic variants have appeared. The consequence of antigenic drift is that new strains do not react well with antisera against older strains, although older strains tend to react well with antibody against the new strain. Antigenic drift is probably due to selective pressures brought about by antibody that favours the emergence of mutants expressing surface antigens sufficiently different as to be unable to combine with existing antibody.

There is a danger that mutants responsible for 'antigen drift' may emerge and dominate as a result of widespread use of vaccination procedures directed against strains responsible for epidemics. In this situation such insusceptible mutants would be 'selected' from the virus population and replace the previously dominant strain.

The phenomenon of 'antigen drift' is not limited to influenza virus and the argument outlined above has been used for not instituting nationwide vaccination as a means of protecting cattle from foot and mouth disease virus. The same difficulties stand in the way of the development of common cold vaccines and vaccines against the AIDS virus. The latter may be mutating at a rate five times faster than the influenza virus.

Immune complexes in viral infections

Formation of immune complexes between microbial antigens and antibodies leads to the neutralization and clearance of many pathogens by phagocytes. This is brought about by interaction of Fc receptors on the phagocyte with exposed Fc regions of the antibody molecule. In certain circumstances, such as when complexes are formed in antigen excess (i.e. with fewer Fc sites available as well as being small and soluble), or in antibody excess that are also small and soluble, clearance is less effective and the complexes may be deposited on filtering membranes (e.g. kidney glomeruli or choroid plexus in the brain) and at sites of turbulence and high pressure in the vasculature (e.g. aortic area). In other situations complexes may themselves be formed on cell surfaces by antibody bound to cell surface antigens that may be endogenous, as in autoimmune disease (p. 246), or exogenous and derived from a microorganism such as viral antigens inserted into a cell membrane. This will lead to cytotoxic effects due to antibody dependent cellular cytotoxicity (ADCC) (see p. 231). Large complexes formed near equivalence (p. 271) not only express Fc regions of the antibody molecules but also fix complement thus leading to effective uptake and clearance by cells of the mononuclear phagocyte system with Kupffer cells of the liver playing a predominant role.

In infectious disease formation of local complexes is rare but circulating complexes can be deposited at various sites, such as the kidney glomeruli, the intima of arteries, synovial membranes of joints and the choroid plexus. This can lead to the release of inflammatory mediators resulting from activation of the complement cascade and by binding of complexes to Fc receptors on platelets, mast cells, monocytes and neutrophils. The enzymes released from the latter two cell types include elastase, collagenase and neutral proteases with damaging effects on connective tissue and activation of the coagulation system.

In viral infections immune complexes are frequently produced and can lead to serious complications in infections such as hepatitis B and Dengue virus infections in humans and in mice in lymphocytic choriomeningitis infection. The pathogenesis of the latter infection is relatively well understood (p. 148) and immune complexes in neonatal mice can be identified in the kidneys, heart, liver, spleen and central nervous system of transplacentally infected mice. The pathogenesis of such neonatal infections contrasts with that in adults where the damage is primarily due to cell mediated cytotoxicity. The immune complex form of the disease in neonatal mice varies from strain to strain and may be related to the amount of C1q (p. 26) that binds to the complexes. The level of C1q is controlled by class three genes of the mouse H-2 locus (see p. 113).

In infections of humans by hepatitis B virus the surface antigens are shed into the blood stream and form complexes with antibody. Persisting levels of hepatitis B antigen can lead to immune complex mediated damage such as polyarteritis nodosa and glomerulonephritis. In acute infections vasculitis, skin rashes and polyarthritis can occur as prodromal symptoms. Whilst the major hepatic damage in the disease is cell mediated, immune complexes are sometimes found in the hepatic sinuses but are probably not responsible for liver damage. Complexes in the synovial membranes with associated depletion of complement components can lead in a proportion of cases (up to one-third) to a self-limiting polyarthritis resembling rheumatoid arthritis. Another way that complexes can contribute to persistence of hepatitis B infection is by blocking ADCC mediated killing of virus infected cells. The complexes by attaching to the Fc receptor of the phagocyte prevent it recognizing antibody on the surface of the virus infected cells.

In Dengue haemorrhagic fever, a disease widespread in southeast Asia, antibody that fails to neutralize Dengue 2 virus forms complexes that, when phagocytosed, appear to enable the monocyte to support viral replication (i.e. for the cells to become permissive). This leads to much enhanced viral replication and viraemia. These consequences occur in only a small proportion of individuals and are believed to be under control of Ir genes (p. 113). Circulating complexes can also be found in the disease and may lead to renal lesions.

Other virus infections in which immune complexes may play a role in the pathogenesis of the disease process are flavovirus infections including yellow fever and West Nile virus infections. In Epstein Barr virus infections viral antigens have been found in immune complexes in the kidneys of patients with Burkitt's lymphoma. Complexes deposited in various tissues may be responsible for some of the symptomatology of many acute virus infections. Deposition of complexes in the choroid plexus has been suggested as underlying behavioural disorders in asymptomatic virus infections.

Cell-mediated immunity

Virus elimination and tissue damage. The humoral immune response is probably the predominant form of immunity responsible for protection from reinfection by viruses. For this reason immunisation procedures aim at producing circulating or mucous membrane antibody. In the case of primary virus infections the position is not very clear but it seems likely to involve some form of cell-mediated immunity. It is known that children with congenital hypogammaglobulinaemia (p. 237) can recover from virus infections without producing any virus-neutralizing antibody. Although it is possible that these children are producing small amounts of neutralizing antibody sufficient to provide immunity, it is significant that the capacity to resist virus infection is associated with normal cell-mediated immune reactions. These subjects are able to develop normal delayed hypersensitivity reactions to bacterial and viral antigens and contact sensitivity to simple chemicals (p. 237). In patients with Swiss-type agammaglobulinaemia (p. 241), who have an additional cell-mediated immune deficiency, susceptibility to virus infection is very great and death often follows the development of severe generalized vaccinia after routine inoculation with live smallpox vaccine.

A laboratory model is available that has enabled the detailed study of the role of cell-mediated immunity in virus infection. Adult mice infected with lymphocytic choriomeningitis virus (LCM virus), which itself is not damaging to cells (non-cytopathic), develop clinical signs (e.g. meningitis) with the onset of an immune response to the virus. If this response is prevented by means of immunosuppressive agents (e.g. antilymphocyte serum, cytotoxic drugs, irradiation or thymectomy) then the disease does not develop. If an infected animal treated in this way is then given spleen cells from an untreated virus-infected animal, the pathological changes characteristic of the disease develop in the recipient. These changes are likely to be brought about by a cytotoxic effect of the transferred spleen cells interacting with infected cells of the recipient. The consequences of this immune response can thus be seen to be twofold: (1) virus-infected cells are destroyed by stimulated spleen cells with the likely elimination of the virus; (2) host cells are themselves damaged and this is responsible for the pathological manifestations of the disease. Whether or not the pathological changes in any human virus infections depend on mechanisms of this type is not clear at present. However, some in vitro experiments in which cells infected with measles or mumps virus are destroyed by incubation with spleen cells of a virus-immunised animal suggest that such phenomena may take place in the disease state itself. In volunteers infected with influenza virus a correlation was found between cytotoxic T cell activity and diminished shedding of virus. MHC restriction (p. 72) applies to the action of Tc cells in virus infection, the Tc cells recognizing viral antigen associated with class 1 MHC antigens on infected cells.

Further evidence that cell-mediated immune reactions are involved in resistance to viruses comes from the finding that, just as in the case of intracellular bacterial agents such as tubercle bacilli and brucellae, cell-mediated reactions of the delayed hypersensitivity type (p. 235) can be demonstrated after many types of virus infection. The best known example of this is the reaction soon after revaccination with vaccinia virus where there is an accelerated reaction (compared to primary vaccination) reaching its maximum at 72 hours with a minimum of tissue damage and a rapid elimination of the infective agent.

An important component of the cell-mediated response is the role of helper T lymphocytes that co-operate with macrophages and B lymphocytes for an optimal antibody response (see Fig. 5.9). Thymectomized animals show an impaired antibody response during virus infection with consequent reduced ability to eliminate virus.

Babies with congenital rubella infection have been shown to excrete virus for periods up to 18 months of age. Such infants can be shown to possess high levels of IgM antirubella antibody, which indicates that they have not developed neonatal tolerance (p. 76) to the virus. Their cell-mediated immune mechanisms seem, however, to be defective due to a direct effect of the virus on lymphocytes. Lymphocytes taken from such an infant do not respond normally to the plant mitogen PHA (p. 106) and normal leucocytes infected in vitro with the virus can be shown to become defective in the same way. **Depression of lymphocyte reactivity** has been associated with a number of virus infections, e.g. rubella, herpes, Newcastle disease virus (causing fowl pest) and hepatitis virus. Certain viruses are able to **replicate** in **macrophages** (e.g. arboviruses, murine hepatitis virus, lactate dehydrogenase virus and herpes simplex virus) and others do so in **lymphocytes** (e.g. lymphocytic choriomeningitis virus, leukaemia viruses and Epstein-Barr virus).

The effects on the activity of the immune system brought about by viral infection have been studied with murine leukaemia viruses. Infection of mice with these viruses usually results in depression of the activity of the immune system affecting both humoral and cell-mediated immunity. In some instances (e.g. Friend virus infection) there is selective depression of a particular class of immunoglobulin (IgG) suggesting an effect on particular populations of lymphocytes. Graft rejection was found to be profoundly depressed in animals infected with gross leukaemia virus.

The mechanisms underlying these effects are not clear. Amongst the proposed mechanisms are: virus-induced changes in the **uptake** and processing of antigens; **destruction** of cells of the immune systems; antigenic **competition** by the virus preventing the host response to other antigens.

The clinical implications include: persistence of virus in the absence of a protective immune response; the development of immune complex disease (p. 145); potentiation of tumour growth as a result of depressed immunological capacity and thus of immune surveillance mechanisms (p. 211).

Acquired immune deficiency syndrome (AIDS)

The last few years have seen an increased interest in the interaction of viruses with the cells of the immune system following the recognition of the human retrovirus called T-lymphotropic retrovirus type III (HTLV III) or lymphadenopathy associated virus (LAV). Recently an international committee has proposed the name human immunodeficiency virus (HIV) for this retrovirus. This virus infects the T helper set of lymphocytes using the T4 (CD4) receptor expressed by these cells as its target receptor. The infected lymphocytes lose their ability to function and are destroyed by the virus. This results in a reversal of the normal ratio of T helper to T suppressor cells. The virus enters the cell by endocytosis whereby the cell membrane engulfs the virus enclosing it in a vesicle and the viral reverse transcriptase becomes active to produce a DNA copy of the viral genetic material that becomes integrated into the genome of the host cell. Transcription of the integrated DNA leads to the synthesis of viral proteins that assemble into new virus that after killing the lymphocyte pass into further cells. Cells of the central nervous system have also been shown to be infected by the virus with resulting neurological symptoms. The effect of the virus on the T helper cells is to interfere with their normal ability to take part in the inductive phase of the immune response described in Chapter 4. Patients with the disease are therefore susceptible to opportunist pathogens, in particular the protozoa *Pneumocystis carinii*. Other infections include tuberculosis, disseminated cryptococcosis, toxoplasmosis and candidiasis. Persistent viruses such as cytomegalovirus, varicella-zoster and adenovirus may be activated and expressed. An unusual type of tumour also can develop — Kaposi's sarcoma.

The antibody response that develops against the virus and enables the detection of the infection appears to be ineffective and it has been proposed that normal neutralizing antibodies do not develop. Such antibodies generally bind to those epitopes of the retrovirus envelope that interact with its target receptor (i.e. the T4 antigen) and it is suggested that the viral epitope and the T4 antigen share antigenic determinants so that a normal immune response does not develop, i.e. molecular mimicry.

Much effort is going into the development of antiviral drugs or vaccines that could prevent or eliminate infection by retroviruses. Among the drugs under test are those active against viral reverse transcriptase such as suramin, antimoniotungstate, azidothymidine (a thymidine analogue) and phosphonoformate. Ribavirin is a guanosine analogue that acts on the capping stage of viral messenger RNA and has been found to be active against a range of infections caused by RNA viruses. Other approaches include the use of alpha interferon that may inhibit the release of the virus from the membrane of the infected cell and the use of monoclonal antibodies against the T4 antigen that may prevent viral attachment. Vaccines against the virus are proving difficult to develop despite detailed knowledge of the virus and its genome. The high degree of glycosylation of the envelope glycoproteins, variability between strains and the possible antigenic relationship with the host T4 antigen may be responsible for these difficulties.

The envelope gene from the AIDS virus has recently been inserted into the vaccinia virus (p. 171) so that it makes the envelope proteins including one that appears to be conserved called gp41. It is hoped that a vaccine made from the altered vaccinia virus might be able to give protection from the HIV (human immunodeficiency virus) (LAV/HTLV III). The situation may be complicated by the possibility suggested by some virologists that AIDS patients are infected by several strains of HIV and that the virus can change its envelope proteins in successive generations supported by recent evidence that some of the virus genes show up to 30% divergence from their common point of ancestry about 20 years ago (see also p. 145). If this is the case the production of an effective vaccine is likely to be difficult.

Hypersensitivity reactions

Recent studies have indicated that the lesions associated with virus infections cannot be explained simply by the cytopathic effects of the virus on cells. The immune response of the host to the viral antigen appears to play a role in producing tissue damage due to the immune complexes (see p. 145), formed by virus and antibody.

Cytotoxic T lymphocytes (Fig. 5.9) will kill histocompatible target cells (see p. 72) infected with a variety of viruses, e.g. LCM and influenza. Another protective mechanism operates through Fc receptor expressing cells such as macrophages that will lyse antibody coated virus infected cells. This is called antibody-dependent cell-mediated cytotoxicity (ADCC) (Fig. 5.9). The mechanism has been shown to be effective against mumps, herpes simplex, vaccinia, and influenza virus infected cells. Another lymphocyte population that cannot be identified as either T or B cells by their surface markers are the so-called natural killer cells or NK cells. These can destroy cells infected with a number of viruses — Epstein-Barr, coxsackie, and LCM viruses — and this ability of NK cells seems to be potentiated by interferon (Fig. 5.9)

Epstein-Barr virus infection is usually a self-limiting disease of adolescents, characterized by fever, pharyngitis, lymphadenopathy, splenomegaly and fatigue. The serological response is dominated by rising antibody titres to the virus capsid antigen and atypical lymphocytes can be found in the blood. The condition usually resolves within one to three months with disappearance of the atypical lymphocytes. Chronic symptomless carriers of the virus are found and occasionally chronic symptomatic cases of the disease have been reported.

If macrophages are rendered inactive by injections of silica, herpes simplex infections have been shown to be potentiated. Macrophages can restrict replication of hepatitis virus in the mouse; this is genetically controlled. The ability of macrophage cultures to resist viral replication in vitro is correlated with in vivo susceptibility or resistance to the virus.

Another way in which a virus can initiate destruction of host cells is by virus-induced changes in the surface antigens of the host cell. The altered surface antigen stimulates an immune response with subsequent destruction of the cell by antibody and complement and possible concomitant release of pharmacologically active mediators of inflammation. Such a phenomenon is not necessarily detrimental only to the host cells as these are virus-infected cells and their elimination would lead also to destruction of the virus. In conclusion it can be seen that the outcome of a virus infection is the result of the **interplay** between **protective** and **hypersensitivity**

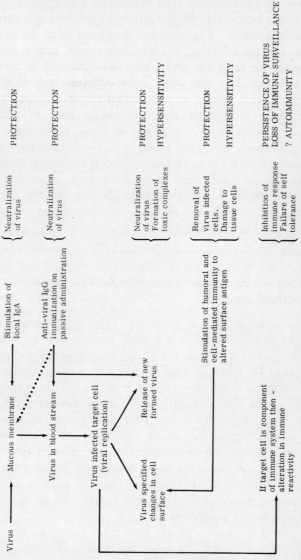

Fig. 5.10 Schematic view of virus infection and immune response, indicating some possible consequences

mechanisms the balance usually settling in favour of protection. Figure 5.10 is an attempt to summarize these complex inter-relationships.

Interferon. A quite distinct type of resistance mechanism in virus infection is the production by the infected host cells of a substance known as 'interferon'. This material interferes with the synthesis of new virus by tissue cells of the host. Interferon, unlike antibody, is not specific for the virus which may have induced its formation but is able to interfere with other quite different species of virus. Interferon probably plays a very important role in eliminating virus in non-immune individuals and the rise in level of interferon appears to coincide with the phase of virus elimination whilst circulating antibody levels are found to rise subsequently to this.

The human interferon gene has now been synthesized. It is the largest gene so far synthesized in the laboratory, consisting of 514 nucleotides. Genetic engineering methods has enabled the gene, after insertion into an *E. coli* plasmid, to produce the substance in large quantities (see Table 4.10).

Susceptibility to virus infections and the role of the major histocompatibility antigens

One of the valuable roles of interferons in antiviral immunity is to increase the expression of class 1 MHC antigens. This is likely to facilitate the interaction between virally infected cells and cytolytic lymphocytes (Tc cells). A possible mechanism the viruses might use to circumvent immune surveillance by Tc cells is to reduce the expression of the class one antigen. Adenoviruses have the ability to diminish messenger RNA levels for class one antigens and also produce a glycoprotein that forms complexes with class one antigens that interferes with its intracellular transport. There appears to be differences in the strength of interaction between the glycoprotein and different HLA types of class one antigen suggesting that the pathogenicity of the virus may be dependent on the HLA type of the infected individual.

In Chapter 4 consideration has been given to the genetic control of the immune response by a specific group of genes called **Ir genes**. These have been shown to be closely related to those genes controlling the major antigenic determinants of graft rejection (MHC genes). A gene product associated with the MHC genes is involved in co-operation between T and B lymphocytes leading to an immune response is noted on page 112. This phenomenon is of interest in view of the known relationship between histocompatibility antigens (determined by the MHC gene complex) and susceptibility to certain virus-induced leukaemias in mice. The susceptibility of mice to lymphocytic-choriomeningitis virus (p. 148) and humans to the SV40 virus may also be determined in this way. The response in vivo in man to certain viral antigens appears to be under HLA control as judged by the response to live vaccines. Poor responses to influenza vaccine has been found in HLA-Bw38 and Bw39 individuals whilst HLA-Bw55 and Bw56 individuals produced high titres to rubella vaccine. *In vitro* lymphocyte responsiveness to tetanus toxoid, vaccinia, PPD and streptococcal antigen show association with HLA, for example B5 persons tended to respond poorly to tetanus toxoid and Cw3 individuals to vaccinia. With increased knowledge of the gene complex controlling histocompatibility antigens and various functions of lymphocytes associated with the immune response, it should be possible in the next few years to elucidate some of the factors that determine susceptibility to virus diseases.

The role of the MHC in graft rejection was the first evidence that the control of the immune response depended on activities of the genes in that area (see p. 195).

It later became apparent that T and B lymphocyte interaction and macrophage T lymphocyte co-operation also required compatibility between the MHC regions of the cell types involved. In this instance surface molecules (Ia antigens) determined by I region genes are those involved and thus are important determinants of immunity to (1) intracellular bacterial infections and (2) in control of cellular interactions in antibody production. The H-2K and H-2D regions control surface molecules involved in cytotoxic T lymphocyte (Tc) activities and thus determine protective immune responses to viruses as well as graft rejection.

Since viruses can infect a large variety of different cell types the ubiquitous distribution of H-2K and H-2D antigens enable Tc cells to deal with virus infections of all cell types. In contrast Ia antigens are more limited in distribution, being found mainly on cells of the immune system including a proportion of macrophages, other inducer cells and B lymphocytes. They are important in generation of protective responses to intracellular bacteria, acting as receptors for signals leading to T cell generated signals for B cell differentiation (see p. 75), such as switching on of Ig production and changes from IgM to IgG.

Immunity to protozoa and helminths

⌐Parasites in this category affect many millions of people in tropical parts of world and are responsible for severe and debilitating disease. Malaria affects some 200 million people and at least one million children die of the disease every year. Schistosomiasis and filariasis fall into the same category as malaria and are responsible for enormous morbidity and mortality.

ℓ Four species of mosquito-borne malaria parasite can infect man: *Plasmodium falciparum*, *P. vivax*, *P. malariae* and *P. ovale*. In many parts of the world the parasites have become resistant to some of the major drugs used for treatment including chloraquine and its derivatives. Each of the malaria parasites have a similar life cycle. After infection by inoculation of sporozoites by anopheline mosquitoes these extracellular forms circulate in the blood for about 30 minutes before penetrating liver parenchymal cells. After asexual multiplication merozoites are released and, after a short extracellular period, infect erythrocytes where a second asexual multiplication cycle occurs. The merozoite becomes a trophozoite that in turn becomes a schizont containing merozoites. Rupture of the infected erythrocyte releases merozoites that go on to infect other erythrocytes. Some merozoites develop into male and female gametocytes that initiate the next phase of the life cycle if ingested by the appropriate mosquito, leading to the sporozoite stage and start of a fresh cycle.

Schistosomiasis is an insidious and debilitating disease caused by small worms (trematodes or flukes) that live in the blood vessels of infected persons. *Schistosoma mansoni* is the most widespread, affects the bowel and is prevalent throughout Africa, the Middle East and parts of South America. Three other species infect man, two infecting the intestine and the other the urinary system. The eggs of the parasite are excreted in the faeces or urine and, after developing into larvae, infect freshwater snails. They multiply and the free-swimming larvae that are subsequently released (cercariae) can penetrate the skin of humans.

Filariasis affecting about 300 million people is transmitted by mosquitoes (and for some species, horse flies and black flies). The parasite, as adult worms, live in the lymphatics and cause obstruction, inflammation and swelling of the arms, legs and genitals (elephantiasis). The most dramatic form of filariasis is river blindness caused by the worm *Onchocera volvulus*, transmitted by the black fly. The worms can reach half a metre in length and can live up to 15 years producing millions of embryos that invade the skin and eyes.

Trypanosomes are flagellate protozoa that appear in different morphological forms in their life cycle. Trypomastigotes are found in mammalian blood and epimastigote and amastigote forms may also occur. The parasite undergoes a complex cycle of development in the tsetse fly before appearing as an infective trypomastigote in the fly's salivary glands. In humans the tsetse fly bite is sometimes associated with the development of a swollen vesiculate lesion (chancre). The patient goes on to develop an acute febrile illness with lymphadenopathy and splenomegaly. The late stage of the disease involves the CNS with increased CSF protein and cells. Progress of the disease is accompanied by anaemia, leucopenia, muscle wasting and myocarditis.

The South American trypanosome *T. cruzi* causes Chagas' disease, affecting 10–12 million people in the region. The disease is transmitted to man by vectors (Reduviid bugs) that live in the cracks of mud huts. The trypomastigote derived from faeces of the vector enters the skin through scratches and infects both smooth and striated muscle, where they transform into amastigotes. The heart muscle may be affected and also the muscle of the alimentary tract. The life cycle of the parasite is completed in the vector after it feeds on the blood of an infected person. An important difference between the South American and African trypanosomes is that the former are intracellular and thus immunity depends upon oxygen-dependent and independent phagocytic defences rather than antibody and complement for the African variety.

The immunopathology of parasitic diseases involve the hypersensitivity reactions described in Chapter 9. IgE antibodies and eosinophilia are the hallmark of parasitic disease and are associated with type 1 antibody mediated hypersensitivity (p. 224). Type 2 autoimmune reactions, directed at antigen on a cell surface with resulting lysis, is frequently found. Blood group substances incorporated into the tissues of the parasite can result in the development of autoantibody against host tissues. Type 3 immune complex-mediated disease occurs in malaria, trypanosomiasis, schistosomiasis and onchoceriasis. Delayed hypersensitivity type 4 reactions are found in toxoplasmosis, leishmaniasis and South American trypanosomiasis. The liver, renal and cardiopulmonary pathology of schistosomiasis is related to cell-mediated responses to the schistosome eggs (see below).

The life cycles of organisms in this category, as noted above, are complicated and the immune response, to be effective, has to interrupt the cycle at a stage when the parasite is accessible to the immune processes.

Protozoa

Malaria infections are initiated by sporozoites and at this stage there is recognizable immunity. The discharge of merozoites from the liver into the peripheral circulation leads to antibodies that are readily detectable in the serum and increase until the crisis seven to 10 days later and then slowly decline. Because these antibodies are able to get access to the parasite only during a relatively short period of its life cycle, immunity is incomplete and the host usually fails to eliminate the parasite completely.

This state in which the organisms persist in small numbers in the tissues in the presence of an immune reaction is called **premunition** by parasitologists.

The IgG class of immunoglobulin is the major antibody class involved in acquired resistance to malaria and there is a considerable rise in the levels of, and rate of synthesis of, the IgG. However, if serum from an infected individual is incubated with parasitized erythrocytes, only a small quantity of the IgG antibody is absorbed. The major part of the IgG probably represents antibody to soluble malarial antigens, and seems unlikely to play a role in protection except perhaps when it is directed against toxic malarial products. Parasitic growth within erythrocytes is unaffected by the presence of immune serum in the culture medium, but invasion of new red cells by merozoites and subsequent parasite multiplication is inhibited. IgG antibodies can bind to Fc receptors on macrophages (p. 75) and it seems likely that phagocytosis of antibody-coated merozoites is an important mechanism of acquired immunity. There is evidence that antibody may act on mature intraerythrocytic forms of the parasite, possibly due to expression of parasite antigen on the surface of the red cells that render the red cells susceptible to attack by antibody.

Considerable experimental evidence exists showing that malarial infection is associated with **immunosuppression**. Depressed responsiveness of T lymphocytes to PHA (p. 106) and B lymphocytes to bacterial lipopolysaccharide can readily be demonstrated, as can diminished antibody responses to certain antigens. In a recent study of a group of patients infected with *Plasmodium falciparum*, peripheral blood lymphocytes, when tested in a lymphocyte proliferation assay, were shown to be unresponsive to antigen prepared from the parasite and in 37.5% of the patients this persisted for more than four weeks. The existence of unresponsiveness was present in all patients and was not related to the degree of parasitaemia or severity of the clinical illness. Suppression of lymphocyte reactivity was also found to an unrelated antigen but was much less profound and only seen in patients with moderately severe disease or with cerebral malaria. The depressed lymphocyte reactivity was associated with a loss of both T helper and T suppressor lymphocytes from the peripheral blood. Once the parasite was cleared from the blood the responses returned to normal.

The efficacy of the immune mechanisms against trypanosomes is complicated by the fact that the parasites can change their surface antigenic constitution from one generation to the next. The number of variants which can be produced by a single strain is at least 20. It is not yet clear how the organism controls the generation of the variants but variation is thought to arise by selection of mutants from a heterogeneous population of parasites.

This complication means that the immune response has great difficulty in keeping up with the antigenic changes in the parasite, and in the case of the trypanosomes responsible for African sleeping sickness, the parasite does not induce an effective immunity. The infected subject develops a progressive infection with invasion of the central nervous system leading to death. Trypanosomiasis is associated with high levels of IgM immunoglobulins in both the blood and CSF. It is not certain if this is due to the repeated new antigenic stimuli resulting from changes in the organism or if the parasite in some way influences directly the cells of the immune system. Increased immunoglobulin production is a common finding in protozoal infections and often affects all classes of immunoglobulins. Because usually less than 5% of the total immunoglobulin appears to react specifically with the inducing parasite, it is probable that protozoa stimulate the lymphoid cells in a non-specific way to overproduce immunoglobulins (i.e. polyclonal B cell activation).

This type of evidence has turned the attention of immunologists away from a direct role for antibody in protection in protozoal infections towards antibody independent cell-mediated immunity. This, as has been noted, takes three forms: direct cytolysis by lymphocytes (class I reactions), soluble lymphocyte products (class II reactions) and natural killer cell (NK) activity. Recent evidence points to a central role for type one direct cytolytic reactions in an important tick-borne cattle disease, theileriosis, caused by several species of *Theileria* prevalent in several parts of Africa and for *T. cruzi* infections that parasitizes heart cells. Tumour necrosis factor (TNF), a cytokine (p. 110) produced by lymphocytes that is known selectively to kill tumour cells both in vitro and in vivo, has recently been shown to be able to inactivate certain species of malaria parasite and *T. cruzi*. TNF has no effect on *Toxoplasma gondii*.

The lymphocyte-mediated cytotoxic reactions against infected cells have the same genetic restriction as virally infected cells in that the effector lymphocytes have to recognize both foreign and self MHC determined antigens simultaneously.

A similar phenomenon has been found in leishmaniasis and points the way to a better understanding of other protozoal infections including those of man.

An interesting example has recently been described of a protozoon that avoids elimination even in the presence of a vigorous immune response. *Entamoeba histolytica* exposed to fresh serum becomes markedly more resistant than untreated colonies to complement-mediated lysis. The effect appears to require active protein synthesis on the part of the protozoa suggesting a possible change in its membrane that resists the effect of activated complement components.

In summary, immunity against protozoal infections seems to be dependent largely on antibody, particularly against those parasites that live in the blood stream or have a blood stream phase as part of their life cycle e.g. malaria or trypanosomes. The effects of antibody are the same as those against other microorganisms including lysis with complement, opsonization, phagocytosis, antibody dependent cell mediated cytotoxicity and limitation of spread. Protection against parasites, once they have become intracellular, in the same way as for intracellular bacteria, depends upon the oxygen dependent and independent microbicidal activities of phagocytes. This in turn depends upon the enhancement of these functions by lymphokines derived as already described by stimulation of Th cells by antigen presenting cells and the subsequent elaboration of lymphokines by Tdh cells (p. 110).

Helminths. Helminths, like protozoa, go through a complex life cycle and protective immune mechanisms appear to act only at an early stage in the cycle. The main stimulus appears to be due to antigens derived from the adult worm and the immunity derived from this acts on new parasites entering the body. A noteworthy feature of these infections is the appearance of IgE (reaginic) anti-bodies (p. 226) with pulmonary eosinophilia, and it seems likely that immediate hypersensitivity reactions of the anaphylactic type (type 1) are involved in the pathogenesis of helminth infection. In *Schistosoma mansoni* infections the pathogenesis appears to be largely due to an **inflammatory granulomatous reaction** around the **schistosome eggs** trapped in the host tissues with a periovular area of necrosis surrounded by inflammatory cells, including many eosinophils. The most severe lesions occur during early infection. Mice in experimental schistosomiasis infections reject 70 to 80% of new infections 12 weeks after their first infection. In baboons a significant reduction in the damage done by the parasite to the host organs was found in pre-immunized animals. The experimental findings suggest a gradual waning of egg hypersensitivity but the mechanism is not understood. The tissues commonly affected are the liver, which shows chronic portal inflammation, the lungs, the kidneys and the spleen. The renal and splenic lesions are not directly related to the presence of worms or eggs, but may in part be due to immune complexes between worm antigens and anti-body. In *Schistosoma haematobium* infection the urinary tract is the primary target and calcification of the bladder can occur in advanced cases. Migration of larvae into the lungs is sometimes associated with eosinophil infiltration and pneumonia which can be fatal.

These worms are believed to be able to protect themselves from host antibody by **incorporating host tissue antigens** in their cell wall. When worms are transferred from mice to monkeys that are immunized against mouse red blood cells, the worms are killed by an antibody-mediated reaction directed at the surface of the para-site. The host antigens acquired by the worms appear to be A, B and H blood group substances (p. 184) and possibly the Lewis antigen.

In many helminth infections there is an association between increased levels of eosinophils in the blood and high IgE levels. If eosinophils are experimentally depleted in mouse schistosome infections, immunity to the parasite is decreased. It is likely that lymphokines produced by T lymphocytes (e.g. eosinophil stimu-lation promotor ESP) control the IgE and eosinophil response and that IgE on mast cells at the site of infection release mediators including chemotactic factor for eosinophils (ECFA). Eosinophils in conjunction with IgG adhere to the schistosomula and eosinophil

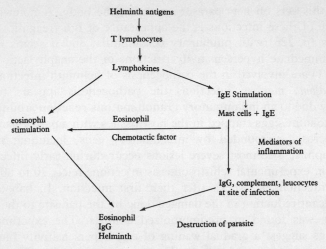

Fig. 5.11 Scheme showing the role of IgE and eosinophils in helminth immunity.

enzymes destroy the parasite. Figure 5.11 illustrates the series of interactions involved. The eosinophil products include peroxidase and a basic protein, which are likely to be involved in the destruction of the parasite as well as enzymes that inactivate the mast cell products histamine and slow reacting substance of anaphylaxis (SRS-A) (see p. 224). Table 5.8 summarizes some of the mechanisms used by parasites to avoid the immune response.

The immunodiagnosis of parasitic infection involves the detection of antibody to current or past infection. The availability of commercial antigens has led to exploitation of immunological procedures such as ELISA (p. 287), fluorescent antibody tests (p. 282) and radioimmunoassays (p. 285).

Fungal infections

The diseases caused by fungi are called mycoses and may involve the skin or mucous membranes — the superficial mycoses; the subcutaneous tissues — the subcutaneous mycoses or systemic or deep mycoses involving the lung, liver or brain. Like other microorganisms, fungi may exist as opportunist pathogens such as *Candida albicans*, or *Aspergillus fumigatus* or as pathogens such as *Histoplasma capsulatum*, or *Coccidioides immitis*.

Susceptibility to superficial fungal infections such as those due to *Candida albicans* is usually the result of an alteration in the

Table 5.8 Parasite escape mechanisms

1. Intracellular habitat	Malaria parasites, trypanosomes and *Leishmania* *E. histolytica* and *T. spiralis*
2. Encystment Resistance to microbicidal products of phagocytes	*Toxoplasma gondi, T. cruzi, Leishmania.*
3. Masking of antigens Variation of antigens	Schistosomes Trypanosomes, malaria parasites
4. Suppression of immune response	Most parasites, e.g. malaria, *T. spiralis, S. mansoni*
5. Interference by antigens Polyclonal activation	Trypanosomes
6. Sharing of antigens between parasite and host — molecular mimicry	Schistosomes
7. Continuous turnover and release of surface antigens of parasite	Schistosomes
8. Exposure to very small numbers of parasites at intervals (trickle infection) so that strong immune response does not develop	

mucous membrane defence mechanisms, commonly following the use of antibiotics that disturb the normal flora, or as a result of hormonal changes. Studies in the author's laboratory have shown that individuals who are non-secretors of blood group substances tend to be more susceptible to infections by *Candida albicans* (see p. 192). It seems likely that the Lewis blood group substance is involved in binding of the organism to its target cells.

Alterations in the host's immune response, for example as a result of immunosuppressive therapy, is the usual cause of systemic fungal infections. Cellular immune mechanisms appear to be important in defence against such systemic infections.

Allergic alveolitis and anaphylaxis

A few examples of pulmonary hypersensitivity to inhaled fungal antigens have been reported in the last few years. The existence of a state of immunity has been confirmed by the finding of precipitating antibodies in the serum. The first of these disorders to be recognized was **farmers' lung** disease in which precipitating antibodies could be demonstrated against antigens derived from

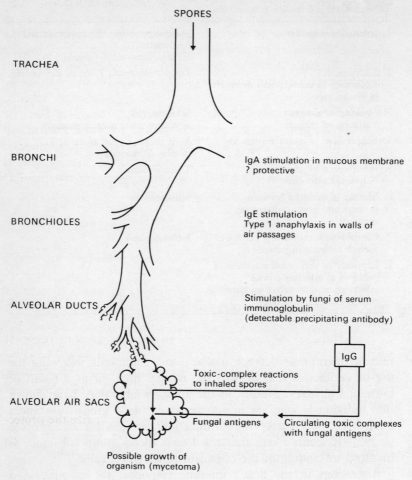

Fig. 5.12 Scheme showing some of the possible consequences that may result from the inhalation of fungal spores

mouldy hay. The antigen has since been found to be *Micromonospora faeni*. Subsequently work in Edinburgh has demonstrated precipitins against *Aspergillus clavatus* in **maltworkers** exposed to high concentrations of *A. clavatus* spores from contaminated barley. Antibodies against *Coniosporum corticale* have been found in the serum of maple bark strippers.

It is likely that following exposure to high concentrations of any of a variety of fungal spores individuals would produce precipitating antibodies and thus this form of pulmonary hypersensitivity, may be more widespread that has so far been identified. The hypersensitivity reaction induced by the presence of precipitating antibodies would be of the toxic-complex (type 3) form inducing a diffuse pulmonary interstitial pneumonitis which has been termed allergic alveolitis. Some of the antigens responsible for this form of hypersensitivity can also provoke in susceptible individuals the anaphylactic (type 1) response exemplified by pulmonary asthma. If growth of the fungus should occur in the lungs, as in the case of *Aspergillus fumigatus*, the metabolic products of the organism will cause further immunisation and increase in precipitating antibodies with the development of an accumulation of inflammatory cells at the site of infection. Figure 5.12 illustrates some of the possible consequences of a fungal respiratory infection.

Conclusions

The interactions between foreign microorganisms and the host's immune system can now be seen as the result of many variables both with respect to the host (e.g. MHC determination of immune response) and the microorganism (e.g. its ability to interfere with the immune response).

It is clear that the development of an acquired immune response to a microorganism is no guarantee that the organism will be eliminated and that whilst often providing protection an immune response can sometimes be disadvantageous to the individual (e.g. immune complex production).

Table 5.9 and Figure 5.13 are attempts to summarize the protective activities of the immune system with general application to the various types of microorganism discussed in this chapter.

COMMON VACCINATION PROCEDURES

Efficacy and hazards

It is generally accepted that one effective way of controlling the spread of infectious disease is by immunization with antigens derived from the appropriate organism. The isolation and bulk preparation of the particular antigens which confer protective immunity is a major difficulty, but success in this field with a number of potentially dangerous microorganisms has radically altered the chances of them causing widespread disease in the population. The use of diphtheria toxoid (inactivated diphtheria

Table 5.9 Summary of immune response to microorganisms

Induction stage
1. Microbe breaks through innate immune mechanisms and is taken up by *inducer* cell (macrophage, dendritic cell)
2. Microbial antigens (processed) associated with MHC product for presentation to T-helper (Th) cells (Th cells have receptors that recognize macrophage associated antigen)
3. Interleukin-1 from macrophage stimulates Th which produce receptors for interleukin-2
4. B-lymphocytes can also present certain types of antigen to Th cells

Effector state — humoral and cell-mediated immunity
1. Macrophage interferon produced — stimulates natural killer cells that attack virus infected cells and prevents viral infection of contiguous cells
2. Interleukin-2 from Th cells stimulates formation of Tc cells that kill virus infected cells and stimulates formation of Tdh cells that produce lymphokines, e.g. chemotactic factor and macrophage activating factor that attract cells and activate macrophages to kill intracellular organisms
3. T cells stimulated to regulate response
4. B cells stimulated by lymphokines (e.g. B cell growth factor) to produce antibody
5. Antibody kills microorganisms with complement, brings about opsonization and phagocytosis and coates the virus infected cell so that cells with Fc receptors (e.g. macrophages and killer cells) can destroy the infected cell (IgG, IgM)
IgA prevents adherence of microorganism to mucosal surfaces and IgE recruits inflammatory cells by releasing mediators from mast cells

---

toxin) is a noteworthy example. In Scotland, notifications of diphtheria averaged about 10 000 cases annually before 1940 when widespread immunization was instituted. The incidence of the disease rapidly decreased thereafter and, with the exception of an outbreak in 1968 involving six cases, none of whom had been fully immunized, the disease can be said to have been virtually eradicated. Sporadic outbreaks of meningococcal meningitis have caused anxiety in the last few years particularly cases infected with the B15 strain that appeared in 1970. Unlike the A and C type meningococci B strains are not readily immunogenic and a suitable vaccine has only recently been developed and is undergoing trials.

Immunization procedures are clearly not the only factor contributing to the decreasing morbidity and mortality from infectious disease. The combined death rate for scarlet fever, diphtheria, whooping cough and measles from 1860 to 1965 for children up to 15 years of age shows that nearly 90% of the total decline over the intervening century had occurred before widespread immunization and the use of antibiotics. Improved environmental con-

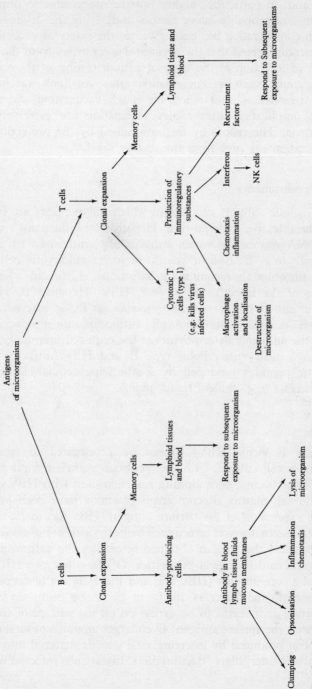

Fig. 5.13 Summary of role of B and T cells in infection

ditions and, in particular, higher host resistance due to improved nutrition, are probably major factors underlying the decline.

Much consideration has been given to the safety of vaccines and it is generally agreed that the greatest danger arises from the introduction of infection at the time of administration of the vaccine. Complications such as encephalitis after smallpox vaccination, febrile convulsions after whooping-cough vaccination and neurological complication after rabies vaccination are extremely rare phenomena. The risk is by far outweighed by the protection that immunization can give from the disease itself.

New developments

These include subunit vaccines in which polypeptides are isolated from the infective material (e.g. Hepatitis B, influenza); recombinant DNA vaccines in which antigens are synthesised by prokaryotic cells (e.g. *E. Coli* or yeasts) or lower eukaryotic cells (e.g. mouse fibroblasts); recombinant infectious vectors in which the genome of the infective agent (e.g. HSV, Hepatitis B, HIV) is inserted into a vector such as vaccinia or BCG; internal image idiotypes in which anti-idiotypic antibodies are produced that mimic the antigenic determinants of the required immunogen (e.g. reovirus, sendai virus, Polio type II and HBs Antigen); finally synthetic peptides produced by synthesizing sequential antigenic determinants (e.g. cholera toxin, polio).

Viruses

Hepatitis B virus (HBV) cannot be propagated in laboratory animals or cell culture. In order to obtain sufficient viral material to use as a vaccine, gene cloning has been used with HBV derived from human plasma. Recombinant plasmids have been prepared for the expression of the surface antigen (HBs Ag) in *E. coli* and the yeast *Saccharomyces cervesiae*. The best yields are obtained from the yeast and the antigen obtained resembles the natural material in physical and biological properties. Of the other two HBV antigens, the core antigen (HBc Ag) and the HBe Ag (a cryptic core component), the latter is likely to be more useful in vaccine production as it seems to be expressed on the surface of the virus along with the surface antigen. Even larger amounts of viral antigen have been produced by inserting viral genetic material into a virus that infects caterpillars (Baculovirus). Insect cells infected with the altered virus are stimulated to produce large amounts of the hepatitis viral antigen that is at present undergoing clinical trials. In another approach, resulting from the sequencing of the amino acids of the HBs Ag, synthetic antigenic material has been prepared and this is being assessed as a potential vaccine.

Immunization against influenza viruses has proved to be a difficult problem because of the variety of subtypes of the virus that exist (p. 144). Disrupted or split influenza A vaccine preparations contain the haemagglutinin and neuraminidase but have proved to be less effective than whole virus vaccines. Protection, however, is of much shorter duration (about one year) than is achieved by natural infection (four or more years). As with the hepatitis antigens, amino acid sequencing techniques have led to the availability of synthetic oligopeptides and it is hoped that common sequences might be found that are present in the different viral subtypes so that cross-reactive immunity could be induced.

Malaria

Much effort is being devoted to the development of a sporozoite vaccine for malaria. The identification and purification of plasmodial antigens has been considerably helped by the use of monoclonal antibodies (p. 80). Identification of protective antigens should lead to their large-scale production and use as a malaria vaccine. As in the case of viral antigens referred to above, the use of recombinant DNA technology and the development of synthetic peptide vaccines is underway. A number of problems remain to be solved, such as the cost of vaccine production, the possible requirement of adjuvants to enhance the immune response (a problem with many vaccine preparations) and the level of immunity required for individuals exposed to infection. Even if only partial immunity was achieved in a population, it is likely that the level of transmission of malaria would decrease.

Leprosy

Knowledge of the molecular biology and genetics of mycobacteria are much less advanced than many other microorganisms. The development of genetically engineered mycobacterial vaccines containing protective antigens has not yet been achieved. Much effort is being expended in cloning T cells from patients with leprosy who show resistance to the disease (i.e. the tuberculoid form) and from individuals vaccinated with a vaccine made in armadillos. The cloned cells from both groups appear to be able to recognize two antigens in particular, but whether or not these antigens are responsible for cell-mediated immunity against the disease has yet to be determined. As about 12 million people suffer from leprosy throughout the world, recognition of the immunizing antigens and the production of a vaccine using recombinant techniques is much needed.

Cholera

Cholera vibrios (and *E. coli* responsible for endotoxin-induced diarrhoea) do not invade the intestinal tissue but remain in the lumen or attached to the epithelium. Thus, secretory IgA provides the main protective role and can be shown to protect mice from intestinal challenge. Research is required to identify the epithelial target material for such microorganisms, which seem likely to be carbohydrate in nature such as fucose associated with blood group substances.

The parenteral whole-cell cholera vaccines available today give only 50–70% protection for three to six months whilst clinical illness provides protection for several years. Vaccination efforts against cholera are directed at stimulating mucosal immunity with non-toxic preparations that contain appropriate protective immunogens such as a combined vaccine containing toxoid and somatic antigens.

Work in Australia in which genes from typhoid and cholera bacteria are cloned in harmless bacteria is hoped to produce more effective and less toxic vaccines than the existing ones derived from dead bacteria.

Trypanosomes

The future development of vaccines against trypanosomes has been aided by studies of *T. cruzi* (responsible for Chagas'disease affecting 10–12 million people in central and south America). The disease is transmitted by blood-sucking insects and blood transfusion (3% of donors in Sao Paulo in Brazil harbour the disease and 10 000–12 000 new cases arise each year as a consequence of blood transfusion). Amongst the glycoprotein surface antigens of the organism, one appears to be involved in the penetration of human cells by a mechanism that depends on the recognition of N-acetyl-

D-glucosamine. The production of monoclonal antibodies to these various surface antigens and their systematic screening for their ability to inhibit interiorization of the parasite should lead to recognition of the protective material for use in recombinant DNA technology and vaccine production.

Other developments

One of the most exciting new developments involves the use of vaccinia virus recombinants that express genes introduced from other infective agents. Tests in mice indicate that protection can be achieved with influenza, herpes, rabies and vesicular stomatitis viruses and against hepatitis B virus in chimpanzees.

The env gene from the AIDS virus that codes for the envelope protein of the virus has been inserted into the vaccinia virus and may prove useful for vaccination against the disease. Even more recently BCG has been modified in the same way to produce an AIDS vaccine.

The advantage of vaccinia virus is that it is simple and economical to manufacture, is relatively hazard free and has a large capacity for foreign DNA to be inserted. It is expected that, by the simultaneous introduction of genes from a variety of organisms, polyvalent vaccines could be produced.

Immunization services are among the least expensive and most effective of all health services. Estimates of the costs of providing a fully-immunized child can be as low as (US) $5 when the coverage is extensive. About 50% of the costs are for personnel salaries, whilst the vaccine itself accounts for about 14%. The remaining costs are for equipment, training and operating costs.

Antigens of microorganisms

Bacterial and viral antigens are in common use in medical practice as a means of inducing immunity to infectious disease such as smallpox, diphtheria, measles, poliomyelitis, typhoid fever and many others. There are four main types of conventional antigen preparations or **vaccines**.

Toxoids

These are the soluble exotoxins of bacteria, such as diphtheria and tetanus bacilli, which have been modified and rendered less toxic by the addition of formalin or gentle heating. They are administered either in solution or precipitated on alum. Many years of useful immunity can be achieved by these procedures.

Killed vaccines

Killed vaccines are cultured organisms killed by heat, usually 60°C for one hour, ultraviolet irradiation or chemicals such as phenol, alcohol or formalin. Protection against whooping-cough, poliomyelitis and perhaps cholera can be achieved in this way.

Antigens isolated from infectious agents

An example of these is the capsular polysaccharide of the pneumococci. A diffusible factor of *B. anthracis* and a cell wall preparation of haemolytic streptococci have been shown to induce immunity, but such preparations are not in general use in medical practice.

Attenuated living vaccines

These are made from strains of organisms that have lost their virulence by growth in culture (e.g. Pasteur's chicken cholera vaccine, p. 6) or in animals when the conditions are not favourable for the growth and proliferation of the virulent strain. Strains emerge which, whilst not able to produce disease, can induce immunity; such strains are known as **attenuated** organisms. The BCG vaccine (Bacille Calmette-Guérin) for tuberculosis and the cowpox vaccine for smallpox are the outstanding examples of this type of vaccine. The oral administration of a strain of poliomyelitis virus induces a powerful immunity without producing the disease. The virus spreads from one individual to another and so is able to produce immunity in a community. An attenuated strain of yellow fever virus has been developed, obtained from the original virulent material by prolonged cultivation in tissue culture. Attenuated strains of measles virus are also used, and it seems likely that rubella virus vaccination will soon reduce the hazard of congenital abnormalities developing in the infants of mothers infected with the virus. See Table 5.10 for examples of common vaccines available for human infections.

In veterinary medicine successful vaccines have been produced against canine distemper, canine hepatitis and Newcastle disease (fowl pest) of chickens.

Table 5.10 Vaccine preparations in use in man

	Viral	Bacterial
Whole organisms Live (attennuated)	Smallpox Measles Rubella Polio Yellow fever Influenza (nasal vaccine)	BCG
Inactivated (heat, u.v. chemicals)	Influenza	Typhoid and paratyphoid
	Typhus	Pertussis Cholera
Products of organisms Toxoids		Diphtheria Tetanus

Routine procedures

The determining factors in the selection of immunization procedures for a particular population must depend on local environmental conditions and epidemiological considerations. In Britain, a child is immunized during its first year of life with a vaccine containing diphtheria and tetanus toxoids in combination with a killed suspension of whooping-cough (*Bordetella pertussis*) organisms. This is known as **triple vaccine** and its efficacy as an immunizing agent is in part due to the adjuvant effect of the pertussis component. This procedure is repeated on two further occasions and at the same time oral polio vaccine is usually given. Vaccination against smallpox is achieved by giving one dose of the vaccinia vaccine during the second year when the chances of developing complications appear to be much decreased. Primary vaccination is not advised after early childhood. The risk of serious complications in early childhood is very small but nevertheless considered to be out of proportion to the risk of being infected with the disease. Thus smallpox vaccination need no longer be recommended as a routine procedure in early childhood. Booster doses of all these vaccines are usually given at five years of age and tetanus, polio and smallpox again between the ages of 15 and 19. Table 5.11 shows the recommended schedules of the Department of Health and Social Security.

In the USA the official recommendation for childhood immunization comprises three primary doses of diph/tet/pert vaccine and oral polio vaccine at intervals of four to six weeks, beginning

Table 5.11 A schedule of vaccination immunization procedures. After Joint Committee on vaccination and immunization (1978)

Age	Vaccine	Interval	Notes
During first year of life 3 months	diph/tet/pert & oral polio vaccine* (first dose)		The first dose triple vaccine together with oral polio vaccine should be given at 3 months. If pertussis vaccine is contraindicated or declined by parents diph/tet should be given
4½–5 months	polio vaccine* (second dose)	preferably after an interval of 6–8 weeks	
8½–11 months	diph/tet/pert & oral polio vaccine* (third dose)	preferably after an interval of 4–6 months	
During second year of life	measles*		
5 years of age or school entry	diph/tet/and oral polio*		
Between 11 and 13 years of age	BCG		For tuberculin-negative children
Girls between 11–13 years of age	rubella*		All girls this age should be offered rubella vaccine
Between 15–19 years of age or on leaving school	polio (oral* or inactivated tetanus)		whether or not there is a past history of the disease

* = live virus vaccines, contraindicated during pregnancy.

(For full details and notes the reader should refer to *Protection and Prevention* 1984 The Wellcome Medical Foundation Ltd.

at the age of two or three months. A booster is given one year after completion of the primary course.

Live vaccines should not be given to persons whose ability to respond to infection is reduced, as for example after radiotherapy, immunosuppressive drugs, steroids or in patients with immune-deficiency states. If a subject has had a local or general reaction to a vaccine, there is a risk of even more marked reactions to the next dose.

Table 5.12 Diseases against which protective immunization may be provided in special circumstances

Hazards to the fetus Rubella	*Hazards associated with occupation or other special circumstances*
Hazards to travellers Enteric fever Yellow fever Cholera Smallpox	Anthrax Influenza Mumps Plague Q fever Rabies Tularaemia Typhus Hepatitis A & B (passive immunization)

Special circumstances

Protective immunization can be performed in situations where a particular hazard exists, such as to the fetus associated with rubella in pregnancy, the infectious hazards of travelling abroad, and the occupational hazards of acquiring certain infections. Table 5.12 shows situations when such immunization procedures may be adopted.

Immunization against rubella

All girls should be immunized just before puberty with the live attenuated virus, regardless of whether they think that they have previously had rubella or not. This avoids the risk of their contracting the disease subsequently when they are pregnant, as rubella in pregnancy may lead to malformations of the fetus.

Female school teachers, nursery staff, and nurses and doctors caring for children in hospital and in clinics may be exposed to rubella; staff working in antenatal clinics may acquire the infection and pass it on to patients in the early stages of pregnancy. These groups should be offered rubella vaccination if preliminary serological tests are negative. However, as the vaccine should not be given during pregnancy, assurances must be sought from women in these groups that they are not pregnant and that they will take precautions against becoming pregnant for at least two months after taking the vaccine.

Immunization of travellers

Travellers are exposed to infectious hazards that vary from country to country. There are national and international regulations which make vaccination against yellow fever, cholera and smallpox statutory for persons travelling to and from countries where the diseases are endemic, or where an epidemic has recently occurred. As the regulations are subject to change, a traveller who is visiting any country where the diseases have occurred in recent years should check from its embassy what certificates of vaccination are necessary, if any.

The traveller is often well advised to seek immunization against other diseases that may be encountered (Table 5.12). Travellers may be unaware that poliomyelitis, diphtheria, tetanus and tuberculosis are still significant risks in some countries; medical students volunteering for work in developing countries should bear these special occupational hazards in mind. It is not yet possible to be artificially actively immunized against infectious hepatitis (hepatitis A), but effective short-term passive protection (up to six months) is conferred by an injection of normal pooled human gamma globulin. International certificates for yellow fever vaccination are valid for 10 years and become valid 10 days after primary vaccination. In contrast, cholera vaccination certificates are valid for only six months, becoming valid six days after primary vaccination. All non-immune children over 10–12 months going to live in the tropics should be vaccinated against measles.

Occupational hazards

Immunization against various infections considered above and also against mumps, Q fever, plague, tularaemia and typhus may be offered to laboratory workers and others at special risk.

In view of the success of the WHO smallpox eradication programme, vaccination against smallpox is no longer required as a routine in many countries. All doctors and nurses, and the staff of bacteriological laboratories and others who may meet previously unrecognized cases of smallpox or come into contact with infected material from them, should be revaccinated at least once every three years. This applies especially to the staff of hospitals for infectious diseases.

High titre hepatitis B immunoglobulin is available for the temporary passive protection of clinical and laboratory workers who sustain a skin-penetrating injury under circumstances associated with a risk of the transmission of the hepatitis B virus; prophylactic immunization should soon become possible using synthetic antigens or those prepared by recombinant DNA techniques (p. 168).

An anthrax vaccine is recommended for those who handle animal hides and bones, etc. Vaccination has similarly been practised against brucellosis and leptospirosis in man, but the protective value of available vaccines against these two occupational hazards is not established.

Notes on special vaccines

Enteric fever. TAB vaccine provides useful protection against typhoid fever, but its protective value against the paratyphoid fevers has not been proved. Tourists, business people and others who travel from countries in northern and western Europe and North America to Mediterranean countries, Africa, Asia and Latin America are advised to be immunized; this is obligatory for members of most armed forces. The paratyphoid components are omitted from **typhoid vaccine** and this is less likely to give the local and systemic reactions that are quite common with TAB vaccine.

Yellow fever vaccine. A preparation of live attenuated virus is given by injection and one dose confers immunity for 10 years.

Cholera vaccine. This vaccine is a preparation of killed cholera vibrios. Two subcutaneous injections with an interval of about 4–6 weeks give a degree of protection against *V. cholerae* and *V. eltor* that is unfortunately only transient.

Vaccination against smallpox. In the mid-1970s WHO announced that smallpox had been virtually eradicated, with only a few pockets of infection remaining in remote mountain villages of Ethiopia. By the end of 1976 Ethiopia seemed to be clear, but smallpox then occurred in Somalia, a non-endemic country which had been free of smallpox since 1963. The problem of the importation of this disease calls for a policy of 'ring vaccination' in which the contacts of any imported case are identified, located and vaccinated, and the population in these locations is offered prompt vaccination to contain the hazard. If follows that health workers who may have to deal at short notice with this emergency should continue to be vaccinated against smallpox, and doctors should know about smallpox vaccination which is given special consideration here.

Active immunity against smallpox is conferred by **vaccinia virus**; its origin is uncertain and it may be derived from variola or cowpox viruses. The vaccine consists of lymph obtained from vesicles produced on the skin of calves or sheep by inoculating the scarified skin with the virus.

The vaccine lymph is supplied in glass capillary tubes or in plastic tubes (which are difficult to handle aseptically). If it is stored frozen, its potency is maintained for about a year at −10°C and it may be kept in a domestic refrigerator for up to two weeks. It is inactivated at room temperature and no vaccine should be used after more than seven days from the date of dispatch, unless it has been kept in a refrigerator. The vaccine is administered intradermally, usually on the upper arm, and the multiple pressure procedure is recommended. A drop of vaccine lymph is spread over an area of skin about 0.5 cm in diameter. The skin must be clean, but no disinfectant should be used. Pressure is applied to the skin through the vaccine with a sterile large flat needle, held so that it is almost parallel to the surface. To introduce the vaccine into the epidermis, the needle is applied quickly, but not so vigorously as to draw blood. From 10 to 30 such 'pressures' are recommended, 10 sufficing usually for a 'take' in primary vaccination. The dermojet, which is recommended when large numbers of vaccinations have to be done, is a small pistol-like injection which squirts a stream of vaccine on to the skin at very high pressure.

After vaccination, excess lymph is wiped off with sterile cotton wool and the site allowed to dry. It is not necessary to apply a dressing at this stage. The patient should be advised to avoid wetting the site and a dry dressing should be applied if a pustule develops.

Three types of reaction may occur:

In the **primary reaction**, seen in persons not previously vaccinated, a red papule appears in 3–4 days. A vesicle develops in 5–6 days, becoming pustular in eight days. After 11 days a dry scab has usually formed and this falls off after about 21 days.

The **accelerated reaction**, occurring only in persons previously vaccinated successfully, is similar but more rapid. The vesicle is formed on the third day and becomes pustular next day and the scab is off within eight days.

An **immediate reaction** consists of an erythematous papule appearing usually within 24 hours and reaching a maximum in 72 hours, when it fades rapidly without the formation of a vesicle. This occurs only in persons previously vaccinated, and is a type IV hypersensitivity reaction. It does not necessarily indicate immunity although it often occurs in immune subjects.

A primary or accelerated reaction is associated with a sore arm during the vesicular and pustular stages. There is usually little or no general malaise, although small children may appear temporarily upset, but some restriction of activity is necessary and children should be forbidden vigorous games. The lesion is infectious at the pustular stage and patients should be advised accordingly.

Serious complications occasionally occur; the incidence of complications is least if primary vaccination is performed during the second year of life. Encephalitis and generalized vaccinia have already been mentioned. In persons with a history of dermatitis, the local reaction may be severe and constitute **eczema vaccinatum**. Necrosis of the skin may occur; this may be progressive in patients with hypogammaglobulinaemia or in patients receiving immunosuppressive drugs and is known as **vaccinia gangrenosa**.

Primary vaccination usually confers a good immunity for 5–10 years. Revaccination every seven years has been the orthodox advice for a long time and this is sensible, but vaccination should have been carried out within three years if an assurance of protection is sought after there has been direct contact with a case of smallpox or during an epidemic. An international certificate of vaccination, which may be needed for travel between some countries, must be renewed every three years.

Influenza. Vaccines containing influenza viruses A and B inactivated with formaldehyde are available, but these are effective only against a limited range of antigenic variants of the virus. As immunization provides little protection against the common small outbreaks of the disease that are due to numerous and often unidentified strains of virus, it is seldom used as a routine. In the event of a major epidemic due to a single strain of virus, a mass immunization programme would be likely to give a large measure of protection to the community, provided that there was no unexpected antigenic change in the causative virus. A case can be made for giving the vaccine to those who are at special risk, for example elderly people in residential establishments, and also doctors and nurses.

Subunit flu vaccines have been developed in which the flu virus has been treated with detergent to release the superficial components of major antigenic significance. These 'split' vaccine preparations seem to be promising (see also p. 169).

Rabies vaccines. These are inactivated preparations of the virus harvested from (1) human or animal cell cultures, (2) duck embryo tissue, or (3) animal CNS tissue after laboratory infection with rabies. Adverse reactions to CNS tissue led to strenuous efforts to develop the less dangerous cell culture and duck embryo preparations. Courses of active immunization given to a person after exposure to the risk of rabies range from 3–21 doses by subcutaneous injection. In cases of severe exposure, passive immunization with rabies antiserum may also be advisable.

Plague and typhus (louse-borne). Vaccines are available for use in the event of an outbreak and are valuable for protection of members of the medical services.

Autogenous vaccines. At one time it was fashionable to treat patients suffering from chronic infections, especially of the skin and upper respiratory tract, with vaccines prepared from organisms isolated from the lesions. Clinical trials were seldom carried out and autogenous vaccines are now rarely made.

Passive immunization

Passive immunity against some diseases can be conferred by injecting specific antibodies obtained from the serum of a convalescent patient or from a previously immunized animal. The extra circulating antibodies, added to those that might be naturally produced, may help to curtail an infection or neutralize a toxin and so moderate the illness. Passive immunization has the disadvantages that it provides only temporary protection and, if an animal serum is used, it is liable to provoke hypersensitivity reactions that range from a minor upset to severe anaphylaxis (p. 232).

In practice, passive immunization has been most effectively exploited in the prophylaxis or treatment of infections caused by bacteria that produce exotoxins, such as diphtheria, botulism, tetanus and gas gangrene. Antisera against other bacteria have been prepared; effective antipneumococcal sera became available just before the introduction of sulphonamides, which proved to be much more effective, less hazardous and cheaper. Today, except for the antitoxic sera, the use of antisera is limited. Passive immunization may be more useful in the future, especially for the prevention or treatment of conditions for which no effective antibiotic therapy is available. Infectious diseases, in which human immunoglobulin can be used in prophylaxis, include hepatitis A and B, rubella, measles, varicella zoster, tetanus and rabies. The amount of antibody required is relatively small and is usually provided by alcohol precipitation of an appropriate serum or pool.

The protection offered by the intramuscular injection of these preparations lasts between three and six months and should be given either before exposure or at least early in the incubation period. In severe septicaemia, patients have been successfully treated with large doses of normal human immunoglobulin given intravenously. Much effort is being directed at improving this form of therapy and identifying the protective bacterial antigens so that appropriate antisera can be selected.

Reactions and contraindications

In general, active immunization with any vaccine should be postponed if the patient is temporarily unwell. If more than one live vaccine is to be given, there should be an interval of at least three weeks between them. Live vaccines should not be given to patients whose defences are compromised by malignant disease, severe chronic disease or immunodeficiency; this includes those receiving steroid therapy or cytotoxic drug therapy. Live viral vaccines, and especially rubella vaccine, should not be given during pregnancy.

Patients should be asked if they have previously reacted adversely to a vaccine and such a history should be taken into account before administering the vaccine again. This is of special importance in relation to pertussis vaccine and in cases of reactions to passive immunization with heterologous antisera when there may be a danger of serious anaphylaxis.

Local erythema and tenderness at the injection site are common minor reactions. Fever, headache and malaise for a day or so occur in some people, especially after endotoxin-containing vaccines such as TAB or after a prolonged series of doses of cholera vaccine. Immune adults tend to react adversely to diphtheria immunization. Children with a history or a family history of neonatal cerebral irritation, or a tendency to convulsions or epilepsy, or a previous reaction to pertussis vaccine should not receive the pertussis component of triple vaccine and should be given only the diphtheria-tetanus toxoids.

FURTHER READING

Ada G L 1981 Controlling influenza epidemics. Immunology Today 2: 219
Bell R, Torrigiani G (eds) 1984 New approaches to vaccine development. World Health Organization. Schwabe, Basel

Blackwell C C, Weir D M 1981 Principles of infection and immunity in patient care. Churchill Livingstone, Edinburgh

Deans J A, Cohen S 1983 Immunology of malaria. Annual Review of Microbiology 37:25

Dick G (ed) 1979 Immunological aspects of infectious disease. London, MTP Press

Fauci A S 1978 Host defence mechanisms against infection Upjohn, Michigan (Scope publication).

Gallin J I, Fauci A S 198?. Advances in host defence mechanisms. Mucosal Immunity

Marchalonis J J 1984 Immunobiology of parasites and parasitic infections. In: Contemporary topics in immunobiology vol 12. Plenum Publishing Corporation, New York

Mimms C A 1982 The pathogenesis of infectious disease 2nd edn. edition, Academic Press, New York and London

Mims C A White D A 1984 Viral pathogenesis and immunology. Blackwell Scientific Publications, Oxford

Torrigiani G, Bell R (eds) 1981 Immunological recognition and effector mechanisms in infections diseases. Schwabe, Basel

Wakelin D 1984 Immunity to parasites: how animals control parasite infections. E J Arnold, London

Youmans G P, Paterson P Y, Somers H M (eds) 1975 The biological and clinical basis of infections diseases. Saunders, Philadelphia

6

Immunohaematology

Objectives

On completion of this section the reader will be able to:

1. Draw up a table of the ABO blood group system indicating the antigens and isohaemagglutinins found in each of the groups A, B, O, and AB.

2. Define 'universal donor'.

3. Describe the phenomenon of Rhesus incompatibility and how the consequences can be abrogated.

4. Describe the antiglobulin test.

5. Outline the consequences of leucocyte incompatibility in transfusion.

6. Give an example of a situation in which platelets may be given by transfusion.

7. Outline the relationship between blood group and secretor state and susceptibility to infection.

Knowledge of blood groups in man and animals has been very closely associated with the development of the science of immunology. Differences between the red blood cells of animals were first noted in goats as early as 1900 when Ehrlich and Morgenroth immunized 'a strong male goat' with nearly a litre of blood obtained from three other goats. The serum which they obtained from the immunized goat lysed the cells of all but one of the nine goats they tested. However, to Ehrlich the most important finding was that the cells of the immunized goat itself were completely unaffected. This proved to him that an animal would not produce autoantibodies against its own tissues and so destroy itself. It was left to Karl Landsteiner, who made the same observations in humans, to take up the detailed study of these antigenic differences. Landsteiner's important work on the immunological determinants of antigenic specificity stems from this period and still stands today as of fundamental value to our understanding of antigens (Chapter 2).

Studies in blood group serology have led to the development of a large variety of techniques which have wide application to immunological problems outside this field. Notable amongst these is the antiglobulin test devised by Coombs and his associates, by means of which enormous advances have been made in many branches of immunology. Study of the development of blood group antibodies in serum has thrown light on the mechanisms underlying the formation of natural antibodies. Apart from these contributions to the understanding of immunological problems, information on blood groups has important implications in genetics and in forensic studies.

As has been noted in Chapter 5 (p. 133), blood group status appears to be associated with susceptibility to infections such as cholera (blood group O), gonorrhoea (blood group B) and *E. coli* infections of the urinary tract (groups B and AB). The reasons for these associations are not clear but may be related to cross-reactions between isohaemagglutinins or isoantibodies (see below) and cell wall antigens of various microorganisms. Such natural antibodies may act by blocking attachment of the bacterium to its target cell (see also p. 192).

Blood groups

ABO antigens and isoantibodies

The ABO blood group system was described as a result of Landsteiner's demonstration of four distinct groups of agglutination reaction between human red blood cells and normal human serum. The differences in agglutination were due to the presence or absence of two antigens A and B on the red cell membrane. The four combinations which result from this are: (1) the presence of A antigen in the absence of B — group A cells; (2) the presence of B antigen in the absence of A — group B cells; (3) the presence of both A and B antigens — group AB cells; and (4) the absence of both A and B antigens — group O cells.

The sera of individuals also contain natural antibodies able to react with, and agglutinate if present in sufficient concentration, the cells of other individuals of different blood group.

These natural antibodies or **isoantibodies** are formed shortly after birth and appear to be stimulated by immunization with A and B antigens derived from the normal bacterial flora of the gut. Antigens with blood group specificity are widely distributed in nature (see also p. 32).

From a consideration of the phenomenon of immunological tolerance and the fact that an individual is tolerant to 'self' antigens (Ch. 9), it can be seen that an individual will respond only to an antigen to which he is not already tolerant. Thus an individual with blood group A cells will be tolerant to the A antigen and will therefore respond only to the B antigen derived from the gut flora. The same holds for blood group B individuals who can respond only to the A antigen.

Thus individuals of blood group A will have isoantibodies of blood group B specificity, i.e. anti-B antibodies, and blood group B individuals will in the same way have anti-A isoantibodies. Blood group O individuals whose immune system will not have developed tolerance to either A or B antigens will have, as would be expected, both anti-A and anti-B isoagglutinins.

The blood group antigens A and B occur not only in the red cells but are widely distributed in the tissues with the exception of the central nervous system. Just under 80% of individuals also have one of these antigens (corresponding to their blood group) in the tissue fluids and secretions (except c.s.f.). Chemical studies on these antigens recovered in quantity from ovarian cyst fluid show them to be glycoproteins and that the difference between A and B substances is determined by the nature of a single saccharide attached to the terminal sugar of the glycoprotein chain. Group O individuals secrete a glycoprotein (H-substance) which is the basic chain structure material from which A and B substances are derived by the addition of the specific saccharides (p. 34).

Blood transfusion in relation to ABO groups

Transfusion of an individual with red cells from an individual of a different group results in exposure of the transfused cells to an isoagglutinin — anti-A or anti-B — and except in the case of O cells which carry neither the A or the B antigen, the cells will be destroyed with resulting haemoglobinaemia and haemoglobinuria. Although it is clearly best to administer blood only of the same group as the recipient, in an emergency group O cells can be given. Although the plasma of a group O individual (sometimes called a **'universal donor'**) contains anti-A and anti-B isoagglutinins, these are so diluted by the recipient's plasma (a pint of blood would be diluted about 1 in 12) to have only a negligible effect except when large quantities of blood have to be administered. Group O individuals whose serum contains anti-A and anti-B isoagglutinins cannot accept blood of any group except O. Since an individual of group AB has neither anti-A nor anti-B isoantibodies he can accept blood of any of the four groups and has therefore been called a **'universal recipient'**.

This relatively straightforward scheme is unfortunately slightly complicated by the existence of a number of subgroups of A (probably five in all). However, only A_1 and A_2 are of importance as far as transfusion is concerned. The frequency of occurrence in Caucasians of the six different ABO groups is shown in Table 6.1.

Table 6.1 Blood group distribution in Caucasians

Blood group	Frequency	Isoantibodies
O	43.5%	Anti-A (+ anti-A_1), anti-B
A_1	34.8%	Anti-B
A_2	9.6%	Anti-B (occasionally anti-A_1)
B	8.5%	Anti-A (+ anti-A_1)
A_1B	2.5%	None
A_2B	0.8%	None (occasionally anti-A_1)

The Rhesus blood group system

This system is the next most important system to the ABO groups. The Rh blood group antigens are present in the red cells of 85% of Caucasians and 94% of Negroes. The most common of the Rhesus antigens are C, c, D, d, E, e, and Table 6.2 shows some of the various combinations which can exist and their frequency in Caucasians.

Table 6.2 Combinations of Rh antigens and frequency in Caucasians

Genotype	Frequency	
CDe/cde	31.7%	
CDe/CDe	16.6%	Rh-positive
CDe/cDe	11.5%	
cDE/cde	10.9%	
cde/cde	15.1%	Rh-negative

The Rhesus group of an individual must be taken into account for transfusion purposes. Of these antigens D is the most potent although immunization by D and at the same time by the C or E antigens can occur. A variant of D named D^u has been described and cells carrying this antigen are not agglutinated by routine anti-

D sera. For transfusion purposes recipients carrying the D^u antigen are considered to be Rh-negative, whilst donors in this category are regarded as Rh-positive.

Rhesus incompatibility

The clinical importance of the Rhesus groups lies in the ability of the red cells of a Rhesus-positive fetus to immunize its Rhesus-negative mother. Immunization usually takes place following the trauma of parturition with the result that the maternal immune response does not develop until a **second** pregnancy. The maternal anti-Rh antibody is passed to the new fetus via the placenta and causes haemolytic destruction of its erythrocytes. This condition is known as **haemolytic disease of the newborn** or erythroblastosis fetalis. Since the original description of the disease it has been found that blood group antigen systems other than the Rh system can be responsible for the condition. For example, a group O mother can occasionally be immunized by fetal antigens if the father is A_1, A_1B or B.

The serious nature of haemolytic disease of the newborn necessitating complete exchange of the infant's blood (exchange transfusion) to remove the maternal antibody, has now been alleviated by a rather ingenious immunological manoeuvre. This is based on the observation that attempted immunization by an antigen in the presence of its specific antibody tends to inhibit synthesis of the antibody to the injected antigen. It is known, for example, that immunization of infants is best delayed for a few months after birth to allow the levels of maternal antibody to fall.

In the case of a recognized Rhesus incompatibility it is now the practice to give a small dose of potent anti-Rh antibody to immunized Rh-negative mothers within three days after delivery of an Rh-positive infant. The antibody appears to inhibit the response to the Rhesus antigen, possibly by diverting the cells carrying the antigen from the antibody-forming tissues or perhaps by a direct 'feedback inhibition' effect on the antibody-forming cells. This treatment has been very successful in clinical trials and the future outlook is very hopeful so that the disease may soon become of only historical interest (Fig. 6.1).

The detection of anti-Rh antibodies

After the recognition of the association between haemolytic disease

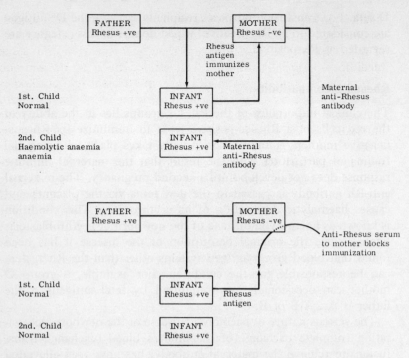

Fig. 6.1 Scheme showing consequence of immunization of Rhesus −ve mother by Rhesus antigen of Rhesus +ve child. Prevention obtained by injection of anti-Rhesus serum after delivery of first child

of the newborn and Rhesus immunization, it soon became apparent that the standard method of demonstrating anti-Rh antibody — by direct agglutination of a saline suspension of Rh-positive cells by serum from an immunized mother — was not able to show up the presence of antibody in one-half to two-thirds of sera tested. A solution to the problem was found by the substitution of a dilute protein solution, e.g. bovine albumen, for the normal saline diluent. Visible agglutination could then be readily demonstrated in the majority of cases. The form of serum antibody responsible for agglutination, demonstrable only in protein diluent, became known as 'incomplete' antibody in contrast to the saline-active 'complete' antibody. The incomplete antibody was thought of initially as univalent, having only one antibody-binding site, but it has now been shown to be IgG antibody of normal bivalent structure (p. 94); the complete anti-red cell antibody, on the other hand, has been shown to be IgM in nature. It seems that the smaller molecular weight IgG antibody is not readily able to link together red cells in suspension unless the mutually repellent effect of red cells, which normally keeps them in suspension in a saline medium, is reduced by altering their surface charge by the addition of protein. In contrast the much larger, multivalent IgM antibodies have a considerably greater chance of bringing about agglutination.

Another very important method for demonstrating incomplete antibodies is the Coombs **antiglobulin test**. An antiserum is prepared in rabbits against human immunoglobulins and this is used to react with Rh-positive cells, coated with human incomplete antibody, bringing about their agglutination simply by linking together the molecules of human globulin still attached to the red cells (p. 279 and Fig. 10.9).

One of the advantages of this method is that it can be used to detect the coating in vivo of Rh-positive cells by small amounts of antibody. After the cells have been thoroughly washed, they are mixed with the anti-human globulin serum which will bring about agglutination of cells with human globulin attached to their surface. This form of the test is known as the 'direct Coombs test'. Another form of the test is used to detect incomplete anti-Rh antibodies in the serum of a patient who has been immunized against Rh antigens. Rh-positive cells are simply mixed with the patient's serum and if anti-Rh antibody is present the cells will be agglutinated by the subsequent addition of an anti-human globulin serum. This variation is known as the 'indirect Coombs test'.

Maternal responses to other fetal antigens

In addition to responding to the Rhesus antigen the mother can respond to other blood group antigens, and mothers lacking the A or B red cell antigen who carry a fetus possessing such antigen will probably develop raised levels of anti-A or anti-B isoagglutinins. Such sera are useful for blood typing purposes, as are sera containing anti-HLA antibodies which are often found in multiparous women and which can be used for leucocyte typing. Spermatozoa, although they carry histocompatibility antigens, rarely seem to immunize. Immunization of the mother to fetal antigen probably occurs following passage of fetal blood (by small haemorrhages) into the maternal bloodstream and occurs more frequently as pregnancy progresses. The fetus represents an allograft containing potentially immunogenic antigens derived from paternal antigens of the major histocompatibility complex (MHC). The mother makes both humoral and cell-mediated responses to these antigens but the fetus survives because the placenta appears to be an immunologically privileged site and does not allow effector cells or antibodies to affect fetal development. The placenta seems to be able to absorb out antifetal antibodies from the maternal blood and H-2K and H-2D antigens of paternal type have been found on the mouse placenta. There is evidence that MHC disaparity is associated with fetal survival. Women who have chronic abortions share more HLA antigens with their husbands than predicted by chance. The placenta is believed to be responsible for balancing the tendency for rejection of the fetus with 'facilitation' that allows the fetus to survive to term. In man (but not mouse) the trophoblast lacks MHC antigens. Maternal antibodies to fetal antigens, where the parents are genetically dissimilar, appear to offer protection to the fetus and this finding has been used with some success to prevent recurrent abortion, where no other obvious abnormality is present, by immunizing mothers against paternal lymphocytes.

A number of pregnancy-associated substances such as alpha-fetoprotein, 17β-oestradiol, prostaglandin synthetase inhibitor and β_1-microglobulin may play a role in regulating the immune response in pregnancy. It has also been found that natural killer cells (p. 64) are absent in neonates. It is becoming apparent that a certain degree of foreignness may actually assist human reproduction and viviparity. An IgG 'blocking factor' has been found in maternal serum that inhibits production of lymphokines by maternal lymphocytes sensitized to antigens on the trophoblast and paternal lymphocytes. Women who undergo recurrent abortions of unknown aetiology lack the blocking factor. Preliminary trials in which 'blocking factor' is induced by immunization with pooled leucocyte infusions have resulted in encouraging results.

Other blood group systems

In 1927 Landsteiner described two human antigens, M and N. The use of antisera against these antigens can divide individuals into three types, half having the MN genotype and 28% and 22% respectively having MM and NN genotypes. A further antigen was later found, the S antigen, and the group is known as the MNS blood group system. This group is of limited clinical importance although a few instances of haemolytic disease of the newborn have been reported due to incompatibility of these antigens.

Landsteiner's P antigen is noteworthy because a naturally occurring anti-P cold agglutinin is found in a large proportion of the 20% of individuals who are P-negative. Amongst a number of blood group systems described including those of Lutheran, Kell, Lewis, Kidd, Duffy and Diego, special mention should be made of the Lewis system because naturally occurring antibodies to Lewis antigens are frequently found in human serum. They sometimes act as cold agglutinins and have been found occasionally to be the cause of haemolytic transfusion reactions. These antigens are unique in that they are not part of the red cell structure but are soluble antigens found in body fluids, which adsorb on to the red cell surface.

Antigens of blood leucocytes and platelets

As will be discussed in the section on transplantation antigens, blood leucocytes in man carry the major histocompatibility antigen system HLA. The appearance of antibodies against donor leucocytes and also platelet antigens is a common finding after blood transfusion. This results in rapid destruction of the transfused cells and although immunization occurs more frequently than anti-red cell immunization the consequences are less dangerous.

Leucocyte and platelet groups fall into two types: those which they share in common with red cells, and those with antigens which are restricted to leucocytes and platelets and other tissue cells. The blood group antigens A and B are the main antigens shared with erythrocytes. The important antigenic group limited to leucocytes, platelets and other tissue cells is the HLA system.

A reaction between antileucocyte isoantibodies and transfused leucocytes often gives rise to febrile transfusion reactions and their incidence can be correlated with the number of transfusions given. Although these reactions are not usually severe they can be a disadvantage to patients for whom repeated transfusions are necessary. In this situation the simplest solution is to remove the majority of leucocytes from the blood by separation of red cells which can be readily sedimented by the addition of gelatin. This is preferable to the complex serological procedures required to assure compatibility of leucocytes.

The transfusion of fresh platelets is of value in patients suffering from haemorrhagic disorders due to thrombocytopenia, and although theoretically, selection of compatible platelets is desirable, in practice platelets are usually obtained from a small number of donors, if possible related to the recipient.

The HLA system of antigens is of considerable current interest to immunologists because of their importance as histocompatibility antigens. Unfortunately the HLA system appears to be a most complex system but with wide implications in immunology. It is the equivalent of the H-2 system in the mouse and of the other main histocompatibility systems known to exist in other mammalian species (see p. 255).

Between 15 and 20 more or less well-defined antigens have been identified in the HLA system, and more than 100 phenotypes have been found within this system. Despite these complexities, as more experience is gained in the grouping procedures (leucoagglutination by a panel of antisera) and supplies of suitable antisera become more widely available, it seems likely that by accumulating a list of available fully typed donors and with improvements in storage and preservation of tissues, it may eventually become possible to select from amongst the many possible variations a suitable donor for each recipient.

ABO blood groups, secretor state and susceptibility to infection

As noted above ABO incompatibility between mother and fetus predisposes to haemolytic disease of the newborn and also to spontaneous abortion. Associations have also been reported between blood group and a wide variety of infective agents. In particular, blood group B is associated with infections of the mucous membranes of the urinary tract, gastrointestinal tract and respiratory tract. ABO blood group substances are secreted in about 75% of individuals into the tissue fluids and other secretions, under control of a dominant gene independent of the genes determining the ABO blood groups. Some populations have a higher proportion of non-secretors, for example Iceland with nearly 50% of non-secretors. Studies in the author's laboratory have shown that non-secretors appear to be immunocompromised. Women with recurrent urinary tract infections have a higher incidence of non-secretion than the general population and the same is true for individuals with oral or vaginal infections caused by *Candida albicans* and *Neisseria meningitidis* infections in Scotland, Iceland and northern Nigeria (p. 133). The reasons for this increased susceptibility of non-secretors to such infections of the mucous membranes have not yet been established, but it is suggested that the blood group antigens of secretors may interfere in some way with the binding of the microorganisms to their target cells. This proposal is supported by the fact that many microorganisms have lectins (sugar recognizing molecules) in their cell wall that interact with carbohydrates, some of which are components of the structure of blood group substances.

FURTHER READING

Bulletin of the World Health Organization 1967 The suppression of Rh-immunization by passively administered human immunoglobulin (IgG) anti-D (anti-Rh_0). Bulletin of WHO 36:467
Dausset J, Colombani J 1967 White cells and platelets in transfusion immunology. In: Cruickshank R, Weir D M (eds) Modern trends in immunology. Butterworth, London, vol 2, p 314
Dodd B E, Lincoln P J 1975 Blood group topics. In: Turk J L (ed) Current topics in immunology. Arnold, London, vol 3
Race R R, Sanger R 1975 Blood groups in man, 6th edn. Blackwell, Oxford
Singh B, Gambel P 1982 Reproduction: protection and prevention! Immunology Today 3:1
Stern C M 1975 Feto-maternal relationships. In: Hobart M J, McConnell I (eds) The immune system. Blackwell, Oxford

7

The immunology of tissue transplantation

Objectives

On completion of this section the reader will be able to:

1. Describe, in outline form, the transplantation antigen systems of man and the mouse and how these antigens are detected.
2. Define 'first set' and 'second set' graft rejection.
3. Outline the role of lymphocytes and humoral antibody in graft rejection.
4. Describe two approaches to immunosuppression.

The tissue cells of animals contain antigens that are specific for the species of origin of the cell, and which if implanted into an animal of another species will induce an immune response. This response rapidly destroys the implanted cells and has the characteristics of the primary and secondary immune response as already described for antigens in general. In addition to species-specific antigens, differences also exist between individual members of the same species so that transfer of tissue cells between members induces a similar immune reaction. The closer the relationship between two individuals of the same species, the more likely are

Table 7.1 Transplantation terminology (older terminology in brackets)

Relationship between donor and recipient	Term applied to relationship	Prefix applied to graft, antigen or antibody
Of different species	Xenogeneic (heterogeneic)	Xeno- (hetero-)
Of same species but different genetic constitution	Allogeneic (homologous)	Allo- (homo-)
Of same inbred strain	Syngeneic (isogeneic) (isologous)	—
Same individual	Autologous	Auto-

implanted cells to survive. In the case of identical twins survival is assured. Inbred strains of animals, particularly mice, have been developed which are genetically identical and these are widely used in experimental work on tissue transplantation immunology.

In man surgical techniques are available to enable transplantation of many organs and tissues but unfortunately a high proportion of organ transplants fail because of rejection by the immune response or because of the side effects of attempts to suppress the immune response, due to toxicity of the drugs or their depressive effect on resistance to infection.

Transplantation antigen systems

The first systematic studies on the antigens carried by cells which determine whether a graft will be rejected or not were carried out in inbred strains of mice of known genetic make-up.

It was found that there were very many antigenic differences between tissues of different strains of mice, the number of separate antigens involved being estimated at between 15 and 500 in different experiments. However, it was found that, just as in the red cell antigenic system, some antigens were very 'strong' and others very weak. The strong transplantation or 'histocompatibility' antigens of the mouse are controlled by the H-2 genetic locus and in man by the HLA locus.

The mouse H-2 system appears to consist of a system of closely linked genes and there are hundreds of possible combinations resulting in different H-2 antigens. H-2 antigens are found in large amounts in epithelium and lymphoid tissues, in very small amounts in kidney or muscle and are virtually absent from brain and testis.

In man, two strong and several weak histocompatibility systems have been found. As mentioned already, the HLA is the strong system with the ABH blood group system next in importance. The major loci are very complex, the antigens being determined by a chromosomal region rather than by a single genetic locus.

Chemical studies on soluble H-2 antigens have shown them to be glycoproteins. Analysis of the amino acid constitution of extracted transplantation antigen of two different inbred strains of guinea-pig indicates that they are distinct.

HLA-A and HLA-B of chromosome 6 (see Fig. 4.19) are the human counterpart of the mouse H-2K and H-2D loci and are the antigens most often used in immune typing. This is done with a panel of various monospecific HLA antisera, often obtained from women who had multiple pregnancies or, increasingly, with monoclonal antibodies prepared against HLA antigens.

The test is carried out with lymphocytes from the individual to be typed incubated with the various antisera and complement. The presence of a particular antigen on the surface of the lymphocyte, in the presence of appropriate antibody and complement, leads to lysis of the lymphocyte. Lysis is detected by the failure of the cell to exclude the dye trypan blue (see p. 285).

Different HLA-A and HLA-B antigens are given numbers, e.g. HLA-B5. No individual has more than two HLA-A antigen specifications and two HLA-B antigen specifications. Thus, an individual heterogenous at each locus can express four major HLA specificities, two from each parent.

A further locus, the HLA-D locus, appears to be the equivalent of the I region in the mouse. As in the mouse it is involved in various lymphocyte activating functions. The HLA-C locus is of lesser importance than HLA-A and HLA-B in graft rejection as it determines relatively weak transplantation antigens.

Grafts between HLA identical siblings are the most successful and have a greater chance of survival than HLA-A and HLA-B matched grafts that are not necessarily identical at other loci.

The structure of the human HLA antigens indicating the two-chain arrangement including β_2 microglobulin are shown in Figure 4.20 (p. 114). The larger component of 44 000 daltons molecular weight contains amino acid sequences that show some homology with the constant domains of the immunoglobulin G molecule.

Leucocyte grouping

The strong antigens of the HLA system are widely distributed in the tissues but absent from the red blood cells which contain only the ABH antigens.

Fortunately blood leucocytes carry all the known HLA antigens and it is therefore possible to test for the presence or absence of antigens of the system using leucocyte agglutination and cytotoxicity tests (p. 285). In principle the leuco-agglutination test is performed with leucocytes separated from the erythrocytes of anti-coagulant-treated blood. Specific antisera for HLA antigens are then used to agglutinate the leucocytes and the tests are read under the microscope. The cytotoxic test is carried out with a purified suspension of blood lymphocytes which are mixed with antisera to

HLA antigens in the presence of complement (p. 25). If the lymphocytes carry the appropriate antigens the antiserum will combine and in the presence of complement will damage the cell membrane. The resulting increased cell membrane permeability is usually detected by dye uptake into the cell. Matching donor and recipient for HLA antigens, including the DR antigens (the human equivalent of the mouse Ia antigens), is normally carried out prior to grafting.

Despite the very great diversity among HLA alleles of unrelated subjects it is encouraging to find that about a third of kidneys from unrelated donors survive for a year or longer although only a third of them show normal kidney function. Although this partial success must be dependent to an extent on the use of immunosuppressive agents, differences in the 'strength' of individual HLA antigens is probably partly responsible.

Mechanisms of graft rejection (Fig. 7.1)

There are two main types of graft rejection process: (a) the so-called 'first set' response which occurs about 10 days after a first graft from an unrelated donor, (b) the 'second set' response occurring in about 7 days in an animal which had previously received a graft from the same unrelated donor. This phenomenon of first and second set rejection can be compared to primary and secondary immunization — the accelerated secondary response being brought about by stimulation of an already sensitized or 'primed' immune system.

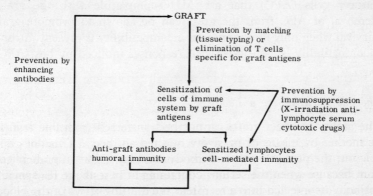

Fig. 7.1 Schematic view of rejection mechanisms and their prevention

The role of lymphoid cells

It can be shown histologically that grafts undergoing rejection are heavily infiltrated with lymphocytes and that there is extensive vascular damage. Other types of cells of the immune system, such as plasma cells and macrophages, are also frequently found in association with graft rejection. The ability to reject grafts can readily be transferred from one animal to another by a process known as **adoptive transfer** of lymphoid cells from an immune animal (i.e. one capable of a second set graft rejection) to a non-immune recipient of the same strain. Lymphoid cells appear to be able to transfer this ability most effectively when taken before the circulating antibody level reaches its peak. Contrary to expectation, it is possible to show, using isotope-labelled cells, that it is not the transferred cells which migrate to the graft but those of the recipient. The donated cells in the main home to the lymphoid organs, as no more are found in the graft than at control sites. It is, however, possible that those few donated cells which settle in the graft area are cells specifically sensitized to the graft antigens whilst those settling out elsewhere are the unsensitized cells.

From what is known about the recirculating lymphocyte pool (p. 67), it seems likely that there is a good chance of cells with a specific ability to react to an antigen coming in contact with such material in a graft during the process of lymphocyte recirculation. Donor lymphocytes carried over as 'passengers' in the vascular bed of the graft are a source of transplantation antigens that can sensitize the host. For a graft to provoke an immune response the transplantation antigens are sometimes presented to the host by inducer cells (APC) that are MHC-compatible with the graft. Removal of APC from the graft can be shown to promote graft survival when only minor antigen incompatibility is present. Strong incompatibility is associated with responses induced by host APC.

The role of circulating antibody

The ability to reject grafts cannot be transferred from one animal to another by means of passively injected antibody. This does not rule out the possibility that antibody can play a part in graft rejection, because when the serum, containing at best about 1% specific antibody, is injected into a recipient the diluting effect of the blood and tissue fluids considerably reduces the possibility of the antibody reaching the graft site in an adequate concentration to influence the viability of the graft. The same antibody-containing serum can readily be shown in vitro to be cytotoxic, in the presence of complement, for cells containing antigens to which the antibody was produced. However, this is an artificial situation and does not take into account the dilution effects discussed above. Kidney grafts which have survived for some time, perhaps months or years, can, it seems, be rejected by serum antibody alone without any evidence of invasion of the graft by lymphoid cells. Deposits of immunoglobulin and complement can be detected particularly in the walls of blood vessels. Although at this stage no antibodies may be detected in the serum, if the rejected kidney is removed they soon appear, suggesting that the antibodies were rapidly removed by combination with kidney antigens. The kidney is rejected by the development of a progressive vasculitis affecting glomerular and other vessels. Attempts have been made to recover antibody by elution from rejected kidneys removed from 27 patients. Seven of the kidneys contained recoverable antibody and this often differed from that found in the patient's serum, supporting the view that grafted incompatible kidneys filter out antibody from the circulation.

Locally produced antibody and non-antibody lymphocyte factors

The possibility is quite strong that antibody made locally in a graft by the infiltrating lymphoid cells is present in a sufficiently high concentration in the area immediately surrounding the antibody-producing cell to damage incompatible cells of the graft. This situation can be compared to the observation made in vitro with the Jerne plaque technique (p. 87) in which lymphocytes can be shown to be producing antibody to sheep red blood cells which produces a surrounding halo of lysis of the red cells in the presence of complement. Indeed, lymphocytes and plasma cells invading grafts can be shown to contain immunoglobulin. Evidence that immunoglobulin is combining with antigen during graft rejection is provided by a detectable fall in the serum complement level.

There are a number of other possible direct ways in which the infiltrating lymphocytes can influence survival of the graft: (a) the antibody which they produce may activate the various pharmacological mediators of immediate hypersensitivity reactions such as histamine (p. 225) and these will bring about changes in the vessels of the graft: (b) the lymphocytes on contact with antigen may release macrophage migration inhibition factor (MIF)

(p. 110) that will cause accumulation of macrophages in the graft; (c) it is known that sensitised lymphocytes can influence non-immune lymphocytes to behave aggressively towards cells in their vicinity and induce cytoxic effects.

Experimental evidence has shown that only a low percentage of the lymphocytes infiltrating a graft are specifically reactive to graft alloantigens. Lymphokines secreted by helper T lymphocytes may be responsible for the migration and proliferation of the majority of the infiltrating inflammatory cells. Graft rejection can be inhibited by in vivo administration of antisera against lymphokines. Adoptive transfer experiments in T lymphocyte-depleted mice indicate that Ly-1 helper T cells are critical to skin-graft rejection in mice. Furthermore, injections of interleukin 2 (a helper T cell product, p. 110) can greatly enhance heart graft rejection in rats.

Other cell types may influence graft rejection and it has been found that monocytes and macrophages accumulate in large numbers early in human renal graft rejection.

It can thus be seen that the reaction against a graft depends upon a complex series of interrelated phenomena, some of which are specifically induced by the foreign nature of graft antigens. Other phenomena are non-specific in the immunological sense and occur as part of an inflammatory process.

Table 7.2 Summary of immune response to incompatible grafts

A. Host factors
Foreign class 1 MHC antigens on grafted cells trigger Th cells.
Th cells induce Tc and Tdth cells
Tc cells recognize and react against graft class 1 MHC antigens
Tdth cells release lymphokines that amplify response (e.g. macrophage infiltration of graft)
Cytotoxic antibodies attack graft, particularly in ABO mismatch (A_1 and B) or class 1 MHC antigen mismatch
Previous donor sensitization by multiple transfusions or grafts results in secondary immune response to graft antigens

B. Graft factors
Class 2 MHC antigens on passenger leucocytes or dendritic cells allow antigen presentation to recipient Th cells and induce immune response to graft
(allogeneic MHC antigens are highly immunogenic and can stimulate recipient Th cells without MHC restriction)
The most immunogenic tissues are those containing dendritic cells or Langerhans cells, e.g. bone marrow and skin

---

Many minor histocompatibility (mH) antigens exist, largely ill defined and difficult to detect. Best known are H-Y antigens of male mice. They induce an MHC restricted T cell response and can induce acute or chronic transplant rejection.

Immunosuppression

Graft rejection, as has been noted, involves a sequence of separate phenomena developing from initial contact of the foreign antigens with the host immunological system through to rejection itself. The steps include establishment of lymphatic drainage, antigen release, its contact with cells of the immune system, proliferation of anti-body-forming cells of the lymphoid tissues, the inflammatory response and release of pharmacological mediators and cytotoxic effects of lymphoid cells and/or antibody on the graft tissues.

Prevention of sensitization; tolerance to graft antigens

Interference with any of these stages would be likely to interfere with the rejection process. One of the most interesting approaches, which is as yet unfortunately only at the experimental stage, is interference with what might be termed the afferent arc of the process of rejection, namely the initial sensitization of the lymphoid cells. If it were possible to induce immune tolerance (p. 83) to the strong histocompatibility antigens of tissue grafts, then immunological rejection would not take place. The tolerant animal, although unable to react against the antigen to which it is tolerant, can still respond to other antigens such as potentially infective agents like bacteria, fungi or viruses; this obviates one of the greatest difficulties associated with immunosuppressive procedures.

As has been noted earlier, Mitchison (using serum protein antigens) has shown that there are two types of tolerance, so-called 'high dose' tolerance where the immune system is overloaded with excess antigen, and 'low dose' tolerance where only minute quantities of antigen are administered. Although the molecular processes underlying these phenomena are not as yet understood, the 'low dose' tolerance phenomena has great potential application to transplantation problems. When it becomes possible to extract purified transplantation antigens from tissue, it should then be possible to prepare an individual for graft acceptance by inducing low dose tolerance to the appropriate antigens.

Some progress has been made recently in the induction of specific tolerance against transplantation antigens in rats by eliminating the T lymphocytes which normally respond to graft antigens. It has been done by preparing antibodies against the T cell receptors for the major histocompatibility antigens. This is achieved by mating two inbred strains of rat; the hybrids would express the histocompatibility antigens of each parent and thus be tolerant to them. The implication is that the T cells would not express receptors for the antigens whilst each of the parents would express receptors for the histocompatibility antigens of the other strain. Thus by injecting the hybrid rats with lymphocytes from a parent the hybrids would not react to the histocompatibility antigen but would react to the receptors for the antigen on the parental cells.

T lymphocytes shed their receptors and it is therefore possible to extract these for the major histocompatibility antigen by binding them to the antibody (attached to an inert particle). The purified T cell receptors are then chemically modified by cross linking with gluteraldehyde (to make them immunogenic). When these are injected into an inbred strain of rats (Lewis) with adjuvant, they are able to slow down the rejection of grafts from another inbred strain (DA). The eventual rejection of the graft in 24 days (compared to 11 days in untreated rats) is probably due to minor histocompatibility differences. The prolongation of graft survival is likely to be due to suppression or elimination of lymphocytes bearing the receptor for the major histocompatibility antigen by the antibodies induced by the chemically modified purified receptor. Another approach that involves T cell receptors is the induction of tolerance by means of anti-idiotypic antibodies against the receptor so that recognition of graft MHC antigens is blocked.

Another approach at inducing transplantation tolerance is the repeated injection of massive doses of serum into neonatal rats. The serum contains small amounts of histocompatibility antigen and this is sufficient in neonatal rats to induce a lasting tolerance to certain skin grafts showing strong histocompatibility differences between donor and recipient. The practical value of this approach is clearly limited by the requirement that tolerance be induced in neonatal animals. Recipients of grafts who have received previous blood transfusions have shown improved graft survival. The mechanism is not understood, but the most significant improvement occurs when the donors and recipients are well matched for MHC antigens.

Another approach that may have important implications for transplantation, so far limited to studies in adult mice, indicates that it is possible to induce tolerance to an antigen without permanently suppressing the total ability of the immune system. This is done by injecting the mice with a monoclonal antibody directed at the T helper cells (anti-T3T4) at the same time as an antigen is injected. After a short period of almost complete immunosuppression the T cell population recovers and the animal is found to be tolerant to both the anti-T3T4 and the antigen that was injected along with it. If this technique can be extended to humans it could provide a way of inducing transplantation tolerance without the loss of other immune functions.

Immunological enhancement

Another phenomenon relevant to the maintenance of incompatible grafts is 'immunological enhancement'. This is brought about by antibody produced against graft antigens that can under certain circumstances protect the graft from attack by cells of the immune system. This system has been used successfully in rats with incompatible kidney grafts, the animals being previously immunized with tissue from the prospective donor. The grafts exhibit normal renal function for a year or more afterwards. The method has been applied in a few instances to human kidney grafts and the results suggest that the method may be of considerable future value. The mechanism may involve coating of the cells of the graft by non-complement-fixing antibody and/or direct inhibition of antibody production by removal of T helper cells coated by immune complexes of antibody and graft antigen. Another suggestion is that enhancing antibody binds to passenger leucocytes in the graft that express alloantigens so that they are removed and fail to stimulate a response against the alloantigens. The danger of the antibody damaging the graft will require the use of antisera (directed against the histocompatibility antigens) that has been treated so as to eliminate any cytotoxic effects. This could be achieved by making use of antibody fragments (Fab) that do not bind complement (p. 94).

Practical approaches

In practice there are at the moment three main approaches to the problem of immunosuppression: (1) X-irradiation to knock out the lymphoid tissues and abolish the immune response; (2) immunosuppressive drugs — antimetabolites and anti-inflammatory agents to prevent proliferation of antibody-forming cells; (3) immunological methods — antilymphocyte serum (ALS) produced, for example, in the horse, to attack the lymphocytes directly and destroy them before they attack the graft.

Whole body X-irradiation used in the early days of organ transplantation has been replaced in the main by immunosuppressive drugs and ALS. Some attention has been given to reducing the lymphocyte count in the peripheral blood by passing it through an extracorporeal shunt and irradiating it outside the body. This method, although tried so far only on a small scale and with a limited degree of success, may be of value in the future. The drugs prednisone and Imuran (azathioprine) in combination are widely used and for immunosuppression are often given together with ALS. These substances in high dosage are toxic but haemodialysis before operation and during rejection crises reduces their toxicity in renal transplant cases. Their effects on dividing cells in other tissues, such as the gut epithelium, are an additional complication. Cyclosporin A, a cyclic undecapeptide from *Trichoderma polysporum*, is now widely used; the drug acts predominantly on the earlier stages of T cell activation. It may not, however, be without toxic effects. Cyclosporin A inhibits the production of interleukin-2 by T cells in vitro but in vivo appears to have a variety of inhibitory effects on cytokine production whilst failing to inhibit T cell proliferation or cytotoxic lymphocyte activity. Thus whilst able to inhibit primary responses to T dependent antigens it fails to prevent secondary responses due to the emergence of drug-resistant memory cells. The drug has also the capacity to cause immune enhancement and exacerbation of experimental autoimmunity.

Any of these regimes clearly carries with it the considerable risk of infection and the commonest cause of death after kidney grafting is not graft rejection but infection with fungi, viruses and bacteria. Another apparent complication noted in the last few years is the small but significant increase in reticulosarcomata following prolonged immunosuppressive therapy. This could conceivably be due to inhibition of the immunological surveillance mechanism (Ch. 8).

Antilymphocyte serum has the advantage of primarily affecting the thymus-dependent lymphocytes of the spleen and lymph nodes, and lymphocytes circulating in the blood. This results in a suppression of the cell-mediated immune response with only a slight effect on the circulating antibody response. Thus, whilst suppressing the graft rejection mechanisms ALS leaves the animal able to produce circulating antibody against infecting microorganisms and their products. However, infections caused by intracellular agents such as viruses in which protection depends on cell-mediated immunity (p. 147) still remain a possible complication in this form of immunosuppression and different preparations of ALS may vary in their effect on the antibody response. Furthermore, ALS can destroy platelets because of shared platelet and leucocyte antigen and may require prior absorption with platelet suspensions. Anaphylactic reactions may occur because of the foreign nature of the protein and severe pain frequently occurs at the injection site.

Trials with monoclonal antibodies to lymphocyte antigens are underway in patients undergoing renal graft rejection. If these continue to prove successful then more specific monoclonal reagents directed at specific T cell subpopulations or to idiotypic determinants on the T cell receptor, may prove to be more useful.

FURTHER READING

Bagshawe K D 1972 Immunosuppression. British Journal of Hospital Medicine 8:677

Baldwin W H 1981 Do cytotoxic T lymphocytes cause transplant rejection? Immunology Today 2:210

Berenabum M C 1967 Transplantation and immunosuppression. In: Cruickshank R, Weir D M (eds) Modern trends in immunology. Butterworth, London, vol 2, p. 292

Carpenter C B 1981 Immunology Today 2:50

James K 1967 Anti-lymphocyte antibody: a review. Clinical and Experimental Immunology 2:615

Merrill J P 1967 Human tissue transplantation. Advances in Immunology 2:615

Perkins H A 1976 Transplantation immunology. In: Fudenberg H H, Stites D P, Caldwell J L, Wells J V (eds) Basic and clinical immunology. Lange, Los Altos

Porter K A 1967 Symposium on tissue and organ transplantation. Journal of Clinical Pathology (supplement) 20:415

Rapaport F T, Dausset J 1968 Human transplantation. Grune and Stratton, New York

8

Malignant disease

Objectives

On completion of this section the reader will be able to:
1. Give two examples implicating deficiency of the immune mechanisms in the development of tumours.
2. Define 'immune surveillance'.
3. Give two examples of the two types of antigenic change found in tumours.
4. Give two examples of agents used in tumour immunotherapy, their mode of action and their possible value.
5. Describe what contribution alpha interferon is likely to make to tumour immunotherapy.
6. Define non-specific tumour immunotherapy.
7. Give two examples of how tumours escape from attack by the immune system.
8. Outline the role of oncogenes in tumorogenesis.

In discussing the general biological significance of immune reactions in maintaining the integrity of the cellular systems of the body, Burnet points out that in man, in whom more than 10^{14} cells are constantly reproducing, there is sufficient evidence to make it likely that at any given genetic locus an error occurs with a frequency in the range of 10^{-5} to 10^{-7} per replication. This means that in the cell population there must be many millions of errors or mutations occurring every day of life. It seems inconceivable that complex and long-lived multicellular animals could have evolved unless some means of dealing with this eventuality had been developed. Recently, however, doubt has been expressed on this view and it has been suggested that 'this daily development of malignant cells is not supported by the experimental evidence, and that spontaneous malignant transformation in vitro appears to be dependent more on cell-to-cell interactions than to be an intrinsic property of single cells.'

The role of immunological mechanisms in the suppression of malignant cells has been appreciated since the work of Paul Ehrlich at the beginning of the century, but it is only in the last 10 years or so that immunologists have begun to unravel the details of the immunological processes underlying the control of tumours, the antigenic changes in tumour cells themselves, and the extent and activities of the immune response arising as a result of these changes.

EVIDENCE FOR THE ROLE OF IMMUNE MECHANISMS

Mention is made in Chapter 5 of the increased incidence in thymectomized mice of tumours induced by chemical carcinogens and viruses. This seems likely to be due to a deficiency of the cell-mediated immune mechanisms which are under the control of the thymus (p. 53). Thus neonatally **thymectomized** animals are unable to reject incompatible tissue grafts and do not give delayed hypersensitivity reactions of the tuberculin type. These activities depend on intact cell-mediated, thymus-dependent immune reactivity and it is the absence of this reactivity which allows tumour cells to grow unhindered.

The experimental evidence in support of this view is conflicting. Thymectomy of mice does appear to increase the incidence of skin tumours to certain chemical carcinogens (polycyclic hydrocarbons) and of tumours induced by DNA viruses. However, early thymectomy seems to have no significant effect on development of spontaneous tumours in mice and there are reports of a decreased incidence of tumours, such as mouse mammary carcinoma, following thymectomy. It thus appears that the effects of thymectomy are variable and depend to some extent on other factors, such as the agent responsible for tumour development.

Another example where deficiency of the cell-mediated immune mechanisms is associated with tumour formation is in a condition known as **graft-versus-host** disease. This condition is produced in mice by injecting spleen cells into an unrelated recipient, the reaction of the spleen cells against the host resulting in destruction of its lymphoid tissues. This can be demonstrated by using two inbred strains of mice, e.g. CBA and C57 Black, and injecting the spleen cells of one of the parents into the offspring of such a mating. CBA cells injected into a CBA/C57B recipient will recognize the C57B component of the host-lymphoid cells as foreign but will not be themselves rejected because the recipient itself carries the CBA antigens.

The destruction of the recipient's lymphoid tissues, and thus its cell-mediated immune response, produces a defect in the control of neoplastic cell proliferation. These mice frequently develop tumours of the lymphoid tissues having many of the features of Hodgkin's disease of the human.

A herpes virus (Epstein-Barr) has been isolated from the human lymphoid tumour known as **Burkitt's lymphoma** and it has been proposed that the tumour is of virus origin. Recent evidence in patients with Burkitt's lymphoma has added considerable support to the significance of cell-mediated immunes mechanisms in the control of the tumour. Only 1 of 12 patients on skin testing with extracts of their own tumour cells had positive delayed hypersensitivity reactions. However, when the tumour growth was suppressed with cyclophosphamide, skin tests became positive in seven of the twelve indicating a recovery of the cell-mediated immune mechanisms which is associated with remission of the tumour.

Serological studies have demonstrated a strong association between the presence of high titres of antibody to EB virus in both Burkitt's lymphoma and postnasal carcinoma. However, antibody to the virus is widespread throughout the world and association can be found with a number of diverse disease states. The virus can be found not only in leucocytes of patients with Burkitt's lymphoma but also in leucocytes of patients with infectious mononucleosis and even in some normal individuals. The virus appears to be able in vitro to **transform** leucocytes into virus-containing cells capable of continuous growth. The virus appears to have a predilection for cells of the lymphoid organs and it cannot yet be excluded that the virus is a 'passenger' trapped within lymphoid cells present in the tumour rather than the prime cause of the tumour. Recent evidence suggests the possibility that the herpes viruses may act indirectly on cells by activating a latent RNA tumour virus. Ultraviolet light irradiated herpes simplex virus, whilst unable to destroy mouse cells, resulted in the activation of an endogenous virus similar to the RNA tumour viruses.

There is as yet no firm evidence that tumours in humans are caused by viruses. The possible involvement of a transmissible viral agent in human sarcomas has been proposed in the last few years. A common surface antigen has been found on sarcoma cells derived from bone, cartilage, fat and muscle and induces a detectable antibody response in patients' serum. This antigen can be transferred to normal human fibroblasts by exposing them to the filtered culture medium from sarcoma cells. That the antigen is transmittable to other individuals is suggested by the finding that cohabitants of sarcoma patients have the anti-sarcoma antibody in their serum.

Retroviruses, oncogenes and tumours

The Rous sarcoma virus (RSV) that induces sarcomas in chickens was the first of the retroviruses to be implicated with tumour formation. It consists of two genetic subunits, one being required for viral replication in the host cell and the other determining its capacity to induce sarcomas. This latter subunit is termed an oncogene — in this case src — and is not required for normal viral growth. Using radioactive DNA probes synthesized from RSV using reverse transcriptase, the src oncogene could be demonstrated in normal chicken cells. Since then oncologists have shown that the src oncogene is present in a wide variety of species. The gene appears to be a normal cellular gene that was in some way picked up by the virus. Its finding has led to the identification of some 20 retroviral oncogenes that can be subdivided into families that share sequences. The way the cellular oncogene is activated so that a virus-infected cell becomes transformed to a tumour cell appears to be by the insertion of proviral DNA that carry sequences that function as control centres for gene expression. The sequences activate the oncogene and lead to overproduction of its protein product and transformation of the cell. Several of the proteins encoded by oncogenes are likely to be abnormal versions of cell surface receptors for growth factors and at least one encodes a portion of a growth factor itself. Several of the proteins are found on the inner surface of the plasma membrane so that they may serve to transduce signals received from growth factors acting outside the cell. Such activation phenomena are likely to happen only rarely in virus infected cells, as viral DNA seems to enter the chromosome of the host cell in a random way. It appears that every human cell contains sets of genes (at least 20 and less than 100) that may become oncogenes when incorporated into retroviruses.

These findings emphasize the need for an understanding of growth factors and their controlling mechanisms so that tumour cell formation can be elucidated. The experimental systems are unfortunately very complex and are ill-understood. Growth factors for various cell types, for example T cell growth factor — interleukin-2 (p. 110), colony stimulating factors and epidermal growth factor have the common features of stimulating DNA synthesis in their target cells. It is significant that transforming retroviruses can substitute for growth factors that are normally essential for maintenance of cell lines in culture. The M-CSF receptor may be identical or closely related to the c-fms proto oncogene.

One of the cellular oncogenes c-myc is joined directly to immunoglobulin genes during chromosomal translocation in B cell tumours and activation of both T lymphocytes and fibroblast proliferation is associated with increased production of c-myc. This area of research is clearly crucial to the detailed understanding of transformation of cells to tumours.

Further understanding of the role of retroviruses in transformation of cells has been achieved by the recent discovery of a gene in one of the retroviruses HTLV-1 (the transacting or tat gene) acting at a distance which appears to be responsible for inducing T lymphocytes to produce both 1L-2 and 1L-2 receptors thus inducing abnormal growth. The HTLV 1 virus has been associated with a form of adult T cell leukaemia found mainly but not exclusively in south western islands of Japan and in the Caribbean basin. The origin of the virus is believed to be Africa where a closely related virus has been found in certain species of monkeys. Spread of the virus to other parts of the world may have been due to trading activities. The lymphocytes from patients with adult T cell leukaemia can be shown in the laboratory to transform T cells from normal infants into cells showing immortal precancerous characteristics and the virus itself can transform T4 cells in culture over a period of five and seven weeks. Such transformed cells when put into hamsters cause malignant tumours. Disease caused by the HTLV-1 virus is rare except in the endemic areas although it is suggested that the virus may be spreading in populations who are at increased risk of infection such as intravenous drug users. The HTLV-2 virus is associated with a less aggressive form of leukaemia known as hairy-cell leukaemia and, like the HTLV-1 virus, can transform cells in culture and shares the same transacting mechanism having been shown to contain a tat gene (tat 2).

In summary, the leukaemia causing retroviruses can be divided into three groups according to their genetic structure and pathogenic mechanism. The chronic leukaemia viruses, such as the mouse leukaemia viruses, contain only the basic viral genome coding for core proteins, reverse transcriptase and the envelope proteins. The acute leukaemia or sarcoma viruses, have another DNA sequence known as the onc gene that regulates cell growth.

The third group, including the HTLV-1 and 2 viruses, contain the tat genes with their ability to induce 1L-2 production in lymphocytes as described above.

Immunity to tumours

Carcinomas of the gastrointestinal tract can be shown to contain an antigen absent from normal adult gut cells but present in those of embryos. The antigen termed **carcinoembryonic antigen** (CEA) has been found in the blood of patients with such tumours and their lymphocytes appear to be able to act in vitro against their cultured tumour cells in contrast to control lymphocytes that have no effect.

A somewhat disturbing result of the use of antilymphocytic serum (ALS) in man for immunosuppression in tissue transplantation (p. 204) is the small but significantly increased incidence of tumours in such individuals; it seems probable that this is due to suppression of immunological surveillance mechanisms. It is also interesting to note that various chemical immunosuppressive drugs and X-rays, acting like ALS on the lymphoid tissues, are in many instances carcinogens as well as immunosuppressive agents. In recent experiments performed to test the effects of immunosuppression by ALS on tumour incidence, once again the results have not been clear-cut. As in the situation with thymectomized mice, local tumour incidence following chemical carcinogens was increased after ALS treatment. In studies of the development of spontaneous leukaemias in ALS treated mice, there are reports of both increased and decreased tumour incidence and the problem so far remains unresolved.

The incidence of cancer in man is highest at the two extremes of life and it is just at these times that the immune system is least efficient. All these observations point to the probable important role played by the intact mechanisms in keeping the body free of undesirable mutant neoplastic cells.

There is considerable discussion amongst immunologists concerning the particular cells of the immune system that may be responsible for 'surveillance' mechanisms to deal with neoplastic cells or host cells altered in other ways. The emphasis has shifted from a central role for the thymus-dependent (T) lymphocyte (partly because of the conflicting experimental evidence discussed above) to a role for the **macrophage** which can readily be shown in vitro to have cytotoxic effects against tumour cells (see Fig. 5.9). Tumours are often heavily infiltrated with macrophages, and transfer of such cells in an activated state to mice with experimental tumours has been shown to lead to tumour suppression. Macrophages undoubtedly have the ability to recognize and bind to their surface (with and without antibody) various foreign materials such as bacteria and altered cells (e.g. red cells), and it is not unreasonable to suppose that this ability might extend to recognition of neoplastic cells.

A view has recently been expressed by some tumour immunologists that offers an alternative approach to the idea of immune surveillance. This is based on a failure of growth and differentiation control rather than escape from immune surveillance. The regulatory mechanisms that determine the self-renewing proliferative capacity of cell populations and their differentiation to mature cells are not fully understood. Knowledge gained from studies on T lymphocyte products indicates that some of them affect a wide range of lymphoid and haemopoietic cells. There is growing evidence that there is reciprocal communication between the immune system and several other cell systems (e.g. the neuroendocrine system, p. 10). Disturbance (destabilization) in these regulatory systems could conceivably disturb normal homeostasis so that the self-renewing proliferative capacity of a particular cell type becomes predominant and differentiation to the mature form is depressed. The consequences of such a series of events could thus lead to uncontrolled proliferation — tumour growth.

TUMOUR ANTIGENS

It can be deduced from the foregoing discussion that for the immunological system to react against tumour cells, these cells must be changed in some way so that they are no longer recognized as self. That this is indeed so is substantiated by many examples of tumours which have been found to develop **new antigens** as part of their cell structure. There are two types of antigenic change: (1) where the specificity of the new antigen is dependent on the inducing agent such as a virus, and (2) tumours induced by chemical carcinogens in which the antigenic change induced by the same carcinogen in two different animals is different in each case. The carcinogen methylcholanthrene has been reported to induce different antigenic changes in cells even in the same animal if the chemical is applied to two separate areas.

There are numerous examples of tumour formation which seem to be associated with these changes. The SV_{40} virus induces tumours in monkeys, the Rous sarcoma virus in chickens and the polyoma virus in mice. The tumours induced in mice by the polyoma virus have recently been shown to consist of two sorts of cells, cells that are malignant on introduction into another mouse and cells that do not survive transplantation. It seems possible that the latter cells are destroyed by the immune system because they carry recognizable foreign antigens on their surface. When cells of the non-transplantable variety are cultured in vitro variants appear which have lost their antigenicity and can thus transfer the tumour. This raises the possibility that attempts to eliminate malignant cells by increasing the immune reaction against them may result in the 'selection' of 'non-antigenic' variants which would allow the tumour to spread.

The tumour-specific antigens are comparable to the weak histo-compatibility antigens (p. 195) and their strength has been found to vary for different aetiological groups. Methylcholanthrene-induced sarcomas in mice have been found to be more strongly antigenic than similar sarcomas induced by dibenzanthracene. Among the virus tumours, Moloney virus-induced lymphomas of the mouse are quite strongly antigenic, whereas the gross agent induces a similar tumour with very weak tumour-specific antigens. Consistent with the finding that the specificity of tumour antigens varies even with one chemical carcinogen is the finding that the strength of these antigens varies also.

Having established that antigenic changes occur in neoplastic cells and that immunological processes are apparently involved in the body's reaction to tumours, the question is, how in fact does any tumour grow and spread throughout the body in the face of the body's immune reaction? Some of the factors which tip the balance in favour of tumour growth have already been discussed in relation to central defects of the immune response.

Another important factor is that the tumour-specific antigens are often not strongly antigenic and the degree of immunity developed is insufficient to cause the rejection of a rapidly growing tumour. In experiments in mice with primary tumours induced by chemical carcinogens, it has been shown that if a mouse is pre-immunized with tumour cells (inactivated by X-irradiation) the animal can then develop a state of immunity to transfer of living tumour cells, provided that the number of transferred cells is not too large to overcome the induced immunity.

The abnormal social behaviour of tumour cells is well known in that they generally fail to form stable intercellular adhesions. It would not be suprising if the interaction between tumour cells and cells of the lymphoid system would likewise be abnormal, leading to escape of the tumour cell from the potentially cytotoxic effects of lymphocytes.

Another way in which tumours could escape the attention of lymphocytes sensitized to the tumour antigens is by the **shedding** from the tumour of excess antigen. Such antigen present in the serum of patients with malignant disease is believed to account for the inhibitory effect of such serum on lymphocyte cytotoxicity for the tumour. Free tumour antigen or antigen-antibody complexes could conceivably 'blindfold' sensitized lymphocytes thus preventing them from identifying and attaching to tumour cells themselves.

Experiments in vitro have shown that complexes of tumour antigen and antibody can interfere with the potentially cytotoxic effects of lymphocytes, presumably by preventing access of the lymphocytes to the tumour cell surface. In a similar way, free tumour antigen can absorb onto the surface of a cytotoxic lymphocyte and be shown to prevent its attaching to the membrane of a tumour cell. The phenomenon in which factors present in the serum block immunes reactions against tumours is known as 'enhancement'. Enhancement does seem to be associated with large progressive tumours. It disappears when the tumour is removed and reappears on recurrence.

Antibody interacting with the surface antigens of tumour cells can induce modulation of expression of the antigen. This leads to shedding of the antigen and redistribution of the antigen in the tumour cell membrane so that it is not available to interact with antibody. Tumour antigens that are carried to a local lymph node may be present in sufficiently large amounts to induce tolerance and also to trap sensitized lymphocytes within the infiltrated node.

The possibility arises that tumour products other than antigens could interfere with immunity, for example prostaglandins are known to reduce the expression of class 2 MHC antigens on inducer cells and can also suppress NK cell activity.

Tumours that are potentially immunogenic can develop in the presence of an intact immune system. This has been ascribed to induction of low-zone tolerance (p. 76) by repeated stimulation of small amounts of antigen. This has been termed 'sneaking through' in which the immune system adapts through a process of selection to tumour growth.

In the last few years attention has been directed at the role of T lymphocyte subpopulations (including helper and suppressor cells, p. 54) in the generation of specific cytotoxic cells and antibodies against tumours. The development of suppressor T lymphocytes can be shown in mice when the tumour burden becomes great. Suppression of immune responses in both mice and humans has also been attributed to the activities of B lymphocytes and macrophages.

The immune response against tumour antigens is thus likely to be modified in a variety of ways with consequences that are very difficult to predict. It is likely that a precise understanding of the role of the immune system in tumour immunity will only be gained when the local response at the site of the tumour is analysed. Thus, for example, in the estimation of the role of suppressor T cells, it may be necessary to take into account only those cells in the local tumour environment.

Table 8.1 Summary of immunity to tumour cells

Natural immunity	Natural killer cells, neutrophil polymorphs, activated macrophages
Acquired immunity Positive effects	Natural killer cells amplified by gamma interferon from T cells activated by tumour antigen
	Macrophages acted on by lymphokines MIF, MAF and chemotactic factor from T cells activated by tumour antigen
	Macrophages and K cells that recognize antibody on tumour cells by their Fc receptors (ADCC)
	Complement components produced in inflammatory response that are chemotactic for neutrophils and cause enzyme release from macrophages
Negative effects	PGE 2 from macrophages and tumour cells suppress NK cell activity

Cytolysins for tumour cells include: natural killer cell cytotoxic factor, perforins, cytolysins, lymphotoxins and tumour necrosis factor. Their mechanisms of action are not understood; perforin in mice, which shows a 27% amino acid homology with C9, has a similar molecular mass and shares antigenic determinants.

IMPLICATIONS IN CANCER THERAPY

The classical treatment for carcinoma of the breast and many other tumours is the radical surgical removal of the neoplastic tissue and much of the surrounding tissue, including the lymph glands of the area.

It is now recognized that this treatment sometimes enhances the spread of secondary deposits, and it is thought that this might be due to removal of lymphoid tissues involved in the immune response to the antigens of the tumour, and possibly also to diminution in the antigenic stimulus to the immune system. The balance is thus tipped in favour of remaining tumour cells which can proliferate unchecked. In addition it should be remembered that mammary carcinogenesis almost certainly also involves the interplay of a variety of non-immunological factors — hormonal, genetic and possibly viral.

Non-specific immunotherapy

Active immunotherapy

Immunization against tumour antigens. As noted above tumour cells are often not very powerful antigens and, even when antigens are present on the tumour cells surface, various escape mechanisms are available to ensure tumour survival. A number of ways are available to enhance tumour immunogenicity, for example myxovirus infected tumour cells have been shown to be more effective immunogens than uninfected cells. The binding of PPD to the tumour cell surface is another approach that has been used to increase immunogenicity and may explain the value of BCG treatment (see below). It is theoretically possible that if T cell clones could be produce in vitro with either helper or cytotoxic activity against tumour cell antigens they may be useful in immunotherapy.

Passive immunotherapy

The most hopeful approach in this form of therapy is the use of tumour specific monoclonal antibodies linked either to toxins such as diptheria toxin or ricin or to agents that suppress cell proliferation such as ^{131}I or cytotoxic drugs. Another possibility with promising preliminary results is the use of anti-idiotypic monoclonal antibodies against B cell lymphomas — the immunoglobulin expressed on the lymphoma being the target.

Agents known to stimulate the cells of the lymphoid tissues in a non-specific manner have come into vogue in the last few years as a form of cancer immunotherapy. This interest derives from the work in France of Mathé who has employed BCG (p. 172) treatment as part of the therapy of acute lymphoblastic leukaemia in children. The length of the remissions in such cases appeared to be prolonged. The possible value of **non-specific stimulation** of the immune system is pointed to by some recent work with such an agent, *Corynebacterium parvum*. Mice injected with *C. parvum* and given vigorous antitumour chemotherapy showed complete remission in up to 70% of mice with a chemically induced sarcoma. The effect was found only when the two treatments were combined. Other experiments in mice showed that BCG was most effective if given a week or more before the injection of tumour cells. This indicated that the treatment is not likely to be effective in the presence of an established tumour unless some steps are taken to reduce the tumour mass by drug or X-ray therapy.

In tumours of mice associated with vertically transmitted viruses such as the Gross virus, there is no evidence of a specific immune response to virus or tumour and it is assumed that the presence of the virus from the early development of the animal leads to immunological tolerance to the virus. Search for a similar situation in human tumours has not been fruitful and histological examination of tumours and associated lymph nodes all point to absence of tolerance.

Non-specific immunodeficiency is often found associated with rapidly growing tumours in humans but it is not clear if this is cause or effect. It appears that patients with early tumours do not usually show lack of immunological competence and that this only appears after fairly extensive tumour growth. This is believed to be due to the appearance of suppressor T lymphocytes and is interpreted to be a consequence of tumour growth rather than a failure of the initial immune surveillance mechanism.

Corynebacterium parvum and BCG injected directly into mouse tumours can be shown dramatically to suppress tumour growth. The effect appears to be largely due to a cell-mediated immune response to the antigens of the microorganisms, in which lymphoid cells are attracted to the injection site in large numbers and appear to act not only on the bacterial antigens but also on the surrounding tumour cells.

Another effect of these organisms is to 'activate' the macrophages of the injected animal in such a way that they can be shown in vitro to become cytotoxic for cultured tumour cells. It is difficult to be sure that this effect operates in vivo but it is possible, at least where tumour cells are circulating in the bloodstream or free in a body cavity, that activated macrophages could capture and destroy them.

Alpha interferon (see Table 4.9)

This interferon is now commercially available in both genetically engineered form and from lymphoblastoid cell lines and is licensed by the Committee on Safety of Medicines for the treatment of a rare form of leukaemia — hairy cell leukaemia. It is under trial for a variety of other tumours including leukaemias and lymphomas and preliminary evidence suggests that it may be valuable for the treatment of non-Hodgkin's lymphomas. It is also being injected into localized tumour sites such as the bladder and peritoneal cavity and it is hoped that trials may establish its value for the treatment of bladder and ovarian tumours. Alpha interferon is also under consideration for use in multiple myeloma and Kaposi's sarcoma. A form of alpha interferon prepared from human leucocytes is extensively used in Cuba for treatment of some viral diseases including dengue fever and for some forms of throat cancer.

The mechanism of action of alpha interferon is not yet established but it is known to exert effects on tumour growth as well as modulating the actions of cells of the immune system. The antiviral effect is believed to be due to interferon-induced changes in intracellular enzymes that block viral replication. In order to reduce the side effects of large doses of interferon, tests are being carried out using conjugates of interferon and monoclonal antibody targetted at colonic tumour cells. A similar procedure proved effective in vitro in preventing proliferation of Epstein Barr virus infected cells. Conjugation of interferon with a cytotoxic drug (cisplatinum) has been shown to be effective against cultured tumour cells from lung cancer.

Other forms of immunotherapy

Human and mouse lymphocytes cultured in the presence of interleukin-2 have been shown to develop cytotoxic activity against a large variety of tumour cells. A preliminary study in humans showed 50% reduction in tumour mass in 11 of 25 patients with various types of tumour. Another approach that has been proposed (based on experiments in mice) involves the injection of small amounts of IL-2 or gamma interferon that are likely to activate cytotoxic T cells and natural killer cells. The NK cell activity does not depend on the expression of antigens by tumour cells and the Tc cells should provide immunological memory to tumours that do express antigens.

In conclusion, it seems possible that immunotherapy may have an important role in the future treatment of malignant disease. It seems likely to be most effective when the tumour mass is small or can be reduced by chemotherapy. The spontaneous disappearance of tumours and complete recovery of patients with widespread cancer does, on rare occasions, happen and is usually explained as divine intervention. A more readily acceptable explanation of such phenomena is that for some other reason the balance between tumour growth and the immune reaction against it has been tipped in favour of the immune response.

The major difficulty confronting the oncologist in the use of immunotherapy is that there is at present such an incomplete understanding of the relationship of tumours with the immune system that it is not possible to make rational decisions on whether immunotherapy will be of value if any particular situation. Present efforts are initiated largely on an empirical basis that in theory might work but the background knowledge is inadequate to provide a proper scientific basis for treatment. In this situation available resources should clearly be allocated to this end and the attractive option of trying out yet another form of immunotheraphy should be resisted. The history of medical progress, however, is full of examples where empirical observations were found to have real therapeutic value. Nevertheless, it is probably true to say that in most instances they occurred before the recent enormous advances in scientific progress in the cell biological and molecular biological sciences, and that it is no longer justifiable to turn aside from a systematic scientific investigation of a disease state.

FURTHER READING

Bengesh-Melnick M, Batel J S 1974 In: Busch H (ed) The molecular biology of cancer. Academic Press, New York

Burnet F M 1962 The integrity of the body. Oxford University Press, London

Burnet F M 1970 Immunological surveillance. Pergamon Press, London

Chirigos M A 1977 Control of neoplasia by modulation of the immune system. Raven Press, New York

Currie G A 1975 Immunology of malignant disease. In: Bagshawe K D (ed) Medical oncology. Blackwell, Oxford

Currie G A 1980 Cancer and the immune response, 2nd edn. Edward Arnold, London

Fenner F 1968 The pathogenesis and ecology of viral infection. Academic Press, New York

Hamilton Fairley G 1971 Immunity to malignant disease in man. British Journal of Hospital Medicine 6:633

Heberman R B 1983 Basic and clinical tumour immunology. Martinus Nijhoff, Boston

Klein G 1985 Viruses as the causative agents of naturally occurring tumors. In: Advances in viral oncology, vol 5. Raven Press, . . .

Lachmann P J, Peters D K (eds) 1982 Clinical aspects of immunology, 4th edn. Blackwell, Oxford

Stutman O 1975 Immunodepression and malignancy. Advances in Cancer Research 22:261

9

Immunopathology

Objectives

On completion of this section the reader will be able to:
1. Distinguish between delayed and immediate type hypersensitivity reactions.
2. Describe anaphylactic (type 1) reactions and the pharmacological mediators involved.
3. Describe cytotoxic (type 2) reactions and antibody-dependent cell-mediated cytotoxicity.
4. Describe toxic complex (type 3) reactions and provide two examples.
5. Outline the lymphocyte-mediated delayed (type 4) reaction and list two common inducing agents.
6. Describe the role of the eosinophil in immunity.
7. Differentiate the two categories of immunodeficiency state.
8. Give three examples of phagocytic defects.
9. Give two examples of complement deficiencies and describe their consequences.
10. Give two examples of each of the following: primary immunodeficiency state and secondary immunodeficiency state. Describe laboratory procedures for diagnosis of each and available therapies.
11. Describe three possible pathogenic mechanisms that might result in autoimmune states.
12. Describe the genetic basis of susceptibility to autoimmune diseases.
13. Describe the possible role of T cell tolerance in the control of autoantibody producing B cells.
14. Provide an example of an autoimmune disease and describe laboratory tests used in its diagnosis.

In the earlier chapters of this section, the immune system has been considered in relation to its role in protection from infection or tumour development and in graft rejection or reaction to transfused blood cells. Such responses can be considered as advantageous to the host in terms of removal of foreign material. As has been noted in Chapter 5, protection is sometimes associated with disadvantageous consequences to the host, as is illustrated by the finding of immune complexes with their effects in the kidneys and elsewhere. In other situations the functioning of the immune system is affected by its exposure to infective agents and in rare instances by inherited defects. In Chapter 4 it was pointed out that in normal individuals self tolerance and the ability to discriminate between self and non-self was an essential feature in the development of the immune system. This ability of the cells of the immune system is not absolute and conditions (largely ill-defined) can arise where self-reactivity, or autoimmunity, occurs. In this chapter an outline is given of these disadvantageous immune responses under the three headings, hypersensitivity, immunodeficiency, and autoimmunity.

HYPERSENSITIVITY

Since immunity was first recognized as a resistant state that followed infection, immunology developed primarily as an aspect of medical bacteriology with emphasis on acquired specific resistance to invasion by microorganisms as a means of protection against infection. Much of the present terminology originates from this early period in the development of immunology. The term immunity, meaning safe or exempt, has now been extended far beyond its early meaning and includes reactions to foreign material such as grafted tissues, blood products and various bland chemical substances none of which bears any relation to infectious agents. Some forms of immune reaction, rather than providing exemption or safety to the affected individual, can produce severe and occasionally fatal results. These are known as 'hypersensitivity reactions' and in the main are due to tissue damage caused by effects of pharmacologically active agents such as histamine which are formed under certain conditions of antigen-antibody combination.

The term **allergy** was originally coined by von Pirquet early this century to describe the altered reactivity of an animal following exposure to a foreign antigen, and included both immunity and hypersensitivity. The term, however, has over the years become restricted to refer only to the hypersensitivity which may be associated with the development of the immune response to a foreign substance.

Immediate and delayed hypersensitivity

There are two main forms of hypersensitivity reaction: **immediate** and **delayed** (Fig. 9.1). The immediate or **antibody-mediated** form appears rapidly and depends on the production of pharmacologically active mediator substances activated by antigen-antibody interaction. The delayed or **cell-mediated** form appears more slowly (usually after 24 hours) and depends on immunologically activated lymphoid cells which, on reaction with antigen, appear to release substances known as lymphokines having a variety of effects on other cells and effects on blood vessel permeability (p. 110).

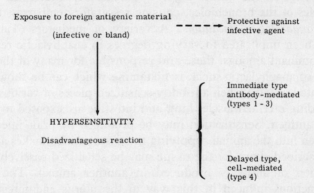

Fig. 9.1 Hypersensitivity reactions

Various classifications of hypersensitivity reactions have been proposed and probably the most widely accepted is that of Coombs and Gell. This recognizes four types or categories of hypersensitivity reactions, three of which come under the heading of immediate antibody-mediated reactions: type 1, anaphylactic reactions: type 2, cytolytic or cytotoxic reactions; and type 3, toxic-complex syndrome. The fourth type is the cell-mediated delayed hypersensitivity form of reaction.

Anaphylactic reactions of type 1

If a guinea-pig is injected with a small dose of an antigen such as egg albumen no adverse effects are noted. If however, a second injection of the egg albumen antigen is given intravenously after an interval of about 10 days a condition known as 'anaphylactic shock' is likely to develop. The animal becomes restless, starts chewing and rubbing its nose with its front paws, respiration becomes laboured, the animal becomes cyanosed and may develop convulsions and die. The initial injection of antigen is termed the **sensitizing dose** and the second injection the **shocking dose**. During the interval between the two injections the animal has formed antibody. Anaphylaxis is the result of interaction of the shocking dose of antigen with antibody which triggers the release of pharmacologically active substances causing increase in capillary permeability and contraction of smooth muscle in many parts of the body. In the guinea-pig this particularly affects the smooth muscles of the bronchioles, causing respiratory embarrassment.

Pharmacological mediators. A variety of mediators (Table 9.1) have been implicated to varying degrees in anaphylactic reactions: Predominant amongst these and responsible for many of the symptoms of anaphylactic shock is **histamine** which can be shown to be liberated in vitro when antibody-sensitized pieces of various tissues including uterine muscle, lung and intestine are exposed to contact with antigen. Sensitization may be produced by prior injection of antigen into the animal supplying the tissue, which makes antibody as described above, or the tissue may be sensitized passively by the addition of antibody produced in another animal. The typical contractions induced in this way in the uterus and intestine are called Schultze-Dale reactions after the originators. The histamine is derived from the granules of mast cells where it exists as its precursor histidine, in combination with heparin; these substances are released by the interaction of antigen with antibody on the surface of mast cells. A leucocyte derived group of substances, the **leukotrienes**, are important in allergy, and account for the activity of a mediator originally called slow-reacting substance of anaphylaxis, SRS-A.

The eosinophil is thought to play an important part in anaphylactic reactions, many of these marrow-derived cells being found in the blood and tissues during an anaphylactic reaction. Eosinophils are attracted to the site of the reaction by an **eosinophil chemotactic factor** that is released following the interaction of antibody

Table 9.1 Mediators from mast cells — triggered by cross-linking of IgE by antigen or anaphylatoxins (C3a or C5a)

Constitutive (preformed in granules)	
Histamine	Initial inflammatory response by increased capillary permeability and vasodilation
Heparin	Acts as anticoagulant
Eosinophil and neutrophil chemotactic factors	Chemotaxis of eosinophils and neutrophils
Platelet activating factor	Formation of microthrombi
Tryptase	Proteolysis
Induced (via arachidonic acid metabolic pathways)	
Leukotrines (LT) LTC4 and LTD4	Early inflammatory response by vasoactive bronchoconstrictive and chemotactic effects
Prostaglandins Thromboxanes	Late inflammatory response Bronchconstrictive and vasodilatory with oedema and mucous secretion

and antigen of the surface of a mast cell. As noted on page 67, eosinophils produce leucotriene C that increases capillary permeability and contracts smooth muscle as well as a factor acting on platelets (PAF). Their ability to kill parasites and tumour cells is probably their main function, with their role in anaphylaxis a disadvantageous side effect.

The other pharmacological mediators of immediate hypersensitivity reactions are: 5-hydroxy-tryptamine or serotonin which causes contraction of plain muscle and increased capillary permeability. It is of uncertain role in anaphylaxis, although it is probably involved in local intestinal food allergies; slow-reacting substance (or SRS-A) has a plain muscle contracting effect acting, unlike histamine, on the larger rather than smaller blood vessels. SRS-A has a particularly marked bronchial constricting effect in man and is probably the predominant pharmacological agent in human asthma. Bradykinins are simple peptides formed from a plasma α globulin (kininogen) by plasma kinin-forming enzymes. They have histamine-like effects on smooth muscle and capillaries, and studies have shown that it is present in the bloodstream in many species in the early stages of an anaphylactic reaction.

Systemic and local forms. In man there are two types of anaphylactic reaction — **systemic** and **local** — and which one of these develops depends on how the shocking dose of antigen enters the body. The systemic form of anaphylaxis is likely to develop if antigen is injected parenterally, as in the case of foreign serum (e.g. horse antitetanus serum), or a drug such as penicillin, or perhaps by the bite of an insect. The symptoms include dyspnoea with bronchospasm and laryngeal oedema, sometimes skin rashes, a fall in blood pressure and occasionally death. If, on the other hand, the antigen comes in contact with respiratory mucous membranes, then in a sensitized individual the local forms of anaphylaxis will develop, i.e. hay fever or asthma. If the intestinal mucous membrane of a susceptible individual comes in contact with the appropriate antigen (e.g. nuts, fish or strawberries), then a mixed form of reaction can develop with intestinal symptoms, skin rashes (urticaria) and sometimes the symptoms of asthma.

The antibodies involved in anaphylactic reactions

The role of IgE. In the human the antibodies which sensitize the tissues for anaphylactic reactions have been known for many years as **reaginic** antibodies. These antibodies have a strong affinity for tissues (cytotrophic) and can readily be detected in the serum of a sensitised individual by injecting a small quantity of the serum into the skin of a normal recipient, and 24 to 48 hours later, introducing the appropriate antigen into the injection site. Within about 20 minutes a weal and flare erythematous reaction develops at the injection site, just like the response to an injection of histamine. This reaction is called the P. K. test after its originators Prausnitz and Küstner.

The nature of reaginic antibody was not finally elucidated until late in 1967 when a hitherto undescribed form of myeloma protein was discovered in Sweden, although work in America suggested the existence of an immunoglobulin distinct from IgG, IgM or IgA. This made it possible (using an antiserum to the myeloma globulin prepared in a sheep) to show in normal human serum a new class of immunoglobulin present in very low concentration (10–130 μg/100 ml of serum, cf. 900–1800 mg of IgG/100 ml serum). The skin-sensitizing activity of reaginic antibody could readily be neutralized by means of the antiserum to this new immunoglobulin which has been named IgE (p. 103). The concentration of IgE in patients with allergic asthma has been found to be much higher than in normal individuals although the level of IgE in the circulation does not correlate with the severity of the allergic symptoms. The comparatively low levels of IgE found in serum presumably reflect the affinity of this immunoglobulin for tissues so that freshly made IgE is very soon removed from serum when it comes in contact with the appropriate cell receptors on mast cells and possibly elsewhere.

IgE appears to have four main activities: (1) the capacity to bind via its Fc fragment to mast cells and basophils; (2) subsequent interaction with antigen that takes place on the cell membrane of the mast cell; (3) resultant triggering of the release of pharmacological mediators; (4) attraction of other cell types — eosinophils. The third of these activities, namely the triggering of the release of pharmacological mediators from mast cells, has been the subject of much recent study and it appears that two adjacent molecules of IgE (attached to Fc receptors on mast cells) must be **bridged** by antigen before degranulation takes place. Monovalent antigens (i.e., with a single antigenic determinant) will block the IgE antibody from further interaction with antigen but will **not** trigger degranulation. The triggering appears to follow the entry of calcium ions into the mast cell, presumably as part of the membrane changes that finally lead to the degranulation or exocytosis process.

Genetic factors in allergy

The IgE levels of normal individuals are low (Table 4.7) and are controlled by a dominant gene. The higher the level the greater the chance of allergic predisposition. Ragweed allergy is closely associated with the DW2 locus of HLA. Immune hyperactivity (associated with HLA-B8 and DW3), particularly of IgE responses to a wide range of antigens, is a feature of allergic individuals. Other factors that are involved include the degree of exposure to allergens, the nutritional state of the individual and the presence of chronic infections or acute viral infections.

Immunological approaches to the prevention of anaphylaxis

Blocking antibody. On consideration of the mechanism of systemic anaphylaxis it would seem likely that if the parenterally injected antigen could be prevented from reaching the tissue-fixed IgE then anaphylaxis would not develop. This desirable state of affairs can be achieved by the simple expedient of injecting frequent small doses of the antigen to which the patient is sensitized. This induces the formation of increasing levels of IgG antibody which, circulating in the blood and tissue fluids, mops up the injected antigen so that it does not reach the tissue-fixed IgE (Fig. 9.2). This IgG antibody has been termed **blocking antibody** and its induction is the basis of desensitization treatment in allergic individuals. As might be expected this method is much more effective in preventing systemic anaphylactic reactions than the local forms where the antigen does not enter the bloodstream. To prevent local anaphylaxis the blocking antibody would need to be present in the mucous secretions and parenteral injection of antigen in hardly the best way to achieve this (see p. 143 for discussion of immunization against influenza virus).

In theory it should be possible, by raising the level of IgE to antigens other than those responsible for the allergic sensitization, to occupy the tissue receptors by non-specific IgE antibodies rather than those formed to the sensitizing antigen. Whether such a procedure is feasible remains to be established. Recent work using rats sensitized to benzylpenicilloyl (a penicillin derivative) raises the possibility that B cell tolerance can be induced to the antigen by repeated injections (subcutaneously or intraperitoneally) of the benzylpenicilloyl linked to a carrier, a random polymer of glutamic acid and lysine (D-GL). Levels of IgE and IgG to the penicillin derivative are markedly reduced for at least six months.

For pollen or seasonal allergies, desensitizing injections are given before the onset of the pollen season. About 70% of cases obtain clinical benefit from the treatment, and with ragweed antigen marked increases in the ratio of blocking IgG to IgE levels have recently been found.

Symptomatic treatment of allergies commonly involves the use of antihistamines and more recently disodium cromoglycate has come into use. This is effective in blocking histamine release if the drug is present before challenge with antigen. Isoprenaline and theophylline, which increase the level of intracellular cyclic-AMP, in turn reduce histamine release from mast cells. Corticosteroids also have a beneficial effect in type 1 allergic disorders, although their mode of action is unclear.

Cytolytic or cytotoxic (type 2) reactions

Cell-associated antigens. Reactions of this type are initiated by an antigenic component either part of a tissue cell or closely associated

ANAPHYLAXIS (Type 1)

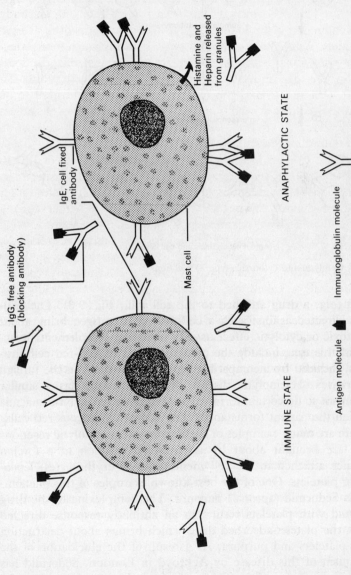

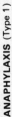

Fig. 9.2 Diagrammatic view of the possible difference between an *'immune state'* (i.e. when immunized animal will not develop anaphylaxis on challenge with antigen) and an *'anaphylactic state'*. Here there is insufficient antibody free in the tissue fluids to mop up the antigen thus allowing it to combine with reaginic antibody (IgE) attached to cell. The interaction triggers the release of histamine and heparine from mast cell granules.

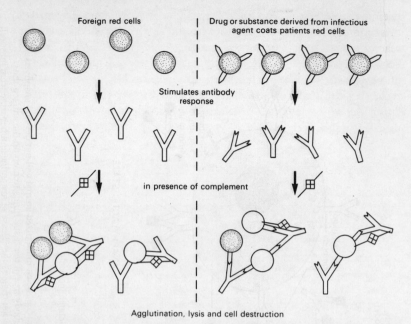

Fig. 9.3 Cytolytic and cytotoxic (type 2) reactions

with it (e.g. a drug attached to the cell wall, Fig. 9.3). The antibodies directed against such a cell-associated antigen bring about a cytotoxic or cytolytic effect usually involving complement. Reactions of this type include the cytolytic effect of anti-red cell antibodies, induced by incompatible blood transfusion, on the foreign erythrocytes. Haemolytic disease of the newborn has a similar mechanism so do certain forms of autoimmune haemolytic anaemia in which the patient forms antibodies against autologous red cells.

There are many examples of these cytotoxic or cytolytic reactions which are brought about by an immune reaction to a foreign substance attached to the cell membranes of erythrocytes, leucocytes or platelets. One of the best known examples of this phenomenon is Sedormid (apronal) purpura. The complexing of the drug Sedormid with platelets results in an antibody response directed against the platelet-adsorbed drug which brings about destruction of the platelets and purpura. As a result of the elucidation of the mechanism of this disease by Ackroyd in London, Sedormid has been withdrawn from use. This type of reaction may be more widespread than is generally suspected. A variety of infectious diseases due to salmonella organisms and mycobacteria are associated with haemolytic anaemia, and there is evidence, particularly in studies in salmonella infections, that the haemolysis is due to an immune reaction against a lipopolysaccharide bacterial endotoxin which becomes coated on to the patient's erythrocytes. A detailed study of *Salmonella gallinarum* infection in chickens has shown conclusively that the red cells are coated, have a shorter life in the circulation due to haemolysis, and that the development of haemolysis directly parallels the level of the antilipopolysaccharide antibody.

Antibody-dependent cell-mediated cytotoxicity

This mixed form of hypersensitivity is mediated by at least two distinct types of non-immune cells acting in conjunction with antibody directed at a target cell.

The non-immune 'killer' cells (or K cells) take two forms:

1. Cells morphologically similar to small or medium-sized lymphocytes without easily demonstrable immunoglobulin on their surface that are not glass adherent (in contrast to macrophages) or phagocytic. They are prominent in human peripheral blood and have receptors for the Fc portion of IgG and sometimes for products of C3. It is believed that these cells are cytotoxic for antibody coated tumour cells (e.g. melanoma cells) and for virus infected cells (e.g. herpes simplex infected cells).

2. A glass adherent cell (possibly a monocyte) that lyses antibody coated red blood cells. This form of lysis takes place without involving the complement system.

These mixed forms of hypersensitivity reaction can readily be demonstrated in vitro and there a number of reports showing cytotoxic effects against various antibody-coated target cells including human tissue cells in certain 'autoimmune' disease states (see p. 246). Whether or not this mixed form of hypersensitivity has its in vivo counterpart remains to be established.

In these reactions, damage to cells is the result of the attachment of antibody to their surface. The consequences include (see Fig. 9.4).

1. Direct lysis of the cell by complement activation
2. Adherence to phagocytes by their Fc and C3 receptors leading to phagocytosis
3. Antibody-dependent cell-mediated cytotoxicity (ADCC), by both phagocytic and non-phagocytic cells (PMNs and macrophages) and cells morphologically similar to lymphocytes but with Fc receptors, referred to as K cells (see p. 64).

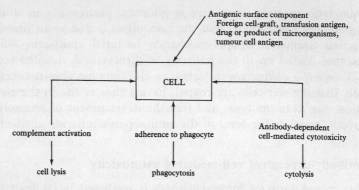

Fig. 9.4 Type II antibody-dependent cytotoxic hypersensitivity

The cytotoxic effects require contact between the effector and target cell and is independent of complement components.

The situations where such cytotoxic reactions develop are the result of the expression of antigen on the surface of a cell that leads to antibody production. Such antigen expression can be initiated in a variety of ways (Fig. 9.4), as already indicated.

Toxic-complex syndrome (type 3) reactions

Serum sickness and Arthus reactions. These reactions are due to the combination of antigen with circulating antibody, with the formation of microprecipitates in and around small blood vessels. This causes inflammation and sometimes mechanical blocking of these vessels which results in interference with the blood supply to surrounding tissues. There are two types of reaction which fall into this category: **serum sickness** which is a systemic form and the **Arthus reaction** which is a local form.

Serum sickness develops, as the name suggests, in individuals injected with foreign serum and was described soon after the introduction of parenteral administration, for therapeutic purposes, of diphtheria antitoxin prepared in the horse. Foreign serum protein is eliminated from the circulation over a period of a few weeks and after the injection of 10 to 20 ml there will still be a large amount present by the time an immune response to the foreign serum protein develops. This results in the formation of antibody-antigen complexes that can cause a wide variety of symptoms ranging form anaphylactic reactions such as asthma or laryngeal oedema when IgE antibody attached to mast cells is involved, to symptoms dependent on the deposition of immune complexes (antigen + IgG antibody) in blood vessels where they activate complement and cause inflammatory changes. Fixation of the first component of complement (p. 25) leads to the formation of anaphylatoxin involved in histamine release. The inflammatory cells are mainly polymorphs attracted by the trimolar C567 complex that has chemotactic activity. Proteolytic enzymes released by polymorphs damage adjacent tissues and plasma kinins are also activated. The intensity of the reaction depends upon the concentration of complexes and on the ability of the antibody to activate complement. IgM, IgG1, IgG2 and IgG3 antibodies have this ability (p. 102) whereas IgG4, IgA and IgE do not. The clinical manifestations depend upon where the immune complexes form or lodge.

On the basis of experimental work in rabbits two forms of reaction have been recognized: (1) following a single large dose of antigen which results in arthritis, glomerulonephritis and coronary artery vasculitis; (2) following daily doses of antigen which results after a few weeks in glomerulonephritis. The first form is complement-dependent whereas the second occurs even in complement-depleted animals. The first form of reaction in humans manifests itself by affecting the kidneys with the development of glomerulonephritis and in severe cases renal failure, the heart, with myocarditis and valvulitis, and the joints which become swollen and painful. Urticaria sometimes develops and the patient becomes pyrexial. The symptoms disappear whenever all the foreign serum protein is eliminated.

Antigens other than serum proteins can cause serum sickness. Nowadays the most likely causes are drugs such as penicillin and sulphonamides. The susceptible patient will develop rashes (urticarial, morbilliform or scarlatinoform), pyrexia, arthralgia, lymphadenopathy and perhaps nephritis some 8 to 12 days after being given the drug. It seems likely that many bacterial and viral infections, include development of hypersensitivity of this type, as rashes, joint pains and sometimes mild haematuria are not uncommon (see Fig. 9.5 and p. 145). In poststreptococcal glomerulonephritis streptococcal antigens have been detected in the glomeruli (see also p. 138). In virus hepatitis circulating immune complexes have been found associated with periarteritis nodosa. Many of the clinical features of the autoimmune disease systemic lupus erythematosus (discussed on p. 253) appear to result from arteritis, and deposits of immunoglobulin and complement (prob-

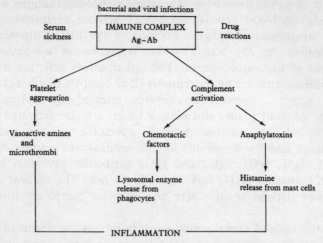

Fig. 9.5 Type III Immune complex hypersensitivity — causes and consequences

ably complexed with DNA) have been found in the skin lesions and glomeruli of patients with the disease.

The Arthus reaction, like serum sickness, is brought about by the formation of antibody-antigen complexes but in this case the phenomenon is a local one at the site of injection of antigen. The Arthus reaction occurs in walls of small blood vessels in the presence of large quantities of IgG antibody forming microprecipitates with antigen. The resulting vasculitis develops a few hours after injection of antigen and persists for 12 to 24 hours. Immune complexes can be shown microscopically in the vessel wall using the fluorescent antibody technique (p. 282) and there is a massive infiltration of granulocytes brought about by a chemotactic effect generated by the antigen-antibody complex. There is activation of the vasoactive amines such as histamine, with resulting increase in vascular permeability and consequent oedema. These reactions may occur in diabetics who have received many injections of insulin and have developed high levels of IgG antibody to antigenic constituents in the insulin preparation.

Arthus reactions in the bronchial or alveolar wall may explain the late asthmatic reactions that occur seven to eight hours after inhalation of antigen. These may be of particular importance in the 'allergic alveolitis' seen in farmers sensitive to mouldy hay antigen (see p. 163) and maltworkers sensitive to *Aspergillus clavatus* of contaminated barley. In some cases of tuberculosis, sarcoidosis, leprosy and streptococcal infections, vascular inflammatory lesions are seen mainly in the legs. These are variously referred to as erythema nodosum, nodular vasculitis and erythema induratum and may be due to the deposition of immune complexes and the development of an Arthus reaction.

Delayed hypersensitivity (type 4) cell-mediated hypersensitivity

Lymphocyte-mediated reactions and 'lymphokines'. These can be defined as specifically provoked, slowly evolving (24 to 48 hours), mixed cellular reactions involving lymphocytes and macrophages. The reaction is not brought about by circulating antibody but by sensitized lymphoid cells and can be transferred in experimental animals by means of such cells but not serum. The classical example of this type of reaction is the tuberculin response which has over the years received detailed study. To induce this response a tuberculin-sensitised individual is given an intradermal injection of 0.1 ml of a 1 in 1000 dilution of a protein extract of tubercle bacilli (purified protein derivative PPD). An indurated inflammatory reaction in the skin, measuring a few millimetres in diameter, appears about 24 hours later and persists for a few weeks. In the human the injection site is infiltrated with large numbers of mono-nuclear cells, mainly lymphocytes, with about 10–20% macrophages. Most of these cells are in and around small blood vessels.

Despite intensive investigation of the delayed hypersensitivity reaction, immunologists are far from understanding the mechanisms underlying this phenomenon. A possible explanation is that, amongst the continuous traffic of lymphocytes passing through the tissues (p. 68), some interact with antigen they meet and influence other lymphocytes and phagocytes to migrate to the area (see also Table 4.10). **Lymphokines** produced by the T cell subpopulation (Tdh) are involved and are discussed on page 110. Their main role appears to be to **recruit** non-sensitized (uncommitted) lymphoid cells to the site of inflammation and to **retain** them at the site where they become activated, thus **amplifying** the immune response. An important factor appears to be responsible for inducing proliferation of lymphocytes at the site of localization and has been termed mitogenic factor. A cytotoxic effect has been demonstrated in tissue culture experiments affecting lymphocytes and other cells (lymphotoxin). Tdh cells proliferate under the influence of IL-2 from Th cells. Tdh cells recognize antigen on inducer cells and secrete lymphokines in the same MHC restricted way as Th cells.

The best known of the lymphokines is the macrophage migration inhibition factor. This effect is readily demonstrated in vitro using peritoneal exudate cells from an animal sensitized to an antigen such as tuberculin. The peritoneal exudate cells, which are mainly macrophages, are collected in a capillary tube that is placed on a glass coverslip in a small tissue culture chamber. After 24 hours macrophages show a fan-shaped area of migration around the end of the capillary tube. If, however, the tuberculin antigen is placed in the tissue culture medium no migration occurs. The effect appears to be due to the release, from the small number of lymphocytes in peritoneal exudate, of a lymphokine known as macrophage migration inhibition factor or MIF. The specificity of the reaction has been shown with several other antigens including bovine gamma globulin, histoplasmin and dinitrophenol. The MIF is released from Tdh cells concerned with the cell-mediated immune state rather than cells concerned with making humoral antibody.

Other lymphocytes modulate phagocyte function including macrophage activating factor (MAF) α and γ interferons, chemotactic factor and leucocyte migration inhibition factor. In vivo the MIF may be responsible for the formation of large aggregates of macrophages in the lymphoid tissues (and perhaps elsewhere), although like the other lymphokines the precise role of MIF in delayed hypersensitivity reactions is not yet clear. Much further work is required to separate and identify the nature and functional activities of the various substances involved. Whether or not macrophages in delayed hypersensitivity reaction sites contribute lysosomal enzymes from their intracellular granules, thus bringing about further inflammatory changes, has yet to be determined.

Inducing agents. Delayed hypersensitivity reactions are characteristically induced by intracellular infectious agents including salmonellae, brucellae, streptococci and a wide range of viruses including measles and mumps viruses, vaccinia and herpes simplex (see also p. 152). Those with most clinical relevance are reactions due to vaccinia — the so-called 'reaction of immunity' occurring 24 to 72 hours after vaccination. This reaction does not proceed like a primary vaccination through the pustular stage and leaves no scar but instead has all the features of a delayed hypersensitivity reaction. The other important reaction is the 'pseudo-Schick' response occurring within 24 hours after the intradermal injection of diphtheria toxoid. This delayed reaction disappears within 6 days and also affects the control injected site (heat-treated toxoid).

Delayed hypersensitivity reactions sometimes develop following sensitisation to a variety of metals such as nickel and chromium, to simple chemical substances such as dyestuffs, potassium dichromate (affecting cement workers), primulin from primula plants, poison ivy and chemicals such as picryl chloride, dinitrochlorobenzene, and paraphenylene diamine (from hair dyes). Penicillin sensitisation is a common clinical complication following the topical application of the antibiotic in ointments or creams. These substances are not themselves antigenic and only become so on combination by covalent bonds with proteins in the skin. The clinical symptoms induced in these 'contact hypersensitivity' reactions (contact dermatitis) include redness, swelling, vesicles, scaling and exudation of fluid.

It is conceivable that, in future, use may be made of the delayed hypersensitivity response in the treatment of tumours. Some recent experiments in man show that certain skin tumours, if painted with a simple chemical antigen as described above, underwent a marked hypersensitivity reaction and then healed with the disappearance of the tumour. One explanation of the effect is that the lymphokine — tumour necrosis factor — is released during the hypersensitivity reaction and destroys the tumour cells. Much more work is clearly required before this can be regarded as a useful clinical procedure.

IMMUNODEFICIENCY STATES

The immunologically competent cells of the lymphoid tissues derived from, renewed and influenced by the activity of the thymus, bone marrow and probably gut-associated lymphoid tissues, can be the subject of disease processes due either to defects in one of the components of the complex itself, or secondarily to some other disease process affecting the normal functioning of some part of the lymphoid tissues. In 1953 Bruton first described hypogammaglobulinaemia in an 8-year-old boy who developed septic arthritis of the knee at 4 years of age followed by numerous attacks of otitis media, pneumococcal sepsis and pneumonia. Electrophoretic analysis of the serum proteins showed almost complete absence of the gammaglobulin fraction. The child appeared unable to give an immune response to typhoid and diphtheria immunization. It is now recognised that this form of deficiency is only one of a group of specific deficiencies affecting the lymphoid tissues which can affect both sexes, manifest themselves at any age and be genetically determined or arise secondarily to some other condition.

Before considering specific defects in the acquired immune response there are a small number of defects that need to be considered in the innate immune mechanisms that possibly involve defects in phagocyte function.

Defective innate immune mechanisms

Defects in phagocytic function take two forms: (1) where there is a **quantitative** deficiency of blood leucocytes which may be **congenital** (e.g. infantile agranulocytosis) or **acquired** as a result of replacement of bone marrow by tumour tissue or the toxic effects of chemicals; (2) where there is a **qualitative** deficiency in the functioning of neutrophil leucocytes which, whilst ingesting bacteria normally, fail, because of an enzymic defect, to digest them. The clinical form of this defect is known as **chronic granulomatous disease** and is a sex-linked recessive condition characterized by increased susceptibility to infection in early life by microorganisms of low virulence to the normal individual. In this condition the monocytes and polymorphs fail to produce H_2O_2 due to a defect in the hexose monophosphate shunt nicotinamide adenine dinucleotide phosphate (NADPH) pathway that is normally activated by phagocytosis (see p. 24). Phagocyte enzyme defects can be detected by the NBT test (p. 301). The ability of the patient's phagocytes to kill bacteria to which they are not normally susceptible is much reduced and organisms can survive for 2 hours or more within the phagocyte.

Other enzyme defects include deficiency of white blood cell glucose 6-phosphate dehydrogenase. In such patients the NBT test may be normal, but the intracellular activity of the phagocytes is reduced. Myeloperoxidase deficiency has also been described. This enzyme is necessary for normal intracellular killing, but the phagocytes from patients with this defect also show normal NBT tests, superoxide and H_2O_2 production.

Defects in the ability of phagocytes to respond to chemotactic stimuli have been described. Such defects include the lazy leucocyte syndrome and Chediak-Higashi syndrome, the latter condition being a multisystem disorder characterized by giant cytoplasmic inclusions in white blood cells and platelets. In this condition the lysosomal granules are structurally and functionally abnormal, and there is an associated reduction in intracellular killing of microorganisms.

The complement system (p. 25) can also suffer from certain defects in function leading to increased susceptibility to infection. The defects that have been described include: C1q deficiency, C1r and C1s deficiency, C2, C3, C6, C7, C8 deficiency, and dysfunction of the C5 component. Many of these disorders, which are very rare, are associated with an increased incidence of autoimmune disease (p. 246).

The most severe abnormalities of host defences occur, as would be expected, if there is a defect in the functioning of C3. Severe deficiency or absence of C3 is associated with increased susceptibility to infection, particularly pneumonia, meningitis, otitis, and pharyngitis. Individuals with inherited C3 deficiency can be shown to have normal C1, C4, and C2 activation. Activation of the alternate pathway or components C5–C9 does not occur. Thus normal chemotactic (C5a) and leucocytosis promoting factors (C3e) are absent.

Individuals with C1, C4, and C2 deficiencies tend not to be particularly susceptible to infections due to their intact alternate pathway mechanisms. C5 dysfunction may lead to deficient phagocyte activity with associated recurrent infections and C6, C7, and C8 deficiency with inability to lyse susceptible bacteria such as *Neisseria*, *Salmonella* and *Haemophilus* organisms.

Diseases in which defects in complement components occur include sickle cell disease and systemic lupus erythematosus (SLE). In sickle cell disease (red cells contain abnormal haemoglobin) there appears to be a defect involving the alternate pathway, and in SLE there is a reduction in levels of the C4 component, sometimes in the C2 component. In addition, persons with SLE appear to have a specific inhibitor of C5-derived chemotactic activity, with the associated susceptibility to infection.

Summary

Defects in the innate immune mechanism may be summarized as follows:

1. Congenital agranulocytosis.
2. Chronic granulomatous disease — due to defect in NADPH pathway of neutrophils, or glucose-6-phosphate dehydrogenase deficiency.

3. Defective phagocyte responses to chemotactic stimuli.

4. Deficiencies of complement components (rare) — most common and severe is C3 deficiency. Sometimes associated with autoimmune diseases.

Primary defects

In the first category are the congenital defects affecting immuno-globulin synthetic mechanisms, cell-mediated immune mechanisms or sometimes both. Deficiency of immunoglobulin synthesis is complete in Bruton type agammaglobulinaemia, an X-linked recessive character found in boys and in which the IgG level is reduced by about a tenth and the IgA and IgM about a hundredth of normal values. Cell-mediated immune mechanisms function normally in these patients, who can reject grafts and develop normal delayed hypersensitivity to tuberculosis. However, they do not give the normal circulating antibody response to bacterial vaccines and are thus very susceptible to pyogenic infections. The lymphoid tissue in the appendix and Peyer's patches is somewhat reduced, and patients do not develop plasma cells and germinal centres in lymph nodes.

Partial defects in immunoglobulin synthesis have been described affecting one or more of the main immunoglobulin classes. For example, (a) the IgG or IgA levels may be reduced and the IgM level raised; (b) the IgA and IgM may be reduced and the IgG level be normal or (c) the IgA level may be reduced and the others normal.

Electrophoresis of serum as shown in Figure 9.6 cannot distinguish between the various immunoglobulin deficiencies and will only show gross changes in total immunoglobulins. Gel diffusion and immunoelectrophoretic techniques (p. 274) using anti-immunoglobulin antisera are required for the detailed analysis of these deficiencies.

In (a), which is inherited as an X-linked recessive character, the lymphoid tissues appear normal histologically although the plasma cells appear to be making predominantly IgM. Patients are susceptible to pyogenic infections and the condition is often associated with anaemia, thrombocytopoenia and neutropenia. In (b) even the IgG which is produced in normal quantity is thought to be abnormal in some way and unable to combine with antigen. Defect (c) occurs in 80% of patients with a condition known as hereditary ataxia telangiectasia who have increased susceptibility to infections

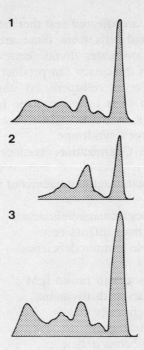

Fig. 9.6 Tracings obtained by ultraviolet scanning of elctrophoretic patterns of human sera. (1) normal serum (2) reduced gamma globulin (antibody deficiency syndrome possible B cell defect) (3) raised gamma globulin (possible myeloma). Peaks right to left: albumin, alpha, beta and gamma globulins (see Fig. 4.15)

of the upper and lower respiratory tract. There is a deficiency in plasma cells in the mucous membranes of the intestinal tract, where IgA is known to be produced in normal individuals, and the disease seems likely to be due to lack of protection at the level of the respiratory mucous membranes normally brought about by IgA secretion.

Both **cell-mediated** immune mechanisms and **immunoglobulin synthesis** are deficient in an X-linked disease of male children known as 'Swiss-type agammaglobulinaemia' or severe combined immunodeficiency. There is almost complete absence of lymphoid tissue in the body, the thymus is very small and the lymphoid tissues of the appendix and Peyer's patches are absent. Children with this condition cannot make antibodies or develop cell-mediated immune ractions, and they suffer from progressive bacterial and/or viral infection and die with in two years of birth.

In another type of defic.ency state only the cell-mediated

immune mechanisms are affected and there is thymic dysplasia and deficiency of lymphoid cells from those areas of the spleen and lymph nodes which are under thymic control. Although children with this rare type of deficiency can produce circulating antibody, their inability to develop cell-mediated immunity renders them highly susceptible to virus infection. One form of this condition associated with thymic dysplasia and absence of parathyroid glands is known as Di George's syndrome.

The World Health Organization classification for antibody deficiencies is as follows:

1. Transient hypogammaglobulinaemia of infancy — as maternal IgG levels fall
2. Congenital hypogammaglobulinaemia — X-linked or autosomal recessive, i.e. male infants only
3. Common variable immunodeficiency — Heterogeneous group of infants or adults
4. Immunodeficiency with raised IgM
5. Immunodeficiency with thymoma
6. Selective IgA deficiency
7. Selective IgM deficiency
8. Selective IgG subclass deficiency

Secondary defects

Acquired deficiencies of the immunological mechanisms can occur secondarily to a number of disease states affecting the lymphoid tissues, such as Hodgkin's disease, multiple myeloma, leukaemia and lymphosarcoma. Deficiency of immunoglobulins can also be brought about by excessive loss of protein through diseased kidneys or via the intestines in protein-losing enteropathy. Malnutrition and iron deficiency can lead to depressed immune responsiveness, particularly in cell-mediated immunity. Viral infections can be immunosuppressive. For example, HIV, measles and other viruses infect cells of the immune system (p. 149). Medical and surgical treatment such as X-rays, cytotoxic drugs, steroids and catheterization can lead to the state referred to as the 'compromised host' in which there is interference with the effectiveness of the innate and acquired immune mechanisms (p. 120).

In contrast to the deficiency states just described, raised immunoglobulin levels are found in certain disorders of plasma cell function, which amount to malignant proliferation of a particular clone or family of plasma cells. In this condition, known as multiple

Table 9.2 A summary of the main primary immune deficiency states affecting T and B lymphocytes

Stem cell defects	Expression	Infections
Haemopoietic stem cell (autosomal recessive)	Severe combined immune deficiency affecting T cells, B cells and phagocytes	Early onset of infections in all systems, e.g. respiratory, alimentary, skin
Lymphocyte stem cell (autosomal recessive, some X-linked)	Diminished numbers of T and B cells	
Adenosine deaminase deficiency		
T cell-defects in development		
Thymus defects	1. Di George's syndrome (congenital but not usually familial) (thymic hypoplasia) with diminished numbers of T cells	Recurrent viral, bacterial, fungal infections, including viral respiratory infections
	2. Ataxia telangiectasia (autosomal recessive) affecting T cells and plasma cells — both reduced	
Defects in T cell sub populations	Variable immunodeficiencies affecting T_s or T_h cells	Viral and bacterial infections
B cell-defects in development		
Arrested development at pre-B-cell level (X-linked)	Infantile agammaglobulinaemia with diminished numbers of B cells	Mainly bacterial infections (occasional viral infections) Infection with pyogenic bacteria, if selective IgM deficiency
Defective terminal differentiation of B cells	Selective deficiency of immunologlobulin classes with reduced numbers of plasma cells, B cells and sometimes T cells	

myeloma, a malignant clone is found to produce one particular class of immunoglobulin, usually IgG or more rarely one of the other classes. The frequency of occurrence among myeloma of particular immunoglobulin classes reflects their relative levels in serum. There is usually a decreased synthesis of normal immuno-globulins associated with a deficient immune response to infective agents. On electrophoresis of serum a distinct band can be seen in the immunoglobulin area, and Figure 9.6 shows an example of the type of pattern found on simple paper elctrophoresis. This abnormal band is produced by the raised levels of the myeloma immunoglobulin which is termed an M-type protein. In about 20–30% of patients with multiple myeloma immunoglobulin light chains are found in the urine. These occur as dimers and are known as Bence-Jones protein. The condition is also associated with excess numbers of plasma cells in the bone marrow and X-ray evidence of myeloma cell deposits in bone. Table 9.3 gives a summary of secondary deficiencies and the types of microorganisms that can infect such patients.

Table 9.3 Summary of secondary immune deficiencies

Defects affecting lymphoid tissues
1. Infections of lymphocytes or macrophages, e.g. severe immunodeficiency in infections with HIV, or the lymphadenopathy associated virus of AIDS. Transient deficiencies in cytomegalovirus infections, infectious mononucleosis, measles, rubella and viral hepatitis. Bacterial infections such as leprosy, tuberculosis and syphilis can induce deficient function of immune system.
2. Malnutrition
3. Lymphoproliferative diseases or secondary tumour deposits
4. Drugs, such as cytotoxic or immunosuppressive agents
5. Drugs that attach to leucocytes and lead to hypersensitivity reaction and leucopenia, e.g. sulphonamides
6. Antibiotics can affect neutrophil and macrophage functions, e.g. chemotactic responses in neutrophils and sometimes the phagocytic function of macrophages

Loss of immunoglobulins
1. Nephrotic syndrome with loss of proteins including antibodies in the urine
2. Protein losing enteropathy — loss of immunoglobulin in the gut. This also occurs in chronic inflammatory bowel disease
3. Burns with severe loss of tissue fluids — sometimes with associated immunodepression

Types of microorganisms involved
1. Viruses — e.g. *Herpes simplex* virus, *Varicella zoster*, cytomegalovirus
2. Bacteria — e.g. *Escherichia coli, Staphylococcus aureus, Streptococcus faecalis, Pseudomonas aeruginosa, Pneumocystis carinii* and others
3. Fungi, e.g. *Candida* spp. *Aspergillus fumigatus*
4. Protozoa, e.g. *Giardia lambia*

Clinical aspects

Increased susceptibility to many types of infection is the outstanding feature of the immunological deficiency states. The age of onset of the congenital types is rarely earlier than three to four months of age due to the protective effects of maternal antibody. The most frequently affected site is the respiratory tract, which is attacked by pyogenic bacteria or fungi. Lack of IgA antibody leads to particular susceptibility to chronic infection of the respiratory tract. Other clinical features frequently associated with immune deficiency states are skin rashes, diarrhoea, growth failure, enlarged liver and spleen and recurrent abscesses or osteomyelitis.

When there is deficiency of the cell-mediated immune mechanisms, resistance to virus infections is diminished and may be recognized by the severe necrosis that will occur at the site of smallpox vaccination. BCG vaccination can lead to generalized tuberculosis infection in such cases.

Investigation of suspected immunological deficiency states should include family studies for any abnormalities of immune function. Lymphocyte function may be assessed by stimulation (a) with nonspecific agents such as PHA or concanavalin A (p. 296) or (b) with a specific bacterial antigen in subjects previously sensitized to the bacterial antigen by natural infection or immunization (e.g. the tubercle bacillus). Quantitative determination of immunoglobulin levels can be made (p. 276) and estimation of the response to immunisation with standard antigens. Peripheral blood counts and X-rays of the thymus region may also prove useful (see also p. 294).

Treatment of deficiency states includes use of an appropriate antibiotic and regular administration of pooled human immunoglobulins. Closely matched sibling bone marrow has been used successfully in some cases and a graft of fetal thymus has been used in the case of thymic aplasia. Bone marrow grafts can be rejected in the same way as other grafts (Ch. 7) unless closely related to the recipient. An additional complication arises in that the graft may attack host cells — a graft versus host (GVH) reaction (p. 207). In immune deficiency states graft rejection is likely to be the lesser of the two problems. Total lymph node irradiation has been found to be preferable to whole-body irradiation in the control of GVH reactions. Pluripotent stem cells (p. 51) of the bone marrow are likely be become tolerant to host antigens and give rise to mature cells that will not react against host cells. This can be made use of as techniques using monoclonal antibodies come into use to separate various subpopulations within the bone marrow.

Below is a summary of the management of immune deficiency states:
1. Immunoglobulin replacement therapy

2. Grafting of immunocompetent cells
3. Genetic counselling
4. Antibiotic therapy
5. Possible use of Interferon and other mediators, such as Interleukin-1 and 2, as they become available through recombinant DNA technology

Table 9.4 gives the indications for, and forms of, immunoglobulin replacement therapy.

Table 9.4 Immunoglobulin replacement therapy

Indications
X-linked agammaglobuinaemia
Common variable agammaglobulinaemia
Severe combined immunodeficiency
Wiskott-Aldrich syndrome

Forms
1. Alcohol-salt fractionated pooled human plasma (immune globulin) for intramuscular use
2. Normal human plasma. Advantages are fewer adverse reactions than immune globulin and less painful injections. Disadvantages are possible hepatitis B or HIV infection
3. Modified (enzyme treated) immune globulin as in (1) for intravenous use. Advantage is that can be given in large doses intramuscularly with rapid action and less painful than (1). Disadvantage — rapid clearance of enzyme treated preparations from blood

AUTOIMMUNITY

A fundamental characteristic of an animal's immune system is that it does not, under normal circumstances, react against its own body constituents. There exists a mechanism which enables the cells of the immune system to recognize what is 'foreign' and what is 'self'. Attempts to explain the absence of reactions against self go back to the early days of immunology when Paul Ehrlich enunciated his well known doctrine of 'horror autotoxicus'. Ehrlich and Morgenroth in 1900, after immunizing a goat with red blood cells of other goats, found that although the animal readily made antibodies against the red cells of other goats these antibodies failed to react with the animal's own red cells. It was thus clear that in some way the immunological response to self antigens was prevented. So powerful was the influence of Paul Ehrlich that it seemed inconceivable that in any circumstances the rule could be broken so that an immunological reaction against self could develop. The view continued to be held despite clinical evidence indicating that diseases existed in which the patient was apparently destroying his own cells.

The main reason that observations of this type failed to achieve the recognition they deserved was the absence of serological techniques capable of demonstrating convincingly the existence of antibodies able to react with tissue cells, or of the presence of such antibodies actually attached to cells. It was not until 1945 that immunologists were provided with this vital tool, when Coombs, Mourant and Race described a technique which detected the presence of antibody globulin on red blood cells by the simple expedient of adding an antiserum against human globulin which, after reacting with the globulin coating the cells, linked the cells together and agglutinated them. This method was particularly valuable for showing antibody globulin adsorbed to cells which was in itself unable to agglutinate the cells.

This technique is commonly known as the 'Coombs' or 'antiglobulin's test (p. 279). The development of the antiglobulin techniques led to the use of antiglobulin sera in a variety of different ways, many of which involved complicated technical operations but which essentially were based on the original antiglobulin method. Amongst the most important of the developments of the method is the fluorescent antibody technique in which one of the most commonly used procedures is to label an antiglobulin serum with a fluorescent marker (fluorescein isothiocyanate) so that the reaction of the labelled antiglobulin with, for example, globulin-coated cells can be visualized under u.v. light microscopy. Under these conditions the sites of attachment of the fluorescein-labelled antiglobulin show up as bright apple-green fluorescent areas (p. 282).

The recognition of autoimmune disease

These methods allowed a breakthrough in the recognition of a variety of human and animal disease in which antibodies could be convincingly demonstrated in serum capable of reacting with a number of different antigens of the individual's own tissues.

The first of these was the demonstration that in some types of haemolytic anaemia in man the red blood cells were coated with antibody globulin. This was soon followed by the finding of an autoantibody serum factor in the blood of patients with a severe connective tissue disease called systemic lupus erythematosus (SLE). This factor appeared to be antibody against the nuclei of tissue cells and was called by the author and his colleagues anti-nuclear factor (ANF). At the same time, workers interested in diseases of the thyroid gland demonstrated the presence of an antibody to thyroglobulin in patients with a particular form of interstitial thyroiditis known as Hashimoto's disease.

The first recognizable clinical description of acquired haemolytic anaemia was given in 1898 in France, and in 1908 haemolytic activity against red cells was found in the serum of patients in whom intense haemolysis was taking place in vivo. These early observations were neglected until 30 years later when Damashek and Schwartz again reported haemolysins in patients suffering from haemolytic anaemia, and with the introduction of the Coombs test in 1945 the immunological basis of the disease was put on a firm foundation.

The effect on immunological theory

Associated with the accumulating evidence on the autoimmune nature of the haemolysins in acute haemolytic anaemia, there arose the need to consider the meaning of foreignness and self-recognition and the mechanisms underlying the ability of the body to diffferentiate between 'self' and 'non-self'. A solution to the problem this created in immunological theory was offered by Burnet and Fenner in 1949. At that time antibody production was envisaged in terms of the antigen acting as a template for modifying the globulin molecules to a form which was complementary to that of antigen (p. 82). It was considered that antigen might act either on the already formed protein chain and bring about a reconfiguration of the chain, or that the antigen induced a chemical rearrangement of the globulin molecule as it was formed.

Burnet and Fenner, whilst accepting this direct template theory, included the notion of 'self-markers' attached to body components by which antibody-forming cells were able to recognize them, rendering them immunologically inert. They also predicted that an equivalent tolerance to foreign antigens should be demonstrable if these had been introduced at an appropriate stage in embryonic life, while the animal's immune system was in the process of learning to recognize the 'self-markers' of its own tissues. This prediction was later confirmed experimentally by Medawar and his colleagues who showed that if neonatal mice were injected with transplantation antigen from another strain of mice, they would later be able to accept skin grafts which an animal not injected neonatally would rapidly reject.

Burnet soon followed his 'self-marker' theory by his rather more plausible **'clonal selection'** theory. This allowed the antigen no part in impressing a pattern on the antibody-producing cells. The capacity to produce a given antibody was regarded as a genetically determined quality of certain clones or families of mesenchymal cells, the function of the antigen being to stimulate cells of these clones to proliferation and antibody production. The theory postulated that in the early stages of embryonic development, mutation of cells led to a variety of **random** arrangements in the globulin molecules so that a very large number of clones were generated which could correspond to potential antigenic determinants (p. 83). To explain the inability of the antibody-forming system to react with self, Burnet proposed that the immature cells could be destroyed if they came across the antigens with which they could react at this early stage. Whenever the antigenic determinants were freely present in the body and accessible to the corresponding immunologically competent cells, such destructive contacts would be inevitable. Tolerance would result from the elimination or inhibition of all cells clones which had the ability to react with antigenic determinants present in the body. After birth, when foreign antigen entered the tissues, antibody to it would be produced by specific stimulation of those cells in clones preadapted to react with the corresponding antigenic determinants. On the basis of this theory Burnet accounted for the development of autoimmune disease as a failure of the destruction of the self-reactive population of antibody-forming cells (see also p. 55).

Possible mechanisms involved in the development of autoimmunity

The question now arises of how the normal controlling mechanism fails with the resulting inability to maintain self-recognition manifested by immune reactions against self.

There are three main ways (Table 9.5) in which this tolerance-maintaining mechanism could conceivably be overcome. The first involves evasion or circumvention of a normally functioning mechanism and the second failure of the mechanism itself. The third possible mechanism involves the stimulation of a pre-existing quiescent self-reactive B lymphocyte population.

Table 9.5 Mechanisms of autoantibody formation

1. **Evasion** of normal tolerance to 'self' antigens
   a. Hidden antigens
   b. Altered antigens — chemicals, drugs, infectious agents
2. **Breakdown** of tolerance mechanism
   a. Agents affecting antibody forming cells — chemicals, drugs, infectious agents
   b. Genetically determined lack of efficiency of tolerance control mechanisms (e.g. by suppressor T cells)
3. **Stimulation** of pre-existing B cell population capable of self-reactivity
   Infectious agents and adjuvants (? effects on suppressor T cells)

In the first category evasion may occur in two possible ways: (1) because a particular body antigen is not accessible to the cells of the immune system as the antigen is hidden within a cell or tissue — these antigens are known as **sequestered** antigens; (2) because a tissue antigen is **altered** in some way by a chemical agent, a drug or an infectious agent.

Sequestered antigens. Hidden or sequestered antigens do seem to exist and the best examples of these are sperm antigens and lens antigen of the eye. Sperm can be shown to acquire an antigen during maturation which is absent from the immature germinal cells. Antibodies can be induced in the guinea-pig by immunising with autologous sperm showing that the immune system fails to recognise the sperm as part of self. Orchitis can be induced by combining the sperm with an adjuvant which gives a boost to the immune response, and at the same time in some way allows the stimulated lymphoid cells and antibody to gain access to the sperm-forming tissues. Orchitis in man is a rare complication of mumps infection in which it is assumed that the virus damages the basement membrane barrier of the seminiferous tubules and the cells of the immune system are thus allowed entry and initiate an immune response.

In the case of the lens it can be shown that if a rabbit is injected with bovine lens material, it develops antibodies which react with its own lens in vitro. Occasionally the surgical extraction of a lens for cataract is succeeded by inflammatory changes in retained lens substance sometimes affecting the other unoperated lens, and the same phenomenon can be induced experimentally in animals.

Interpretation of observations of this type is fraught with complications and can be regarded at present only as speculative evidence to support the concept of sequestered antigens as an initiating factor in autoimmune disease.

Altered antigens. Evidence in support of the second way in which normal tolerance mechanisms are circumvented is more concrete. Experimental studies of tolerance evasion by altered antigens have been carried out with purified proteins, conjugates of hapten and protein, and with cellular antigens. Some of the most definitive work is that carried out in America by Weigle who showed that rabbits made tolerant to bovine serum albumen (BSA) and then immunized with the cross-reacting antigen human serum albumen (HSA) eventually made antibodies which could react with BSA. The same result was obtained with chemically modified BSA. A closer approximation to autoimmune disease is provided by experiments using thyroglobulin in rabbits; not only are anti-rabbit thyroglobulin antibodies induced by injection of altered thyroglobulin but inflammatory lesions are also found in their thyroid glands.

Shared antigens. There has been considerable interest in the last few years in the role of microorganisms as a source of cross-reacting antigens sharing antigenic determinants with tissue components. The ability of viruses to bring about alterations of cell membranes has been suggested by studies on the effect of herpes and rabies viruses on tissue culture cells. New cell surface antigens (neoantigens), which appear to act as transplantation antigens, have been found in mouse cells infected with herpes and also with polyoma viruses.

There is an antigen in human colon extractable even from sterile fetal human colon, which is similar to a polysaccharide antigen present in *E. coli* 014. It is conceivable that the inflammatory condition of the colon known as ulcerative colitis, in which anti-colon antibodies are found, is due to an immune reaction initiated by the cross-reacting bacterial antigen. Similarly the group A streptococci, which are closely associated with rheumatic fever, have a antigen in common with a human heart antigen. Heart lesions are a common finding in rheumatic fever and anti-heart antibody is found in just over 50% of patients with the condition.

Nephritogenic strains of type 12 group A streptococci carry surface antigens similar to those found in human glomeruli and infection by these organisms has been associated with the development of acute nephritis. ·

Drugs as haptens. Drugs can act as haptens (p. 257) which bind to tissue proteins. The resulting complex may be antigenic and result in an immune reaction which damages cells coated with the drug. An example of this is a metabolic breakdown product of the drug α-methyldopa (used in the treatment of hypertension). The immune response generated by these drug-altered cells can then result in haemolysis of the affected cells and α-methyldopa is thought to have the effect of altering or exposing normally hidden red cell antigens. The antibody which results has been found to combine with Rhesus antigens present on the surface of the patient's own normal erythrocytes. One hypothesis is that the α-methyldopa is incorporated into the Rhesus antigen when the red cell is being made and the change this induces prevents the antigen being recognized as self (see also discussion of the effects of the drug Sedormid, p. 230).

Disturbed immunological mechanisms

The second main category of mechanisms by means of which autoimmune reactions may develop (Table 9.5) are those due to alteration in the cellular processes on which maintenance of normal tolerance depends. One way in which this might occur is by the direct effect of a chemical, a drug or an infectious agent on the lymphoid tissues. Alternatively, it is conceivable that the loss of normal tolerance control might be due to an inherited defect or lack of efficiency in the lymphoid cell population. The existence of a T lymphocyte population (suppressor T cells) the controls B lymphocyte activity has been noted on page 54. Suppressor T cells may prevent development of autoimmunity in the normal animal by recognizing idiotypic determinants (p. 77, 99) of anti-self immunoglobulins expressed on the B cell surface. It is conceivable that a defect (inherited or induced) of such suppressor T cells might allow B cells of this type to escape and produce anti-self immunoglobulin. The recent recognition of a subpopulation of B cells expressing a surface marker (CD5) that are increased in patients with rheumatoid arthritis has led to the suggestion that CD5 positive cells escape the control of Ts cells and produce rheumatoid factor.

There is much speculation amongst immunologists and clinicians on the role of infectious agents acting **directly** on the lymphoid tissues as a cause of autoimmune disease. This stems from the experimental evidence on the induction of autoimmune disease using tissue antigens combined with Freund's complete adjuvant. This water-in-oil emulsion owes its powerful stimulating effect on the lymphoid tissues, to killed mycobacteria which are incorporated in the oil. Without the mycobacterial component, tissue antigens are much less effective in disturbing the tolerance mechanisms. Rabbits injected with *Mycobacterium tuberculosis* alone have been shown to develop autoantibodies against a wide range of autologous tissues. The same phenomenon is found in a number of chronic infections in the human such as syphilis, actinomycosis and chronic tuberculosis. Infection with *Mycoplasma pneumoniae*, responsible for a disease known as primary atypical pneumonia, is associated with the development of IgM agglutinins in the patient's serum, which in the cold will react with the patient's own red cells.

A leukaemia virus has in the last few years been found in a strain of mice (New Zealand Black or NZB mice) characterized by the early development of autoimmune disease including autoimmune haemolytic anaemia and immune complex nephritis. The virus has been found in many body tissues and in the blood and can be seen in lymphoid organs, attached to the surface of lymphocytes. Similar virus particles have been found in embryos of the NZB strain, suggesting that it is passed through the placenta or is associated with the germ cells. The association of the virus with lymphocyte membranes has attracted the attention of immunologists and there has been speculation that the presence of the virus might interfere with normal lymphocyte reactivity no antigens. It is known (p. 141) that antigens can react with the lymphocyte surface and that this is probably one stimulus to immune transformation of these cells. The virus could conceivably upset the mechanisms controlling lymphocyte reactivity so that they respond abnormally to antigens to which they should remain tolerant. This idea receives some support from experiments in which animals stimulated with certain microorganisms (e.g. tubercle bacilli or corynebacteria) or the products of organisms (e.g. bacterial endotoxin) do not develop the expected immune tolerance when these antigens are administered in a way which would induce tolerance in the absence of the microbial product.

The human autoimmune disease systemic lupus erythematosus is characterised by anti-DNA antibodies and immune complexes containing DNA present in the kidneys (Fig. 9.7). Tubular structures resembling the nucleocapsids of myxo- or paramyxoviruses have been found by electron microscopy in the endothelial cells of renal glomeruli and occasionally in the lymphocytes and joint tissues. Similar particles have been found in the tissues of patients with a number of other diseases in which autoantibodies are found (thyroiditis, myasthenia gravis, scleroderma and dermatomyositis). A relationship between these findings and the pathogenesis of these diseases has not yet been established and is complicated by the difficulty in distinguishing between immune reactions directed

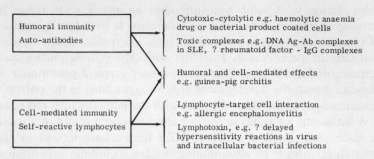

Fig. 9.7 Scheme showing pathogenic mechanisms in autoimmune disease with examples of disease states in each category

against virus specified antigens and host antigens (autoantigens). Raised titres of antibody to various DNA and RNA viruses have been detected in patients with rheumatoid arthritis. Amongst these is the finding of an abnormally high incidence and titres of antibodies to the herpes virus, Epstein-Barr virus (EBV) and more recently human parvovirus (a very small single-stranded DNA virus). Evidence with EBV suggests that there is a defect in the control by T lymphocytes of the expression of the virus by infected cells. Lymphocytes from RA patients, on exposure to EBV in vitro, transform more readily than do normal lymphocytes into EBV-containing lymphoblastoid cell lines secreting immunoglobulin. This immunoglobulin, if produced over a long period, would be likely to result in an anti-immunoglobulin response, some of which might be anti-idiotypic in nature (see p. 99). The anti-immunoglobulin rheumatoid factor could conceivably originate in this way.

Stimulation of pre-existing B cells

Another explanation for the development of auto-antibodies has recently been put forward (Table 9.5) — stimulation of a pre-existing population of lymphocytes (B cells) capable of making anti-self antibodies. In the mouse, cells making anti-red cell autoantibodies can be induced to proliferate by the administration of substances with adjuvant activity (p. 91) e.g. certain corynebacteria and *B. pertussis*. Evidence indicating the presence of such lymphocytes was provided some years ago by a number of immunologists including the author, who described a variety of naturally occurring autoantibodies in the serum of rodents. The availability of techniques such as immunocyto-adherence and localized haemolysis in gel (p. 87) have now allowed the identification of the lymphocytes producing the autoantibodies and thus put the earlier observations on a much firmer footing. It is a matter of speculation at present whether any human autoimmune state is a result of stimulation of these anti-self reactive lymphocytes. B lymphocytes capable of producing autoantibodies may increase in numbers with age. It is likely that in the normal individual proliferation of autoantibody producing B lymphocytes are held in check by immunoregulatory T lymphocytes.

There is little evidence that autoreactive T cells are present in the normal person. The possibility has been suggested that the autoreactive B cells are produced as a reaction to gut-derived antigens cross-reactive with self antigens. In a mouse model, autoantibody has been shown to first occur in lymph nodes draining the intestinal tract. If the mice were thymectomized neonatally, the autoantibodies did not appear, indicating the need for some T cell help. As indicated above, there is much evidence linking autoimmunity with exposure to a wide variety of infectious agents. It is possible that such agents can interfere with T cell regulation of autoreactive B lymphocytes without the direct participation of autoantigen in triggering the response.

Recent evidence suggests that B cells lose tolerance more readily than T cells and that T cells tolerant to self may be bypassed by presenting autoantigens to B cells in a sufficiently immunogenic form perhaps combined with adjuvants as discussed above. If, as seems possible, the antibodies produced were of low affinity this would favour the development of toxic complexes with results as described on page 259.

HLA, immune response genes and disease susceptibility

The human leucocyte antigen system (HLA system), consisting of several hundred genes on the short arm of chromosome six, is described on page 113.

In Chapter 4 the important role performed by HLA-associated immune response genes is discussed in relation to the expression of acquired immunity. There has also been an extensive search for associations between the expression of these genes and disease states.

In mice, some histocompatibility-associated Ir genes appear to predispose to autoimmune thyroiditis and susceptibility to viral meningitis infection. This suggests that products of these genes, expressed as receptors on lymphocytes, may be important in genetic susceptibility or resistance to autoimmune diseases, infection and neoplasia.

The MHC locus can be thought of as a genetic locus which codes for cell surface structures important in various cell–cell interactions. Certain of the surface structures may provide selective advantages in providing protection against certain potentially dangerous disease states but, at the same time, may predispose to a limited number of somewhat rare diseases. In other words, such predisposition may be a minor inconvenience of a gene that confers a protective advantage.

There are a number of different categories of association between the HLA complex and disease states. The first is a series of disease associations with different loci within the MHC, called the A, B, C and D loci. The best example is the association between ankylosing spondylitis and HLA-B27. However, the frequency of this locus in the population is about 8%, whilst the disease has a frequency of less than 0.1%. In those individuals who develop the disease and are not HLA-B27 there is a possible increase in HLA-A2 frequency. There is also a preponderance of males with the disease. A second category appears to be linked to the presence of two HLA-B loci, as in the case of juvenile-onset diabetes when there is an association with HLA-B8 and — BW15 loci. A third category is the incidence of, for example, sensitivity to ragweed allergen where a particular haplotype is inherited within a given family and appears to carry disease susceptibility. The implicated haplotype may vary from family to family, and the HLA identity only extends to siblings with the disease.

Table 9.6 shows that there are associations between specific HLA types and various chronic diseases, and that the association is much closer in some cases than in others. The fact that the association is not absolute may be due to the presence of other genes not linked to the HLA system. In support of this, multiple sclerosis has a much closer association (70% as against 15% of controls) with the MLC (mixed lymphocyte culture reaction) gene complex than with HLA types. Associations of diseases with individual HLA types imply that either increased resistance or susceptibility to the disease has been conferred by the HLA type. Positive associations suggest increased susceptibility, but an excess of a particular HLA type among the survivors of a disease with a high mortality suggests heightened resistance. One view explains the association by linking

Table 9.6 Some examples of disease associations with HLA types

Disease	HLA type	Relative risk*
Hodgkin's disease	A1	1.4
Idiopathic haemochromatosis	A3	8.3
Ankylosing spondylitis	⎫	87.4
Reiter's disease	⎬ B27	37.0
Acute anterior uveitis	⎭	10.4
Bechet's disease	B5	10.1
Subacute thyroiditis	B35	13.7
Psoriasis vulgaris	CW6	13.3
Dermatitis herpetiformis	⎫	10.8
Coeliac disease	⎮	14.3
Sicca syndrome	⎮	9.7
Idiopathic Addison's disease	⎬ DR3	6.3
Graves disease	⎮	3.7
SLE	⎮	5.8
Insulin-dependent diabetes	⎭	3.3
Insulin-dependent diabetes	DR4	6.4
Insulin-dependent diabetes	DR2	0.2
Multiple sclerosis	DR2	4.1
Rheumatoid arthritis	DR4	4.2
Hashimoto's thyroiditis	⎫ DR5	3.2
Pernicious anaemia	⎭	5.4

* Relative risk is a measure of the increased chance of developing the disease for individuals of particular HLA antigen type relative to those lacking the antigen.

the Ir genes which are part of the MHC with the pathogenesis of those diseases in which an immune response is implicated. Another view is that HLA antigens or very closely linked gene products act as viral receptors or in other ways influence the pathogenesis of the condition. Environmental factors such as exposure to viruses may also be required for a susceptible individual to develop the disease, and the disease itself may have more than one aetiology (p. 133).

Some recent work has provided further information on this difficult area that should make it possible to predict which women will develop autoimmune complications (SLE-like) if treated with Hydralazine, an antihypertensive drug. Women who are HLA DR4 positive and are slow acetylators always develop the autoimmune complication. Another development showing how a combination of apparently unrelated genetic markers can be used for accurate identification of a population at risk is the finding that a combination of HLA-B2/DR3 and a particular immunoglobulin allotype marker (p. 99) was associated with a 40-fold greater relative risk of developing chronic active hepatitis than if neither marker was present. Relapses in Graves' disease of the thyroid, associated with

B27 can be accurately predicted by a combined analysis of HLA-DR3 status and Gm allotype. It therefore seems that investigation of genes for HLA antigen and immunoglobulin genes may lead to some useful information on susceptibility to disease. There is a tendency for some of the antigens of the HLA loci to occur together more often on the same chromosome than is expected by chance. Such non-random associations are termed linkage disequilibrium. This is calculated by the difference between the observed frequency of the haplotype and the frequency that would be expected if the association occurred randomly (the random frequency is the product of the separate allele frequencies of the antigen). It is not known if the HLA types that show disease associations as shown in Table 9.6 are causally involved or are the markers of as yet unknown antigens occurring in linkage disequilibrium with the known antigen. The HLA disease associations whilst showing in inherited component, do not follow simple Mendelian segregation. It is clear that environmental factors play a role in bringing about the incomplete penetrance of the inherited component.

There is little doubt that as further knowledge is gained of the HLA system, especially of the associated immune response genes (p. 44) and their role in the immune response itself, more insight will be gained into resistance or susceptibility to a variety of neoplastic, autoimmune and infectious diseases of man (see p. 133).

The pathogenesis of autoimmune disease

There is even more uncertainty in this area than exists with respect to the underlying abnormalities and stimuli that induce the autoimmune response.

Autoimmune diseases can be classified as **hypersensitivity** reactions on the basis of the definitions given above (p. 223). These immune reactions, in contrast to those involved in protection from infectious disease, actually bring about severe and sometimes fatal reactions affecting the individual's own tissues and cells. The hypersensitivity reactions are divided into four types and three of these encompass autoimmune reactions.

Cytolytic or cytotoxic (type 2) reactions

The foremost of the autoimmune conditions in this category is autoimmune haemolytic anaemia. Here the antibodies are of two main types: (1) antibodies of the IgM class which agglutinate the patient's own red cells in the cold; (2) antibodies of the IgG class which do not usually bring about direct agglutination of the red cells but can be detected by the Coombs test (p. 279) using an antiglobulin serum.

The anaemia is caused largely by the removal of antibody-coated cells in the spleen or the liver. Only rarely does lysis or agglutination take place to any extent in the circulation and involve the uptake of serum complement. Whilst normal red cells survive with a half-life in the circulation of just over three weeks, in this form of anaemia they are unlikely to have a half-life of more than one week.

Other forms of haemolytic anaemia exist including drug-induced types and those involving infective agents such as mycoplasma. Drugs involved include penicillin, phenacetin, quinine and α-methyldopa. The anaemia is brought about by the reaction of antibody with the drug linked as a hapten to the red cell surface, resulting in haemolysis. The precise details of the haptenic groups responsible for antigenic stimulation and their linkage to the red cell surface are uncertain. In mycoplasma infections the IgM cold agglutinins react with a widely distributed red cell antigen known as the I antigen.

Drug-induced agranulocytosis and thrombocytopoenia have also been described in which the leucocytes or platelets are destroyed by antibody directed at a complex of the drug and cell surface structures. Sedormid purpura has already been mentioned (p. 230).

Toxic-complex (type 3) reactions

Complexes of antibody and tissues antigens, particularly nuclear antigens (Fig. 9.7) are the cause of glomerulonephritis in a number of diseases where a wide range of anti-tissue antibodies is found, and in the similar type of disease of NZB mice. Complexes of antinuclear antibody and nuclear antigen, together with complement, can readily be demonstrated in the glomerular capillaries. The glomerular basement membranes become thickened and secondary changes develop in the renal tubules with progressive renal failure. The role of toxic complexes has been extensively studied in mice infected with lymphocytic choriomeningitis virus (see p. 148). Some strains of mice develop toxic complex nephritis whilst others do not. Current evidence suggests that toxic-complex reactions are most likely to occur in strains of mice that produce low affinity antibodies and thus fail to eliminate antigen effectively. Clearance of immune complexes has been shown in rabbits and monkeys to be related to the number of antigen and antibody molecules in the complex. In strains of mice prone to develop toxic-complex nephritis low affinity antibodies are produced and thus the complexes would have poor lattice structure (p. 272) and would not be cleared from the circulation by phagocytic cells as effectively as larger aggregates.

The mononuclear phagocyte system can remove circulating complexes at the rate of 300 μg/h and tissue fixed complexes within 24 h. The Fc and C3 receptors on the phagocytes bind the complexes and remove them. Another way complexes are removed is by a solubilization by C3b and C4b enzymes. In rheumatoid arthritis such large quantities of complexes are formed in the inflamed synovial membranes that the removal system is over-whelmed. A chronic inflammatory state is thus maintained with infiltration of inflammatory cells and release of mediators such as collagenase and other proteases that damage that joint. Recent work in Edinburgh has identified tumour necrosis factor (TNF) in the synovial fluids in patients with inflammatory joint disease. The various biological activities of the factor (p. 110) may contribute to the pathogenesis of the joint disease.

Cell-mediated (type 4) reactions

There is no doubt that in both man and experimental animals the development of a number of autoimmune states is paralleled by the finding of cell-mediated reactions of the delayed hypersensitivity type as demonstrated by skin tests using tissue antigens. Whether the diseases are actually caused by immune reactions mediated by lymphoid cells is a matter of conjecture. Support for the role of such cells in the disease process comes from studies in an experimental autoimmune disease known as autoimmune allergic encephalomyelitis. This is brought about by immunisation of animals with brain homogenate in Freund's complete adjuvant and paralysis follows demyelination of motor nerve fibres. The disease can be transferred in inbred strains of rats by the injection of lymphoid cells from affected animals to normal animals. The same type of transfer has been performed in autoimmune thyroiditis. In the latter condition it is proposed that the sensitised lymphocytes produce a surface injury to the cells of the thyroid acini and this allows the cytotoxic antibody, frequently present in the serum of affected subjects, to enter the cell and react with intracellular antigens.

That there may be an interaction between cell-mediated immunity and a humoral antibody is emphasized by work on autoimmune orchitis in guinea-pigs. Animals injected with a purified testis homogenate in Freund's complete adjuvant develop cell-mediated immunity (as shown by the development of delayed hypersensitivity on skin testing) but no circulating antibody or testicular lesion. When these animals are injected with anti-testis antibody (from a guinea-pig injected with testis homogenate in incomplete Freund's adjuvant, i.e. without tubercle bacilli) orchitis can be shown to develop. This interpretation is supported by the finding that anti-testis antibody enters the seminiferous tubules (as shown by the indirect fluorescent antibody method, p. 282) at the same time as cell-mediated immunity first appears. Antibody-dependent cell-mediated cytotoxicity is described on page 231. The possibility that this form of reaction occurs in autoimmune states is supported by *in vitro* experimental work, but its role *in vivo* remains to be established.

Other diseases associated with autoimmune states

There is a large reservoir of diseases in which some form of auto-antibody has been found but where neither the stimulus for auto-antibody formation nor the role, if any, of immune reactions has been elucidated.

Among these conditions is rheumatoid arthritis in which an IgM antibody called rheumatoid factor is present in the serum. This antibody is detected in vitro by its ability to agglutinate red cells or latex particles which have been coated with IgG globulin (p. 294). The rheumatoid factor does not appear to be directly involved in the pathogenesis of the disease and no satisfactory explanation has been offered to account for its pathogenesis. The possibility has been suggested that infective agents are involved, such as mycoplasma or chronic infective bacterial agents, and there are reports of the isolation of such agents from rheumatoid joints in man and in arthritis in a number of other species. One suggestion is that the infective agent may modify the lymphoid tissues so that there is a failure of the normal tolerance control mechanisms (see also p. 252 and 254). Experimental arthritis can be induced in rats by the injection of Freund's complete adjuvant containing killed tubercle bacilli. This is a polyarthritis with mononuclear cell infiltration similar to the arthritis found in a human illness known as Reiter's syndrome, the main features of which are urethritis and arthritis and which may occur in the presence of a mycoplasma infection.

Recent evidence suggests that there may be a IgG form of rheumatoid factor present in both the blood and joint fluid of rheumatoid patients as well as the IgM type and that injection of autologous purified IgG into previously unaffected joints can induce actue arthritis. Further evidence suggesting that an antigen-antibody reaction is taking place is provided by the low complement levels found in patient's joint fluid and the presence of immune complexes.

Rheumatoid factors react with the C γ 2 domain of the Fc fragment of IgG (rabbit or human) but not with the Fab fragment. Rheumatoid factors are sometimes found in patients with diseases other than rheumatoid arthritis. These include systemic lupus erythematosus, Sjögren's syndrome, scleroderma, lymphoproliferative disease and in certain persistent bacterial, protozoal and viral infections. Even healthy subjects sometimes have low titres of the factor in their serum, particularly in the older age groups.

The mechanism underlying the appearance of these rheumatoid (anti-globulin) factors is not clear. In chronic infections it is conceivable that the factor is a response to antigenic determinants on the IgG molecule that are exposed when IgG antibody complexes with the infective agent. In the healthy individual a low titre of rheumatoid factor may perhaps serve a physiological function as a way of clearing degraded immunoglobulin molecules arising during infective or inflammatory processes. HLA-B27 individuals who become infected with *Salmonella*, *Yersinia*, *Shigella* and gonococci often develop arthritis, suggesting that HLA-B27 acts in conjunction with the bacterial infection to cause the development of autoantibodies.

Diabetes mellitus of the insulin-dependent type is believed to involve both an inherited susceptibility (p. 133) and environmental factors in the pathogenesis. The details of these interacting factors and their role are poorly understood. Susceptibility to the disease shows linkage to HLA haplotype inheritance within families, whatever the actual HLA phenotypes may be. A child that is of identical HLA phenotype to a diabetic sibling is likely to be susceptible. Autoantibody against pancreatic islet cells is found in 50–80% of these individuals, and when it is of the complement-fixing type, seems to lead to islet cell damage. The antibody appears early in the disease before clinically obvious diabetes and serves as a marker of islet cell damage before progression to insulin insufficiency. This suggests the possibility for development of measures to arrest islet cell destruction before diabetes occurs. More recently an insulin autoantibody has also been found in the prediabetic preinsulin treatment phase.

Multiple sclerosis (MS), another disease believed to have an autoimmune basis, is associated with a variety of HLA antigens (A3, B7, DR2) with DR2 showing the highest relative risk of 4.1 compared with approximately two for each of the other antigens. Subgroups of DR2 also appear to be involved. In a large survey of Canadian MS patients over half were DR2 compared to 28% in controls. Relative risk rates have been estimated as above 5% for siblings of patients and for their parents aunts and uncles. In contrast, it is about 1% for children of patients compared with 0.1% for the population at large. The multifactorial basis of the disease is emphasized by the finding that Lapps and gypsies, over 50% of whom are DR2, have a very low incidence of MS. The increased prevalence of the disease at higher latitudes appears to be accounted for by the percentage of the population of Scandanavian ancestry. Like rheumatoid arthritis the nature of the initiating event is unknown. A number of viruses produce demyelinating disease in animals, such as canine distemper virus, visna virus in sheep and goats and murine encephalitis viruses. This had led to the suggestion that molecular mimicry between viral antigens and host tissue antigens may exist and be responsible for autoimmunization. In a recent report, HTLV-like viral RNA has been found in cells cultured from the c.s.f. of MS patients. The disease in characterized by perivascular cellular infiltrates and demyelination of the white matter of the central nervous system. The plaques that are formed show a depletion of oligodendroglial cells and proliferation of astrocytes. Evidence for a possible immune pathogenesis comes from the finding of macrophage-like cells with lipid inclusions and lymphoid cells in these lesions. Identification of the cell types has become possible using monoclonal antibodies to a variety of cell surface markers. Large numbers of cells bearing HLA-DR (la) antigens are present at the edges of the plaques decreasing towards the centre. T helper, T cytotoxic and T suppressor cells have also been found both around and within the plaques but no ,B cells. These findings, along with the additional presence of interleukin-1 and prostaglandin E2, suggest that an active immune process is taking place in the lesions of multiple sclerosis. These findings in humans are supported by extensive evidence from work with animal models of the disease in which demyelination can be induced by immunization with myelin basic protein and in which susceptibility can be transferred to normal animals by spleen cells of the immunized donors. More recently, T cell clones have been developed with specificity for myelin basic protein that produce typical disease in rats.

Myasthenia gravis associated with HLA B8 and DRw3, relative risk 3.4 and 3.0 respectively, is a neuromuscular disease characterized by muscle weakness and fatigability. There is a marked reduction of acetylcholine receptors at the postsynaptic membrane that is associated with antibody to the receptor acting together with complement. In experimental models of the disease in mice, monoclonal antibodies to L3T4 murine helper T lymphocytes suppressed established disease and prevented loss of acetyl choline receptors. Similar approaches have been applied to mouse models of systemic lupus, experimental autoimmune encephalomyelitis and collagen-induced arthritis. An interesting development is the use of monoclonal antibodies against a single T cell clone specific for myelin basic protein that appears to protect rats from the development of experimental autoimmune encephalitis.

Although the possible side effects of therapy that is directed at lymphocyte subpopulations (e.g. susceptibility to infection) are unknown it seems likely that this approach will be tested in patients with severe life-threatening forms of autoimmune disease in which other forms of therapy have proved ineffective.

Table 9.7 Examples of autoantibodies in disease

Disease	Autoantibody specificity
Autoimmune haemolytic anaemia	erythrocytes
Thrombocytopenic purpura	platelets
Systemic lupus erythematosus	nuclear antigens and antigens of various tissues and blood cells
Rheumatoid arthritis	immunoglobulin G
Primary biliary cirrhosis	mitochondria
Ulcerative colitis	colon lipopolysaccharide
Hashimoto's thyroiditis	thyroglobulin
Thyrotoxicosis	Cell surface thyroid stimulating hormone (TSH) receptors
Pernicious anaemia	intrinsic factor
Myasthenia gravis	acetylcholine receptors (and certain muscle tissue)
Juvenile diabetes (type 1)	islet cell surface

Table 9.7 gives some examples of autoimmune diseases and the autoantibodies found.

Antibodies as a consequence of tissue damage

In considering the role of autoantibodies as a possible cause of autoimmune disease it should be remembered that antibodies of IgM type, directed at subcellular antigens, can be readily induced by various forms of tissue damage. These arise secondarily to the damage and appear to have no role in perpetuating it. Antibodies of this type have been shown in the author's laboratory and can readily be induced in rats by the injection of the hepatotoxic agent carbon tetrachloride. It was subsequently found that normal rats, mice and hamsters have some IgM anti-tissue antibody in their serum. A possible physiological role for these antibodies is suggested by the finding in vitro of a chemotactic effect on rat polymorphs of a mixture of the antitissue antibody and its antigen. Thus the antibody might be responsible for initiating a phagocytic cell clearing process to deal with the breakdown products of normal cell turnover.

Recent evidence indicates that IgG antibody existing in the normal individual seems to be able to recognise glycoprotein determinants which appear on aged red blood cells. These determinants are exposed following the loss of sialic acid groups from the outside of the cells on ageing. Their exposure can be reproduced experimentally by treatment with neuraminidase. The IgG antibodies bind to the exposed glycoprotein and enable the attachment of the red cell to the Fc receptors on a macrophage. The aged red cell is then phagocytosed and destroyed by the lysosomal enzymes of the macrophage.

All autoantibodies are therefore not necessarily autoregressive, although the history of immunity and protection inculcates the idea of antibodies acting solely as aggressive agents.

FURTHER READING

Hypersensitivity states
Austen F J, Block K J 1972 Biochemistry of acute allergic reactions. Blackwell, Oxford
Brostoff J 1973 Atopic allergy. British Journal of Hospital Medicine 9:29
Cream J J 1973 Immune complex diseases. British Journal of Hospital Medicine 9:8
Cochrane C G, Koffler D 1973 Immune complex disease in experimental animals and man. Advances in Immunology 18:185

Dale M M, Foreman J C 1984 Textbook of immunopharmacology. Blackwell Scientific Publications, Oxford

Ishizaka K 1984 Mast cell activation and mediator release. Progress in Allergy, vol 34. Karger, Basle

Lachmann P J, Peters D K 1982 Clinical aspects of immunology, 4th edn. Blackwell, Oxford.

Turk J L 1967a Delayed hypersensitivity. In: Neuberger A, Tatum E L (eds) Frontiers in biology. North Holland, Amsterdam, vol 4

Turk J L 1967b Delayed hypersensitivity — specific cell-mediated immunity. British Medical Bulletin 23(1)

Turk J L 1969 Immunology in clinical medicine. Heinemann, London

Uhr J W 1966 Delayed hypersensitivity. Physiological Review 46:359

Immune deficiency states

Ammann A J, Fudenberg H H 1976 In: Fudenberg H H, Stites D P, Caldwell J L, Wells J V (eds) Basic and clinical immunology. Lange, Los Altos

Asherson G L, Webster A D B 1980 Diagnosis and treatment of immunodeficiency diseases. Blackwell, Oxford

Lachmann P J, Peters D K 1982 Clinical aspects of immunology, 4th edn. Blackwell, Oxford

Martin N H 1970 The paraproteinaemias. British Journal of Hospital Medicine 3:662

Turk J L 1969 Immunology in clinical medicine. Heinemann, London

Waldenstrom J G 1968 Monoclonal and polyclonal hypergammaglobulinemia — clinical and biological significance. Cambridge University Press

Autoimmunity

Asherson G L 1968a The role of microorganisms in autoimmune responses. Progress in Allergy 12:192

Asherson G L 1968a Autoantibody production as a breakdown of immune tolerance. In: Cinader B (ed) Regulation of the antibody response. Thomas, Springfield, Illinois, p 68

Burnet F M 1959 The clonal selection theory of acquired immunity. Cambridge University Press

Chapel H, Maeney M 1984 Essentials of clinical immunology. Blackwell Scientific Publications, Oxford

Cudworth A G 1980 Current concepts in the aetiology of type 1 (insulin-dependent) diabetes mellitus. In: Bellingham A J (ed) Advanced medicine 16. Pitman, London, p 123

Freedman S O, Gold P 1979 Clinical immunology, 2nd edn. Harper and Row, London

Gupta S, Talal N 1986 Immunology of rheumatic diseases. Plenum Publishing Corporation, New York

Holborow E J (ed) 1981 Clinics in immunology and allergy. Autoimmunity. W B Saunders, Philadelphia

Irvine W J (ed) 1979 Medicial immunology. Teviot Scientific Publications, Edinburgh

Lachmann P J, Peters D K (eds) 1982 Clinical aspects of immunology. Blackwell, Oxford

Levy J A 1974 Autoimmunity and neoplasia: the possible role of C-type viruses. American Journal of Clinical Pathology 62:258

McDevitt H C, Bodmer F 1974 HL-A, immune response genes and disease. Lancet 1:1269

Marmion B P 1976 A microbiologist's view of investigative rheumatology. In: Dumonde D C (ed) Infection and immunology in the rheumatic diseases. Blackwell Oxford, p 245

Marmion B P, MacKay J M K 1977 Rheumatoid arthritis and the viral hypothesis. Bayer symposium VI: Experimental models of chronic inflammatory diseases. Springer-Verlag, Berlin, p 188

Moller G 1975 HLA and disease. Transplant Review 22:2

Samter M 1965 Immunologic diseases. Little Brown, Boston

Talal N, Fyek M 1976 Autoimmunity. In: Fudenberg H H, Stites D P, Caldwell J L, Wells J V (eds) Basic and clinical immunology. Lange, Los Altos

Taussig M J 1984 Processes in pathology and microbiology, 2nd edn. Blackwell Scientific Publications, Oxford

Trentin J J 1967 Cross-reacting antigens and neo-antigens (with implications for autoimmunity and cancer immunity). Williams and Wilkins, Baltimore

Turk J L 1969 Immunology in clinical medicine. Heinemann, London

Weir D M, Elson C J 1969 Anti-tissue antibodies and immunological tolerance to self. Arthritis and Rheumatism 12:254

Willoughby D A, Giroud J P (eds) 1980 Inflammation mechanisms and treatment. MTP Press, London

World Health Organisation 1977 Immune complexes in disease. Report of a WHO scientific group. WHO, Technical report series no. 606

10

Interaction of antibody with antigen and applications in laboratory investigations

Objectives

On completion of this section the reader will be able to:

1. Describe the difference between the primary interaction of antigen and antibody and the secondary effects of this union.

2. With the aid of a diagram, describe a precipitation reaction in terms of optimal proportions.

3. Give two examples of immunodiffusion in gels.

4. Describe agglutination and give three examples of practical applications.

5. Outline the stages in a complement fixation test.

6. Describe an antiglobulin test and explain how the same principle is used in the fluorescent antibody techniques and the ELISA test.

7. Describe the principle of radioimmunoassay.

8. Give four examples of the use of antibody-antigen reactions in the clinical laboratory.

9. Describe, with examples, the investigation of immune deficiency states.

10 Give two methods for the detection of immune complexes.

An antibody, as has been pointed out, is an immunoglobulin molecule secreted into the tissue fluids from lymphoid cells which have been exposed to a foreign substance — an antigen. An antigen may be potentially harmful, such as bacterium or virus, or it may be a harmless bland substance such as foreign serum protein. The antibody can combine only with antigen which is identical or nearly identical with the inducing antigen and not with unrelated antigens. When molecules of antibody and antigen are brought together in solution, they interact with each other by the formation of a link between an antigen-binding site on the immunoglobulin molecule — part of the Fab fragment — and the particular chemical groupings which make up what is termed the antigenic determinant of the antigen molecule. The molecules are held together by **non-covalent intermolecular forces** which are effective only when the antigen-binding site and the antigenic determinant group are able to make close contact. The better the fit, the closer the contact and the stronger the antigen-antibody bond. These factors determine what is often called the **affinity** of the antibody molecule. Antibodies of varying combining quality exist and the overall tendency to combine with antigen is the average ability of the antibodies to combine with antigen or the average intrinsic association constant. This can be calculated experimentally by application of the concepts of chemical equilibria to antigen-antibody interactions. Studies of this type have shown that the affinity of antibodies increases as immunization proceeds and that the dose of antigen can influence the quality of antibody (see p. 84).

The methods used for the detection of antigen-antibody reactions in the laboratory fall in two functional groups: first, procedures designed to elucidate the cytodynamics of antibody formation which involve the study of the behaviour of single cells or small populations of cells; the second group, which is the subject of the present discussion, concerns the detection and quantitation of **secreted antibody** circulating in the blood or present in the tissue fluids.

The methods used here range in their application from highly specialized studies of the physico-chemical aspects of antigen-antibody interaction to widely used procedures designed to aid in the diagnosis of disease.

PRIMARY INTERACTION AND SECONDARY EFFECTS

In practical terms, the union of antibody with antigen can be detected at two different levels. The first level is that following **primary union** of the two reactants and usually requires that one or other reactant is labelled with a suitable marker such as a fluorescent dye or a radioactive isotope. A simple example of this is the microscopic localization in a tissue of a particular microorganism utilising an antiserum prepared against the microorganism and labelled with a dye that fluoresces under u.v. light. A widely used method in experimental immunology makes use of the fact that immunoglobulins are insoluble in 50% saturated ammonium sulphate. The test developed by Farr uses antigen labelled with ^{131}I

that is mixed with antibody-containing serum and left to equilibrate. Ammonium sulphate solution is then added to the mixture resulting in the precipitation of the antibody together with any labelled antigen bound to it. The unbound antigen remains in solution (only antigens that are themselves soluble in 50% ammonium sulphate can be used in this form of the test). The quantity of isotope-labelled antigen bound to the salt-precipitated antibody is then estimated by placing the washed precipitate in radioactive counting equipment. This sensitive and useful technique is a measure of the capacity of an antiserum to bind antigen.

The second level at which antigen-antibody combination can be detected depends on the development, after primary union, of certain changes in the physical state of the complex, resulting in precipitation or agglutination of the components or, alternatively, in the activation of non-antibody components such as serum complement or histamine from mast cells. Reactions of this type occurring subsequent to primary union are termed **secondary phenomena**. This discussion is concerned with the principles of a few of these secondary phenomena that are in common use.

Secondary effects; interpretation and applications

Before considering these reactions individually, it is important to be aware of the difficulties in interpreting results of such tests. The initiation and development of the secondary phenomena constitute a complicated series of events involving many variables such as the type of antibody taking part, the relative proportions of antibody and antigen, characteristics of the antigen molecule, presence of electrolytes, inhibitory substances and unstable components.

Despite these formidable difficulties, the widely and long-used secondary phenomena such as precipitation, agglutination and complement fixation have an important role to play as aids in the diagnosis of disease and in the identification of microorganisms.

The secondary phenomena can bring about several readily observable changes when carried out in vitro. These are used in tests to demonstrate the presence of antibody in the sera of patients suffering from infectious disease, or producing an antibody response to cell antigens as might, for example, occur after incompatible blood transfusion, tissue grafting or in autoimmune states.

Reactions of this type can also be used to identify antigens in the tissues or body fluids and, for example, would be utilized for blood grouping, tissue typing or the identification of microorganisms.

Among the most important of these reactions are **precipitation,** which occurs between antibody and antigen molecules in soluble form; **agglutination,** in which the antibodies directed against surface antigens of particulate materials such as microorganisms or erythrocytes, link them together in large clumps or aggregates; and **complement fixation** in which antibody molecules, after reaction with antigen, activate the complex blood components that make up serum complement.

In addition to these widely used serological tests, a number of other effects of antigen-antibody interaction are of medical importance. These include **neutralization** tests used for example in virus identification, **immobilization** tests with bacteria and protozoa and **skin tests** for the reaginic antibody characteristic of anaphylactic states.

Precipitation

Optimal proportions

As a result of the interaction of antibody and antigen molecules in solution, complexes of the two types of molecule will form and precipitation may occur depending on the relative concentration of the two reactants. If a series of tubes is set up (Fig. 10.1), each containing a constant amount of antiserum, and decreasing amounts of antigen are added to the tubes in the row, a haziness will start to appear in the tubes gradually increasing to clearly visible **aggregates** or **precipitates**. The amount of precipitation will

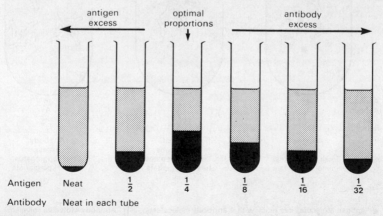

| | antigen excess | | | optimal proportions ↓ | | antibody excess | | |

| Antigen | Neat | $\frac{1}{2}$ | | $\frac{1}{4}$ | $\frac{1}{8}$ | $\frac{1}{16}$ | $\frac{1}{32}$ |
| Antibody | Neat in each tube | | | | | | |

Fig. 10.1

be seen to increase along the row, reaching a maximum and then falling off with the lower antigen concentration. The tubes where most precipitate appears contain the **optimal proportions** of antigen and antibody for precipitation. The composition of the precipitate varies with the original proportions of the antibody and antigen; if antigen is in excess the precipitate will contain relatively more of this component and similarly more antibody if it is present in excess. As can be seen from Figure 10.2, on the antigen excess side of optimal proportions less precipitate appears. This is due to the inability of the antigen-antibody complexes formed to link up to other complexes and so makes a large aggregate or lattice which will appear as a visible precipitate (tube 1, Fig. 10.2). Large aggregates of antibody and antigen can form best under conditions of optimal proportions where the antibody and antigen proportions are such that after initial combination of the molecules, free antigen-binding sites and antigen determinant groups remain, enabling the complexes to link up into a large lattice formation (as in tube 2 of Fig. 10.2). In antibody excess all the free determinants of the antigen molecule are soon taken up with antibody, so that very little linking can take place between the complexes (as in tube 3 of Fig. 10.2).

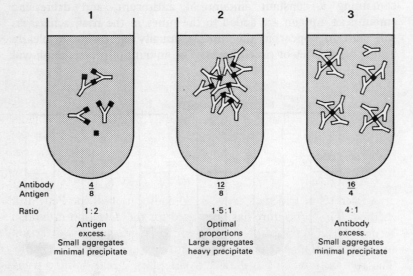

	1	2	3
Antibody	4	12	16
Antigen	8	8	4
Ratio	1:2	1·5:1	4:1
	Antigen excess. Small aggregates minimal precipitate	Optimal proportions Large aggregates heavy precipitate	Antibody excess. Small aggregates minimal precipitate

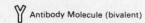

■ Antigen Molecule (can react with 4 antibody molecules)   Ɏ Antibody Molecule (bivalent)

Fig. 10.2

Applications

The precipitin test can be carried out in a quantitative manner by estimating the protein content of the precipitate at optimal proportions. The qualitative test is much more widely used and is of considerable value in detecting and identifying antigens, having applications in the typing of streptococci or pneumococci. This is done by layering an extract of the organism over antiserum. After a short while, a ring of precipitate forms at the interface (this is called the ring test). The technique is also used in forensic studies and in detecting adulteration of foodstuffs. A modification of the test in which precipitation is allowed to occur in **agar gel** is very widely used for detecting the presence of antibody in serum or antigen in unknown preparations, and is valuable for showing the identity of different antigen preparations (Fig. 10.3). A concentration gradient forms in the gel, the concentration of a substance decreasing as the molecules diffuse away from the well in which they were placed. **Precipitin bands** form in the gel in the position where the antigen and antibody molecules reach optimal proportions after diffusion.

When a large number of different antigens are present in a solution, it is difficult to separate the precipitin bands for each of the antigen-antibody reactions by the simple gel-diffusion method just described. In such a situation, a variation of this method can be used to identify the individual components. This modification is particularly valuable in analysing a multicomponent system such as serum. The individual components of serum are first separated by electrophoresis in agar gel and an antiserum, prepared against the serum, is allowed to diffuse towards the separated components, resulting in the formation of precipitin bands (Fig. 10.4). This method, known as **immunoelectrophoresis**, is particularly valuable for showing the presence of abnormal globulin constituents in the serum of patients with myelomatosis and other serum protein abnormalities.

A microimmunodiffusion test with wells cut in a layer of agar on a microscope slide is a convenient modification of the Petri dish method. This procedure has been used for the detection in human serum of the **hepatitis B antigen** which is associated with serum hepatitis although a radioimmunoassay (see below) is now available. The routine screening of blood products by this technique using specific antisera prepared in animals is likely to become an important laboratory test in the prevention of serum hepatitis outbreaks.

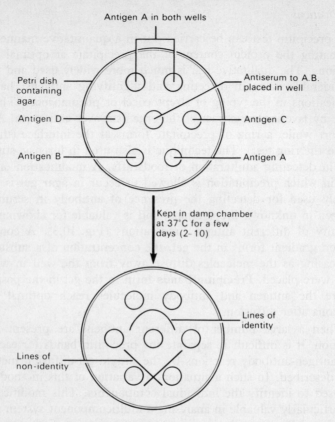

Fig. 10.3 Immunodiffusion or gel diffusion test. Wells are cut in a layer of agar in a Petri dish. Antiserum and antigen solutions are placed opposite each other in the wells and after allowing a few days for diffusion to take place precipitin bands will form where antibody and antigen meet in suitable proportions (optimal proportions). No reactions take place with antigens C and D as the antiserum in the central well contains antibodies only for antigens A and B. Lines of identity as formed between the two A wells enable the technique to be used for identifying unknown antigens

Instead of placing antibody and antigen in separate wells and allowing them to diffuse towards each other, the antibody can be incorporated in the agar and the antigen placed in wells. This technique is known as **single radial immunodiffusion** and depends upon diffusion of antigen from the well until a point is reached where the concentration is optimal for precipitation to occur. Close to the antigen well the concentration of antigen will be high and although the antigen will combine with antibody in the agar, the

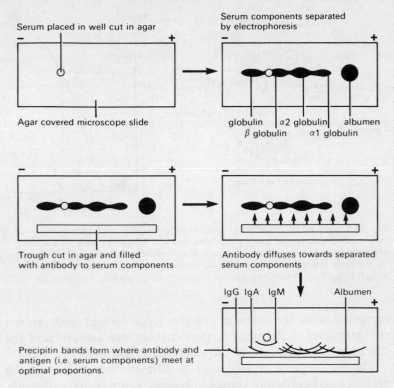

Serum placed in well cut in agar

Agar covered microscope slide

Serum components separated by electrophoresis

globulin | α2 globulin | albumen
β globulin | α1 globulin

Trough cut in agar and filled with antibody to serum components

Antibody diffuses towards separated serum components

IgG IgA IgM Albumen

Precipitin bands form where antibody and antigen (i.e. serum components) meet at optimal proportions.

Fig. 10.4 Immunoelectrophoresis. The antigen, for example, serum, is placed in a small well cut in a layer of agar on a microscope slide. A direct current is applied and differential migration of the serum components takes place. (They are not normally visible in the agar and will show up only if suitably stained.) After electrophoresis for an hour or so, a trough is cut longitudinally in the agar and an antiserum against the electrophoresed antigen is placed in the trough. The two components diffuse towards each other and precipitin bands form. These can be shown up more clearly by staining with a protein stain. This is a very powerful analytic technique and can show up about 30 different components in human serum compared with 4 or 5 by electrophoresis

complexes will be unable to form the large lattice structure necessary for precipitation to take place (Fig. 10.2) and will thus remain as soluble complexes. The precipitin band that forms at optimal proportions of antigen and antibody will show up as a ring around the antigen well. The distance the ring forms from the antigen well will be dependent on the concentration of the antigen in the well. In practice the **diameter** of the ring is measured around a well containing an unknown concentration of antigen and this is

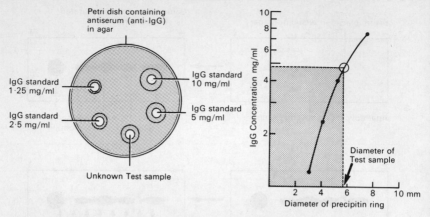

Fig. 10.5 Diagram of single radial immunodiffusion plate with antiserum incorporated in agar and antigen dilutions and test sample in wells. Reference graph drawn using three concentrations of antigen standard showing the diameter of precipitin ring obtained with each concentration (●). Diameter of unknown sample (○) when plotted enables determination of its antigen concentration

compared with the diameter of the rings formed with known concentrations of the antigen, thus enabling the estimation of the concentration of antigen in the unknown preparation.

This technique is widely used to estimate the quantity of the various immunoglobulin classes in human serum samples. An antiserum to a particular immunologloglobulin class (e.g. IgG) is incorporated in the agar and test serum sample is placed in a well. The diameter of the precipitation band that forms after incubation is then compared to the diameter obtained with standard IgG preparations of known concentration. The diameters of the rings with the **standard** IgG preparations (e.g. three or four dilutions of a known concentration) can be plotted graphically against the concentration of IgG and the diameter obtained with the unknown sample can be read of against concentration on this reference graph (Fig. 10.5)

Agglutination

In this reaction the antigen is part of the surface of some particulate material such as a red cell, bacterium or perhaps an inorganic particle (e.g. polystyrene latex) which has been coated with antigen. Antibody added to a suspension of such particles combines with the surface antigens and links them together to form clearly-

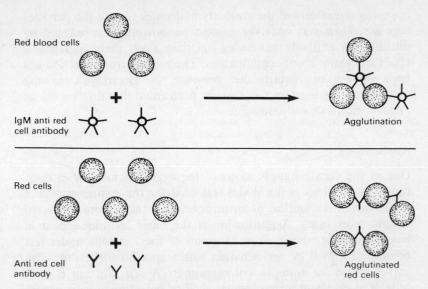

Fig. 10.6 Agglutination reaction. The IgM molecule, with at least five antigen-binding sites, is particularly effective in bringing about agglutination

visible aggregates or **agglutinates** (Fig. 10.6). In its simplest form an agglutination test is set up in round-bottomed test tubes or perspex plates with round-bottomed wells and doubling dilutions of the antiserum are made up in the tubes (neat, 1:2, 1:4, 1:8, etc). The particulate antigen in then added and after incubation at 37°C agglutination is seen in the bottom of the tubes. The last tube showing clearly visible agglutination is the end point of the test. The reciprocal of the antiserum at the end point, e.g. 1/256, is known as the the **titre** of the antiserum and is a measure of the number of antibody units per unit volume of serum, e.g. if the end point occurs at a 1/256 dilution of the antiserum and if the test has been carried out in 1 ml volumes, the titre of the serum in 256 units per ml of serum.

One practical difficulty of importance in agglutination tests is the occasional inhibition of agglutination in the first tubes of an anti-serum dilution series, agglutination occurring only in those tubes containing more dilute antiserum. This is known as the **prozone phenomenon** and is probably, in part, due to the stabilising effects of high protein concentration on the particles. The protein coats the particles, increases their net charge and so brings about increased electrostatic repulsion between individual particles, thus opposing the efforts of the antibody molecules to link the particles together. However, once the protein concentration is reduced by dilution the antibody molecules can then exert their aggregating effect and bring about agglutination. The agglutination reaction has been shown to require the presence of electrolytes in the suspending medium and is usually performed for this reason at physiological salt concentration.

Applications

One of the classical applications of the agglutination test in diagnostic bacteriology is the **Widal test** used for the demonstration of antibodies to salmonellae in serum specimens taken from suspected enteric fever cases. Agglutination is the basic technique used in blood grouping, the A, B or O group of the red cells under test being determined by agglutination with a specific antiserum — an anti-A serum for example will agglutinate A cells but not B or O cells. Red cells and inert particles such as polystyrene latex can be coated with various antigens and suitably coated particles are used in a variety of diagnostic tests such as thyroid antibody tests using thyroglobulin-coated cells or latex particles. Hormone-coated red cells or inert particles are used in many hormone assay procedures which are based on the inhibition of the antibody-induced agglutination of the hormone-coated particles by hormone added in the sample under test (Fig. 10.7). Tests of this type are in wide use in pregnancy diagnosis.

Certain viruses, e.g. the myxoviruses causing influenza and mumps, have the property of bringing about agglutination of red cells (haemagglutination). **Inhibition of haemagglutination** by antibody in patient's serum is a widely-used diagnostic procedure. The presence of antibody in the patient's serum is thus detected by its ability to link with virus particles and prevent them from bringing about agglutination of the red cells (Fig. 10.8).

IgM antibodies capable of agglutinating human red cells (including those of the individual producing the antibody) between 0° and 4°C are sometimes found in certain human diseases including primary atypical pneumonia, malaria, trypanosomiasis and acquired haemolytic anaemia.

The presence of antibody globulin on a red cell many not result in direct agglutination of the cells, for example in some Rh-negative mothers with Rh-positive infants or in acquired haemolytic

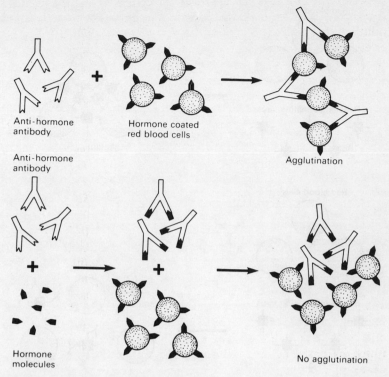

Fig. 10.7 Principle of hormone assay by agglutination inhibition. Red cells coated with hormone are agglutinable by anti-hormone antibody. The addition to the antiserum of a test sample containing free hormone will block the antigen-binding sites and prevent agglutination. The test can be carried out quantitatively by comparing the activity of a known standard hormone preparation with the test sample

anaemia. It is, however, possible to show that the red cells are coated with antibody by using an **antiglobulin** serum (produced in the rabbit by injecting human globulin) which will bring about agglutination of the cells (Fig. 10.9). This is the basis of the Coombs test which is a very widely used serological procedure. The coagulation test depends on the presence of protein A (p. 125) on *Staph. aureus* (Cowan strain 1) that binds to the Fc region of IgG leaving the Fab sites free. Staphylococci with specific antibody attached in this way can be used to detect bacteria in serum or urine or microbial antigens in such fluids. Clumping of the staphylococci indicates a positive test.

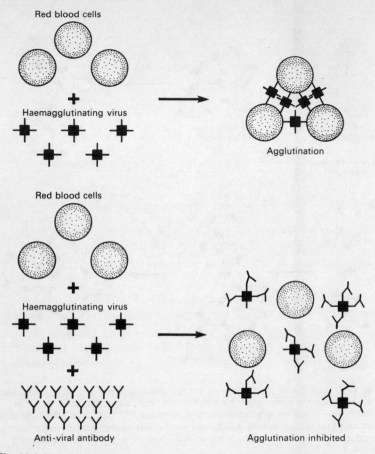

Fig. 10.8 Virus haemagglutination inhibition test. Red cell agglutination is brought about by a variety of viruses (see text). This can be inhibited by mixing the virus with anti-viral antibody as shown in the diagram. The test can be quantitated by comparison of serial dilutions of virus alone and virus-antibody mixture

Complement fixation

The fact that antibody, once it combines with antigen, is able to activate the complement system is used as a way of showing the presence of a particular antibody in a serum, e.g. the **Wassermann** antibody in syphilis, or in identifying an antigen such as a virus.

The complement of most species will react with antibody derived from other species and guinea-pig serum is a common laboratory source of complement. Some of the components of complement are heat-labile are destroyed by heating at 56°C for 20 to 30 minutes.

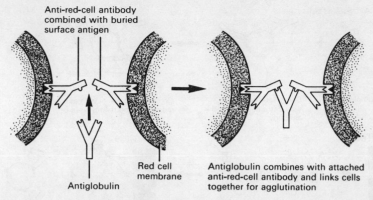

Anti-red-cell antibody
combined with buried
surface antigen

Antiglobulin

Red cell
membrane

Antiglobulin combines with attached
anti-red-cell antibody and links cells
together for agglutination

Fig. 10.9 Coombs antiglobulin test. The red cell antibody, probably because it is directed against an antigen situated deep in the cell wall, cannot link two red cells together for agglutination. The addition of an antiglobulin serum brings about agglutination by linking two attached immunoglobulins to one another

The individual components of the complement system are taken up by the antigen-antibody complex in a particular order and destruction of the heat-labile components which are taken up early prevents the remaining components from taking part (see p. 25).

For most antigens the reaction of the complement system with the antigen-antibody complex causes in itself no visible effect, and it is necessary to use an indicator system consisting of sheep red cells coated with anti-sheep red cell antibody. Complement has the ability to lyse the antibody-coated cells, probably by virtue of the esterase activity of one of the components acting on the red cell membrane. In a test the antibody, complement and antigen are first mixed together and after a period of incubation the indicator system, antibody-coated sheep cells, are added. The complement will, however, have been taken up during the incubation stage by the original antibody-antigen complex and will not be available to lyse the red cells. Thus, a **positive** complement fixation test is indicated by **absence of lysis** of the red cells whilst a negative test, with unused complement, is shown by lysis of the red cells (Fig. 10.10).

Applications

The classical complement fixation test is the Wassermann reaction used in the diagnosis of syphilis. The test system consists of Wassermann antigen mixed with dilutions of the patient's serum in the presence of guinea-pig complement. After the antigen and

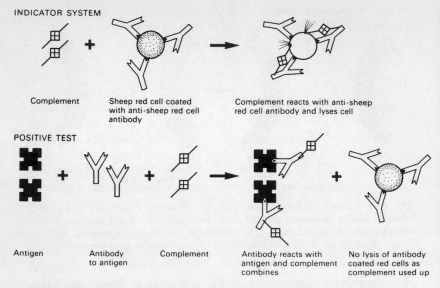

INDICATOR SYSTEM

Complement | Sheep red cell coated with anti-sheep red cell antibody | Complement reacts with anti-sheep red cell antibody and lyses cell

POSITIVE TEST

Antigen | Antibody to antigen | Complement | Antibody reacts with antigen and complement combines | No lysis of antibody coated red cells as complement used up

Fig. 10.10 Complement-fixation test. The indicator system (sheep red cells coated with antibody to sheep red cells) is normally lysed in the presence of complement (fresh guinea-pig serum) — top. If another antibody-antigen system is first mixed with the complement it will no longer be available to lyse the indicator system — bottom

patient's serum have had time to react and take up the limited amount of complement available in the system, the indicator system is added to show whether or not there is free complement. Controls are included to ensure that none of the reagents are anti-complementary (able to take up complement nonspecifically as might, for example, occur with contaminated serum) and positive and negative control sera are tested in parallel. Complement fixation tests are used routinely for detecting viruses in tissue cultures which have been inoculated with specimens of blood or tissue fluids from humans with probable virus infections.

Antigen-antibody reactions using fluorescent labels

The precise localization of tissue antigens or the antigens of infecting organisms in the body, of anti-tissue antibody and of antigen-antibody complexes was achieved by the introduction of the use of fluorochrome-labelled proteins by Coons and Kaplan in 1950. The adsorption of ultraviolet light between 290 and 495 nm by fluorescein and its emission of longer wavelength green light (525 nm) is used to visualize protein labelled with this dye. The technique is more sensitive than precipitation or complement fixation techniques, and fluorescent protein tracers can be detected at a concentration of the order of 1 μg protein per ml body fluid.

Applications

Some of the uses to which the technique has been put include the localization of the origin of a variety of serum protein components, for example immunoglobulin production by plasma cells and other lymphoid cells. The demonstration and localization in the tissues of antibody globulin in a variety of autoimmune conditions has been shown, including an antinuclear antibody in the serum of patients with systemic lupus erythematosus and thyroid autoantibodies in the sera of patients with Hashimoto's thyroiditis. In the diagnostic field most human pathogens can be demonstrated by immunofluorescence and a tentative diagnosis may be made much sooner than by cultivation. The fluorescent method at present can be used to supplement rather then replace conventional methods.

There are two main procedures in use, the direct and indirect methods (Fig. 10.11). The **direct method** consists of bringing fluorescein-tagged antibodies into contact with antigens fixed on a

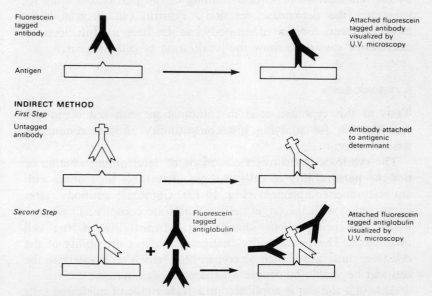

Fig. 10.11 Fluorescent antibody technique — direct and indirect methods. The indirect method can be seen to be more sensitive as two or more fluorescein-tagged antiglobulin molecules can be attached to each immunoglobulin molecule bound to its antigen

slide (e.g. in the form of a tissue section or a smear of an organism), allowing them to react, washing off excess antibody and examining under the u.v. light microscope. The site of union of the labelled antibody with its antigen can be seen by the apple-green fluorescent areas on the slide. The **indirect method** can be used both for detecting specific antibodies in sera or other body fluids and also for identifying antigens. This method differs from the direct method in the use of a non-labelled antiserum which is layered on first, in the same way as described above. Whether or not this antiserum has reacted with the material on the slide is shown by means of a fluorescein-tagged **antiglobulin serum** specific for the globulin of the serum applied first. Such an antiglobulin serum can be used to detect antibody globulin in sera to a variety of different antigens which gives it a considerable advantage over the direct test; it is also more sensitive.

Other types of labelled antibody test have been developed on the same principles as the fluorescent methods. Horseradish peroxidase can readily be linked to antibody leaving the antibody still able to combine with its antigen. After this has occurred (e.g. in a tissue section layered with the peroxidase-labelled antibody and then washed) the site of localization of the antibody can be visualized by conventional histochemical staining of the peroxidase using its substrate (the peroxidase reaction). Ferritin (an electron-dense blood pigment) conjugated antibody has also been used in electron-microscope studies to show the localization of cell antigens.

Cytotoxic tests

Tests of this type are used in combination with red blood cell agglutination for studying histocompatibility antigen systems in tissue typing.

The cytotoxic test consists essentially of determining whether or not the **permeability** of cells changes after their incubation with antibody and complement (Fig. 10.12). Cytotoxic antibody, after combination with the target cell, will activate complement compo-nents and bring about changes in permeability of the cell membrane. The permeability changes can affect the ability of the cell to exclude a dye such as trypan blue which will penetrate the cell and be visible by simple microscopic examination.

Although the test is applicable to a wide range of nucleated cells and is the test of choice with blood leucocytes, it is rather less sensitive than the red cell haemagglutination tests and more labori-ous to perform.

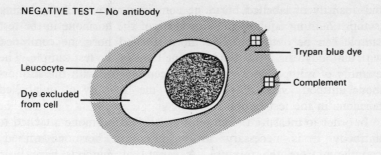

NEGATIVE TEST—No antibody

Leucocyte

Dye excluded from cell

Trypan blue dye

Complement

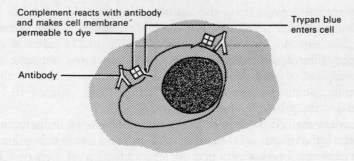

POSITIVE TEST—Antibody present

Complement reacts with antibody and makes cell membrane permeable to dye

Antibody

Trypan blue enters cell

Fig. 10.12 Cytotoxic test

Radioimmunoassay methods

Increasing use has been made over the last few years of immuno-logically based assay methods for the accurate quantitative estimation of **polypeptide hormones**. These methods offer a unique combination of specificity, precision and simplicity and are already available for the assay of some 14 of the 20 or so polypeptide hormones in man. Monoclonal antibodies are now used extensively in the tests.

The principle of the assay methods is that radio-iodine labelled (purified) hormone competes with the non-labelled hormone of a sample under test, for the antihormone antibody with which the labelled and non-labelled hormone are mixed. The more of the hormone in the test sample the less chance the labelled hormone has of combining with the limited number of antibody molecules that are available in the antihormone serum. Thus by measuring the quantity of labelled hormone combined with antibody (using isotope counting equipment) a measure of the hormone in the test sample can be obtained. The more labelled hormone combined with antibody, the lower the hormone level in the test sample. The quantity of isotope labelled hormone complexing with the antihormone antibody varies inversely with the quantity of unlabelled hormone in the test sample.

In order to measure the amount of labelled hormone attached to antibody it is necessary to separate the hormone-antibody complexes from the mixture. A variety of methods have been developed to achieve this, perhaps the most common being electrophoretic separation. Provided the **free** hormone has a different electrophoretic mobility from the antibody globulin then separation of hormone **bound** to antibody is straightforward. Other methods of separation depend upon the antibody being linked to an insoluble support (e.g. cellulose). The insoluble complex is then mixed with labelled and test hormone (tube 1, Fig. 10.13), allowed to interact (tube 2, Fig. 10.13) and later the unreacted hormone is removed and the amount of labelled hormone attached to the insoluble complex is measured (tube 3, Fig. 10.13). Figure 10.14 illustrates the principle of these assays.

An assay for IgE levels in serum has been developed using iodine labelled IgE and anti-IgE linked to cellulose, and assays using these principles are being developed for the detection of hepatitis B antigen in human serum.

Immunoassays using enzyme-linked antibody or antigen

Enzyme-linked immunosorbent assay (ELISA)

Labels other than radioactive isotopes and fluorescent dyes can be linked on to antibody or antigen molecules. There has been recent interest in the use of enzymes such as horseradish peroxidase or alkaline phosphatase linked to antibody or antigen molecules. The presence of the enzyme linked molecule is detected by means of the enzyme substrate and can be measured by spectrophotometry. Either the labelled antigen or the antibody can be attached to an insoluble support, such as plastic beads or plastic agglutination plates. After the material has attached and the excess has been washed away, enzyme-linked antigen or antibody is added, together with the test substance. The antigen or antibody (whichever is

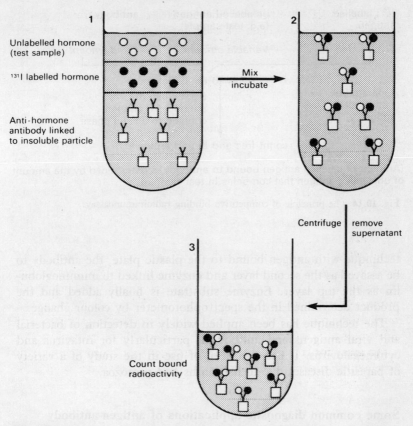

Fig. 10.13 Illustration of the use of antihormone antibody linked to an insoluble particle for the assay of the amount of hormone in a test sample. The quantity of ^{131}I labelled hormone complexing with the anti-hormone antibody varies inversely with the amount of unlabelled hormone in the test sample. A standard curve can be prepared using known concentrations of purified hormone in the same way as illustrated in Fig. 10.5. This will enable the result obtained with the test sample to be plotted and its concentration obtained

being measured) in the test solution competes with the added labelled antigen or antibody reagent for the material attached to the plastic plates. The amount of enzyme-labelled reagent can then be estimated by the addition of enzyme substrate. The product of the reaction between enzyme and substrate is finally determined by spectrophotometry.

There are a number of variations of the technique similar to those used with fluorescent antibodies. These include a sandwich

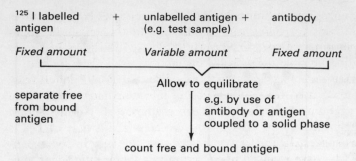

count free and bound antigen

(Amount of labelled antigen bound to antibody is determined by the amount of unlabelled antigen that competes in test sample)

Fig. 10.14 The principle of competitive binding radioimmunoassay.

technique with antigen bound to the plastic plate, the antibody to be assayed as the second layer and enzyme linked to immunoglobulin as the top layer. Enzyme substrate is finally added and the product determined in the spectrophotometer by colour change.

The technique has been applied widely in detection of bacterial and viral antigens and antibodies, particularly for rotavirus and cytomegalovirus. It has also been of use in the study of a variety of parasitic diseases due to helminths and protozoa.

Some common diagnostic applications of antigen-antibody reactions in medical microbiology

Agglutination tests

The agglutination tests already referred to for the serodiagnosis of salmonella infections is known as the Widal test. It is usual to test dilutions of the patient's serum against standard suspensions of somatic (O) antigen and flagellar (H) antigen of each organism likely to be encountered in the patient's environment. The test usually becomes positive with both suspensions a week after the onset of the illness but may be weakly positive with one of the antigens even earlier. The titre in an acute infection rises to a maximum by the end of the third week. Complications in interpretation of the results may arise in patients who have been immunized with typhoid-paratyphoid vaccine (TAB). A **rising titre** may be of some help in diagnosing an infection; furthermore, some months after immunization the titre of O agglutinins tends to fall off leaving only H agglutinins. Normal sera sometimes have low titres of agglutinins for *Salmonella* organisms and this varies in populations in different parts of the world. These difficulties make the test of questionable diagnostic value and its use is now limited.

Another widely used agglutination test is the **Paul-Bunnell** reaction. This is used for the diagnosis of infectious mononucleosis in which agglutinins develop for sheep erythrocytes. Normal serum may agglutinate sheep cells in low dilutions and a titre of 128 is taken as suggestive and 256 as positive for the test. In some individuals who have received horse serum as a therapeutic agent (e.g. anti-tetanus serum) agglutinins develop for sheep cells because of the presence in the horse serum of an antigen very widespread in nature, known as the **Forssman** antigen. This antigen is present in the red cells of sheep and the cells of a number of other species, including the guinea-pig. The usual way of differentiating the two types of antibody is to mix the serum with minced guinea-pig tissue (usually kidney). This treatment will absorb out the anti-Forssman antibody leaving the anti-sheep cell antibody unaffected. Ox red cells, which contain both the Forssman antigen and an antigen similar to that on sheep cells which reacts with the Paul-Bunnell antibody, will absorb out both types of antibody.

Complement fixation tests

These tests, described on page 279, have wide application in the diagnosis of bacterial and viral infections. One of the most commonly used methods is the Wassermann test used in the diagnosis of **syphilis**. This reaction depends upon the fixation of complement by the patient's antibody after it has reacted with cardiolipin, an alcoholic extract (a phosphatide lipoid) from normal animal tissues, usually ox heart. Why antibodies against this material develop in syphilis is not clear. Some workers suggest that it results from autoimmunisation with host lipids made antigenic in some way by the spirochaete (*Trep. pallidum*) responsible for syphilis, whilst others believe that the spirochaete contains a cell wall antigen related to the tissue antigen (p. 33).

Interpretation of the results of the Wassermann test is difficult and a final assessment depends on the results of both this and other serological tests and the clinical findings. False-positive reactions are sometimes found in leprosy, malaria, sleeping sickness, tuberculosis, infectious mononucleosis and other febrile diseases. Persistent **false-positive** reactions are sometimes found in autoimmune haemolytic anaemia, systemic lupus erythematosus and liver cirrhosis. A commonly performed test is a slide flocculation test using cardiolipin mixed with the patient's serum. This test is preferred by many laboratories because of its simplicity, as an alternative to the Wassermann test. It is known as the VDRL (Venereal Diseases Research Laboratory) slide test. When there is doubt a more specific test may have to be exmployed, e.g. the treponemal immobilization test, in which motile treponemata can be seen to be immobilized when examined microscopically after exposure to patient's serum. This test is, however, technically complicated and has largely been replaced by an indirect fluorescent antibody (p. 282) test (fluorescent treponemal antibody absorbed, FTA-ABS test). The test is highly specific and sensitive; it is able to detect antibody at all stages of syphilitic infection. The enzyme-linked immunosorbent assay (ELISA) described on page 286 has the potential for large-scale application in syphilis serology.

Complement fixation tests are used widely in the diagnosis of virus diseases. The source of the antigen is usually the infected tissues of animals, or eggs, or infected tissue cultures. The virus is usually extracted from the tissues or cells by differential centrifugation or sometimes by purifying the virus by adsorbing it on to red cells and then eluting it later.

Haemagglutination-inhibition tests

Another useful procedure for the diagnosis of some types of virus disease is the **haemagglutination-inhibition** test. This depends on the fact that certain viruses, e.g. those of influenza, mumps and parainfluenza, will agglutinate chicken, human and guinea-pig red cells (Fig. 10.8). Other viruses, e.g. the adenoviruses, agglutinate rat or monkey red cells; the reoviruses and many enteroviruses agglutinate human red cells. The test is performed by mixing the virus with the appropriate red cells in the presence of patient's serum. If antibodies to the virus are present the virus will be unable to bring about haemagglutination. These tests are very valuable because of their extreme specificity and their ability to distinguish antibodies to various substrains and variants of viruses, e.g. the influenza virus. The complement fixation test on the other hand is less valuable for detecting these fine differences.

LABORATORY INVESTIGATIONS IN CLINICAL IMMUNOLOGY

Increasing attention is now being paid in the clinical laboratory to the investigation of the role of immune reactions in the **pathogenesis** of disease and to methods of assessing the **functional status** of the immune system in situations where apparent immune dysfunction exists.

Many of the disease states in which immune reactions are believed to be involved in disease pathogenesis have been considered briefly in preceding sections on hypersensitivity reactions and autoimmune states. Immune deficiency states are referred to in Chapter 9. This text is not to be intented to replace the many excellent text-books dealing with the laboratory aspects of clinical immunology but to provide a simple outline of the main principles of this complex and difficult subject.

Investigation of hypersensitivity states

Antibodies in anaphylactic states

Hay fever and asthma sufferers characteristically have IgE antibodies in their blood. In 1921 Prausnitz and Küstner described a method for the detection of such 'reaginic' antibody performed by injecting a small quantity of serum from the hay fever patient into the skin of a normal subject. The IgE antibody fixes to the cells of the recipient close to the site of injection and when the antigen (or allergen) to which the patient is sensitive (e.g. a pollen extract) is injected at the site, an inflammatory response takes place due to the release of histamine from mast cells (see p. 225). The same type of reaction can be elicited in the patient by introducing a small quantity of dilute antigen into the skin (Prick test).

IgE antibodies can be quantitated by the radial immunodiffusion technique described on page 276. IgE directed at particular antigens can be assayed by coupling antigen to an insoluble material and mixing the complex with the patient's serum containing IgE antibody against the antigen. After allowing the binding of the IgE antibodies with antigen to take place, unbound serum proteins are washed away and the bound IgE antibody is detected with radiolabelled (^{125}I) anti-IgE antiserum.

Another procedure that can be used to detect sensitization to a particular antigen is to collect peripheral blood leucocytes from the patient and mix them with antigen. The lymphocytes will bind the antigen by their cell membrane receptors, as described on page 84, and the cells will be stimulated to transform in the way described on page 107. Macrophage migration inhibition tests have also been applied on detect sensitization to antigens. This procedure is described on page 296.

Another laboratory procedure as yet little- used in clinical practice is the determination of the histocompatibility antigen type (p. 284) of the peripheral blood leucocytes. In studies in the United States an association has been found between the occurrence of allergy to ragweed antigen (antigen E) and HLA haplotypes. These studies have been confined so far to a small number of families. The association has been found to occur within particular families, making it possible to identify within a particular family the members at risk and likely to develop the particular ragweed allergy. If these studies are confirmed leucocyte typing may become a useful laboratory aid to the clinician.

Antibodies to inhaled organic material

A condition called 'extrinsic alveolitis' has been recognised in persons who inhale organic material such as fungal spores, dust from various birds or dust from mouldy hay or barley. The lung changes appear to be associated with IgG antibodies formed against the inhaled material and these antibodies are detected by gel diffusion precipitin tests, as described on page 274.

Pulmonary aspergillosis due to inhalation of spores of *Aspergillus fumigatus* sometimes develops in patients with asthma or with an old healed tuberculous cavity, and precipitating antibodies can be detected in their serum. *Candida albicans* respiratory infections can also result in similar antibodies.

Inhalation of *Micromonospora faeni* from mouldy hay can result in a form of alveolitis known as farmer's lung disease, and mouldy barley containing *Aspergillus clavatus* can result in maltworker's lung disease. Gel diffusion tests for precipitating antibodies against antigenic extracts of the microorganisms have proved useful in the diagnosis of the conditions (see also p. 163).

Inhalation of antigens from birds is responsible for bird fancier's lung disease, and here again precipitating IgG antibodies can be detected against avian antigens. The antigens are present in bird serum, feathers and droppings and for the most reliable results material should be used from the particular species of bird to which the patient has been exposed — chickens, pigeons, budgerigars, parrots, and so on.

Antibodies against self-constitutents (autoantibodies)

Organ (or tissue) specific autoantibodies

Autoantibodies against organ-specific antigens or non-organ-specific antigens are found in a wide range of disease states, as described in Chapter 9. Whilst their role, if any, in the disease process itself is not clear, their presence can be a useful guide as an aid in clinical diagnosis.

Amongst the more common organ-specific autoantibodies are those found in autoimmune haemolytic anaemia. Two main types of antibody have been found: (1) So-called 'warm antibodies' that combine at body temperature with red cells. These are usually of IgG class in contrast to IgM anti-red cell autoantibodies responsible for 'cold antibody' haemolytic anaemia that can be shown to agglutinate red cells at 4°C. The detection of these antibodies usually depends on the use of the Coombs antiglobulin test described on page 281. (2) Leucocyte and platelet autoantibodies have also been described in some rare disease states and are occasionally induced by drugs that combine with these blood components (p. 230).

Organ-specific autoantibodies have been described in the serum of patients with thyroiditis, adrenal disease, pernicious anaemia and disease of the salivary glands (Sjögren's syndrome). The main test here is the fluorescent antibody method (p. 282) with tissue sections of the appropriate tissue; but passive haemagglutination (p. 276) or gel diffusion tests are sometimes used in which red cells are coated with the tissue antigen or the antigen is placed in the wells for the immunodiffusion test (p. 274) with the patient's serum in opposite wells.

Non-organ specific antibodies

In certain disease states such as rheumatoid arthritis and systemic lupus erythematosus (discussed in Ch. 9) autoantibodies are found in widely distributed antigens not restricted to any one organ or tissue. Autoantibodies in this category are also found in various forms of chronic liver disease.

An agglutination test is widely used for the diagnosis of rheumatoid arthritis; the sera of 70 to 80% of patients with this disease contain an IgM antibody which is able to combine with the IgG globulin from various species. Detection of the antibody depends on the agglutination of sheep red cells or inert particles (polystyrene latex) coated with IgG globulin. Sheep red cells, for example, may be coated with specific rabbit antibody and will then be agglutinated by the IgM antibody in the rheumatoid patient's serum. The antibody is known as **rheumatoid factor**. Occasional low titres (less than 16) are found in normal sera (2 to 5%) and the test is not entirely specific for rheumatoid arthritis.

The fluorescent antibody tests is the most commonly used method for the detection of the **antinuclear factor** (ANF) found in the majority of cases of systemic lupus erythematosus. Sections of tissue, e.g. rat liver, are used as the substrate and are layered with patient's serum. Binding of ANF to the liver cell nuclei is detected with fluorescein-labelled antihuman immunoglobulin (see p. 282).

In a liver disease known as primary biliary cirrhosis most patients have antibodies against mitochondrial antigens. These are detected by the fluorescent antibody test with unfixed tissue sections or sometimes by complement fixation tests with rat liver mitochondria. In chronic active hepatitis, and transiently in just over half of patients with infective hepatitis, antibodies are found against smooth muscle actinomyosin. The fluorescent antibody test is the method of choice using unfixed sections of rat stomach.

Immune deficiency states

The clinical and immunological aspects of these states are discussed in Chapter 9 and can be seen to involve one or more of the different components of the immune system: (1) the cells responsible for making circulating immunoglobulins; (2) the cells concerned with the cell-mediated immune response; and (3) the bone marrow stem cells. A wide range of laboratory tests are available to investigate the various forms of deficiency.

Immunoglobulin production. Assay of circulating immunoglobulins can be assessed qualitatively by electrophoresis and quantitatively by immunodiffusion tests. These latter tests are capable of identifying deficiencies of particular classes of immunoglobulin, as described on page 276.

The ability of the patient to make specific immunoglobulin can be tested by **active immunization** with, for example, a bacterial antigen such as tetanus toxoid and the antibody response measured by a tube precipitation test (p. 273).

The presence of the cells involved in the humoral immune response can be assayed by making use of the fact that the particular cells concerned — the B lymphocytes — have receptors on their surface for the Fc component of the Ig molecule and for the C3 complement component. In the test, sheep red blood cells coated with anti-sheep red cell antibody and complement (in non-lytic quantities) are mixed with peripheral blood leucocytes. The sheep red cells become attached to B lymphocytes by means of the Fc and C3 receptors (that combine with the antibody and comp-lement on the red cell) forming 'rosettes' (p. 87). The proportion of leucocytes forming such rosettes gives an estimate of the number of B lymphocytes and is normally about 25% of the lymphocytes in human peripheral blood.

Tests of the function of the cell-mediated immune system

Skin tests. The classical method for testing the responsiveness of the cells involved in cell-mediated immunity is the **delayed hyper-sensitivity skin test** described on page 235. The tuberculin response is the best known example. It is induced by the intrad-ermal injection of 0.1 ml of a 1:1000 dilution (or a greater dilution in a highly sensitive individual) of a protein extract of tubercle bacilli (purified protein derivative, PPD). The reaction is described on page 235; it is only one of a number of similar tests of delayed hypersensitivity such as that using lepromin (in leprosy) and brucellin (in brucellosis). One of the main uses of tests of this type is to detect sensitisation to the relevant microorganism, as for example prior to the use of the BCG vaccine (p. 172) in the prevention of tuberculosis. Clearly in the presence of a positive tuberculin test immunization with the vaccine will not be called for. A negative reaction in an adult, particularly in one known to have previously shown a positive test, raises the possibility of a defect of the cell-mediated immune system, which in the adult would be likely to be secondary to some disease state affecting the lymphoid tissues such as Hodgkin's disease, multiple myeloma, leukaemia and lymphosarcoma.

Lymphocyte function tests. The thymus-dependent (T) lymphocyte has been pointed to as the main effector cell in cell-mediated immune reactions (Ch. 4). The presence of the T lymphocyte in the peripheral blood can be detected very much in the same way as B lymphocytes can be detected. Instead of using antibody and complement-coated sheep red blood cells as is required for B cells, sheep cells alone are all that is required. T lymphocytes have receptors for sheep erythrocytes and can thus form rosettes when the two types of cell are mixed together. Between 40% and 60% of the human peripheral blood lymphocytes can form rosettes of this type. Monoclonal antibodies against T and B cell differentiation antigens are now widely used and can be used to estimate subclasses of T cells and T and B cell ratios as in AIDS patients.

Lymphocyte transformation. A particularly useful and widely used assay of lymphocyte function is the lymphocyte transformation test. This is usually carried out using plant phytohaemagglutinin (PHA) as the stimulating agent; the process is described in some detail on page 107. In other situations a transformation test may be performed with specific antigens to which the individual is believed to be sensitized (e.g. tuberculin). In contrast to the use of PHA, which stimulated a high proportion of T lymphocytes, specific antigen will only stimulate those lymphocytes that are specifically 'committed' to the antigen in question and this is usually only a small portion of the total T lymphocytes. A low level of lymphocyte transformation (when compared with control subjects), either with PHA or specific antigen, indicates impaired cell-mediated immunity (or perhaps absence of previous exposure to the antigen used), whilst increased transformation in the presence of a specific antigen may occur in certain hypersensitivity states, e.g. drug allegies (p. 236).

Migration inhibition. A modification of the macrophage migration inhibition test using human peripheral blood leucocytes (instead of guinea-pig peritoneal macrophages) can be used in the assessment of cell-mediated immunity. Peripheral blood leucocytes are collected in a small capillary tube in the same way as for the macrophage inhibition test and, when put in a culture chamber, grow out of the end of the tube in a fan shape. If, however, antigen, to which the cell donor has previously be sensitized, is put into the chamber the leucocytes fail to grow out of the tube. This inhibitory effect is due to a 'lymphokine' produced by the sensitized lymphocytes on exposure to antigen. This form of assessment of lymphocyte function has very much the same value as the transformation tests referred to above.

Tests of phagocytic cell activity. Defective phagocytic mechanisms are discussed in Chapter 9 and can be assayed in a variety of ways in the laboratory:

1. The ability of phagocytes to respond to a chemotactic agent (e.g. antigen-antibody complexes in fresh serum) can be measured by inducing the phagocytes to migrate from a chamber through a millipore membrane towards an outer chamber containing the Ag — Ab complexes and serum. The number of phagocytes that respond can be estimated by removing the membrane, staining it with a suitable stain and, under the microscope, counting the number of cells either in the process of passing through the membrane or on the outer side of the membrane.

2. The ability of phagocytes to ingest and kill microorganisms (e.g. staphylococci) or ingest inert particles such as latex or oil droplets can be determined by microscopic examination of cell preparations mixed with the microorganism or inert particle. Killing of microorgansims within phagocytes can be estimated by disrupting the cells (e.g. by distilled water) and counting the colonies of microorganisms that can be grown on a suitable nutrient agar plate.

3. The normal functioning of phagocyte lysosomal enzyme activity can be assessed by a dye reduction test using tetrazolium nitroblue. A defect on the part of the patient's cells can be detected by a failure of the leucocytes to reoxidize the reduced colourless dye to its blue colour. A deficiency of this function is characteristic of chronic granulomatous disease (p. 238).

The complement system. Changes in the levels of this complex group of serum protein constituents (see Ch. 2) are often a reflection of an underlying disease process. **Raised** levels of the components are frequently found in acute inflammatory and infective disease states in conjunction with raised levels of 'acute phase proteins' such as C reactive protein.

Reduction in complement levels is a more useful guide to the understanding of disease pathogenesis and fall into two categories: (1) primary deficiencies — genetically determined deficiencies of complement components; and (2) secondary deficiencies — as a consequence of complement consuming antibody-antigen interactions or associated with renal or liver disease.

The genetically determined deficiencies are rare conditions, the best known of which is the deficiency of C1 esterase inhibitor (see p. 27). Very rare deficiencies of other components (C3, C1, C5) have been described.

The secondary deficiencies are much more frequently found and most often occur in renal disease such as poststreptococcal nephritis, in the nephritis of systemic lupus erythematosis and in chronic membrano-proliferative glomerulonephritis. Low levels also occur in serum sickness (immune complex disease), bacterial septicaemia, malaria and in various forms of liver disease.

In the laboratory two main type of assay are available: (1) functional tests of the haemolytic activity of the complement system; and (2) immunochemical estimation of the levels of individual complement components.

Haemolytic activity of the complement system is usually assayed by the method described by Mayer, which measures the number of 'units' of complement per ml of serum. A unit of complement is defined as the quantity required to lyse 50% of a standard sheep cell suspension, optimally sensitized with anti-sheep cell antibody. The volume, buffer components and incubation conditions are likewise defined. The test is sometimes referred to as a CH50 assay.

Estimation of individual components, whilst possible by assays of their functional activity, is usually performed by immunochemical methods utilising specific antisera against individual components. The method of choice is the quantitative radial immunodiffusion test (p. 276) in which the antisera are incorporated in the agar and the serum specimens are placed in the wells. Commercially prepared plates are available for a wide range of complement components.

Immune complex detection. In the circulation the potentially pathogenic complexes are those found in antigen excess. There is now convincing evidence that they play a role in the pathogenesis of rheumatoid arthritis, glomerulonephritis, polyarteritis, rheumatic fever and a number of infective states discussed in Chapter 5. Detection of complexes is valuable in the diagnosis of bacterial endocarditis. In most instances, complement activation seems likely to be responsible for the inflammatory changes that occur, with chemotaxis of neutrophils and release of lysosomal enzymes as the prime factors involved (see Ch. 2, p. 24).

The following detection methods in general require specialized laboratory facilities:

1. Electron-microscopic demonstration of complexes in tissues, such as those found in the liver of patients with hepatitis B virus infections.

2. Precipitation of complexes in the cold, cryoprecipitation, and subsequent identification of microbial antigens, e.g. hepatitis B antigens.

3. Detection of bound complement component (e.g. C1q) in the complexes, often after precipitation by polyethylene glycol. The

principle of the assay is that the naturally bound C1q is removed with Na_2EDTA, a radiolabelled C1q is then added, followed by polyethylene glycol to precipitate the complexes. The C1q remaining in the supernatant is then measured, allowing the estimation of the bound C1q. A similar test commercially available involves the binding of bovine conglutinin to the bound complement.

4. Immunobiological tests such as aggregation of platelets and inhibition of antibody-mediated cytotoxicity. The latter test is quite widely used and involves inhibition of the killing by non-sensitized lymphocytes of target cells (e.g. Chang cells, a line of human liver cells) coated with antibody. If immune complexes are added to the lymphocytes, their Fc receptors are blocked by the antibody in the complexes so that the receptors cannot bind the antibody on the target cell.

Other tests

A number of miscellaneous clinical immunological investigations are sometimes called for and include examination of biopsy material for deposits of antibody or complement by immunofluorescence, estimation of cryoglobulins, radioimmunoassay for the presence of hepatitis B antigen and characterization of monoclonal antibodies by immunoelectrophoresis or examination of bone marrow by immunofluorescence. In diagnosis of virus infection speed is important, enabling public health control measures to be started and more immediate care for the patient.

The ELISA assay has been discussed and is likely to have wide applications. Assay of specific IgM may be helpful in atypical measles or mumps and in certain arbovirus infections. Electron microscopic examination is widely used for biopsy material as well as the fluorescent antibody technique.

Most of these procedures required specilized laboratory facilities not generally available in the routine clinical pathology laboratory.

Summary of clinical applications

Quantitation of serum immunoglobulin levels

1. Patients with severe or repeated infection, e.g. actinomycosis, subacute bacterial endocarditis, infectious mononucleosis.
   2. Liver disease.

3. To monitor immunotherapy of patients with immunoproliferative disorders, e.g. monoclonal gammopathies of IgG, IgA or IgM (Ch. 9).

4. To distinguish transient changes, such as those following burns and in primary immunodeficiencies.

5. Estimation of immune responses following natural infection or immunization — IgA levels in patients with infections of mucosal surfaces or IgE levels in patients with allergies.

6. Levels of antibodies in cerebral spinal fluid of patients with infections or in demyelinating diseases.

7. To detect free heavy or light chains of immunoglobulins in the urine of patients with multiple myeloma.

Detection of levels of C reactive proteins

Used to follow the progress of treatment for an infection.

Detection of autoantibodies (Ch. 9)

Using immunofluorescence in tissue sections — thyroid sections for antithyroid antibodies; commercial assay kits for rheumatoid factor in rheumatoid arthritis; and an antinuclear factor in systemic lupus erythematosus.

Detection of immune complexes in type 3 hypersensitivity states (Ch. 9)

Many methods are available — cryoprecipitation; precipitation by polyethylene glycol; and detection of complement, if it is bound to the complexes.

Unfortunately the results tend to be variable and difficult to interpret. Valuable in bacterial endocarditis.

Skin tests for type I and type 4 hypersensitivity states (Ch. 9)

There are various forms of the skin test:
1. **Intradermal injection** of dilute antigen (allergen).
2. **Prick tests**, in which test material is placed on the skin and needle pricks are made through the material.
3. **Patch tests**, in which the material is placed in absorbent materials and placed on the skin — particularly used for type 4 hypersensitivity contact dermatitis.

Estimation of complement components

The most common procedure in the past was to measure total complement levels, but individual components can be measured more conveniently with commercially available immunodiffusion plates.

Tests of lymphocyte function

1. **Lymphocyte tranformation test** (see above) used for in vitro test of cell mediated immunity in suspected immunodeficiency.
2. **Macrophage (leukocyte) migration inhibition test.** This is less commonly used than the transformation test above.

Tests of phagocyte function

For suspected chronic granulomatous disease in patients with unresolving infections:
1. **Intracellular enzyme activity** the ability to reduce the dye nitrobluetetrazolium (NBT) as an indicator of the activity of oxygen-dependent bactericidal activities.
2. **Phagocytosis** — ability to ingest inert particles (yeast or latex), opsonized red cells or bacteria to test for Fc receptor function.
3. **Chemotaxis** — ability to be attracted by a chemoattractant through a membrane filter.
4. **Chemiluminescence** — emission of light by phagocytes as a test for their ability to be activated.

Diagnosis of infection

Many of the assays described above can be used to help in the diagnosis of infection. The availability of monoclonal antibodies has brought rapid progress to this area and they can be used, for example, to identify specific microorganisms in culture or in tissues and fluids from infected patients. Complement fixation tests, virus neuralization tests, ELISA assays, coagglutination tests, radioimmunoassay and immunofluorescence are widely used in the diagnostic laboratory. Immune complex detection can be valuable in diagnosis of bacterial endocarditis. The development of simple and highly sensitive methods for detection of nucleic acids is now being applied to diagnosis of infection using nucleic acid hybridization and are likely to provide a valuable additional aid to immunoassays in the diagnostic laboratory.

FURTHER READING

Duguid J P, Marmion B P, Swain R H A 1978 Mackie and McCartney; medical microbiology. 13th edn. Churchill Livingstone, Edinburgh

Glynn L E, Reading C A 1981 Immunological investigation of connective tissue diseases. Churchill Livingstone, Edinburgh

Hudson L, Hay F C 1980 Practical immunology, 2nd edn. Blackwell, Oxford

Rose N R, Friedman H, Fahey J L (eds) 1986 Manual of clinical laboratory immunology. American Association for Microbiology, Washington.

Thompson R A (ed) 1981 Techniques in clinical immunology, 2nd edn. Blackwell, Oxford

Weir D M, Herzenberg L A, Blackwell C C (eds) 1986 Handbook of experimental immunology, 4th edn. Blackwell Scientific Publications, Oxford

Williams C A, Chase M W 1968 Methods in immunology and immunochemistry. Academic Press, New York

World Health Organization 1981 Technical report series no. 661: Rapid laboratory techniques for the diagnosis of viral infections. WHO, Geneva

Index

ABO
  antigens, 184
  blood group system, 7
Abortions chronic, 190
Acquired cellular immunity, 139
  immune deficiency, 150
Acute infection, 132
  phase proteins, 109
  phase substances, 19
ADCC, 146, 152, 231
Adjuvant, 89, 90, 91
  bacterial, 92
  depot, 92
Adjuvanticity, 38
Adoptive transfer, 198
Adrenal dysfunction, 6
Affinity, 44, 84
Agglutination, 102, 271, 276
  tests, 288
Aggressins, 125, 126
AIDS, 150
  candidiasis, 150
  cryptococcosis, 150
  envelope gene, 151
  Kaposi's sarcoma, 151
  receptor, 151
  tuberculosis, 150
  virus, 150, 171, 210
Alkaline gaps, 17
Allergic alveolitis, 234
Allergy, 222
  genetic factors, 227
Allergic alveolitis, 163
Allotype, Gm, 258
Allotypes Gm, Km, Am, 99
Alpha 1 anti-trypsin, 19
Alpha 2 macroglobulin, 19
Alpha interferon, 218
Altered antigens, 251
Alternative pathway, 27
  evolution, 50
Anamnestic response, 44

Anaphylatoxins, 26, 29, 131
Anaphylaxis, 224
  IgE, 226
  prevention, 227
  tests, 291
ANF, 248
Anthrax, 25
  vaccination for, 176
Anti-DNA antibodies, 253
Anti-Rh detection, 187
Anti-idiotypic antibody, 81
Anti-lymphocyte serum, 204
Antibacterial immunity, 136
Antibiotics, 20
Antibodies
  cold, 293
  monoclonal, 79
  warm, 293
Antibody
  blocking, 228, 227
  complete, 188
  diversity, 86
  mediated immunity, 142
  incomplete, 188
  reaginic, 226
  variability, 85
Antibody-antigen reactions, 268
Antigen
  binding site, 97
  localization, 69
  presenting cells, 75
  processing of, 75
  properties of, 71
  trapping, 56
Antigenic determinants, 32, 34
  drift, 145
  specificity, 32, 35
Antigens, 31, 36
  ABO, 184
  acidic groups, 36
  basic groups, 36
  carbohydrate, 33

Antigens (*contd*)
  charge, 38
  Forssman, 32
  heterophile, 0
  high molecular, 37
  leukocytes, 191
  lipids, 33
  membrane, 53
  MHC, 72
  microbial, 171
  nucleic acids, 33
  particle size, 38
  persistance, 39
  physical state, 38
  platelets, 191
  proteins, 33
  shape, 38
  T dependent, 72
  T independent, 72
  thy, 54
  toxoids, 171
  tumor, 212
Antiglobulin serum, 284
Antilymphocyte serum, 211
Antimicrobial activity, 24
Antinuclear factor, 247
  test, 294
Antitoxins, 132, 133
Antiviral drugs, 151
Appendix, 63
Arthus reaction, 232, 234
Aspergillus fumigatus, 165, 292
Aspergillus clavatus, 164, 234, 292
Attenuated flu virus, 143
Attenutation, 6
Atypical pneumonia, 253
Autoantibodies, 264
  in diagnosis, 293
Autoantibody
  formation, 84
  detection, 300
Autogenous vaccines, 180
Autoimmune, 11
  pathogenesis, 258
  type 2 reactions, 258
  type 4 reactions, 260
  type 3 reactions, 259
Autoimmunity, 246
  mechanisms, 249
  sequestered antigens, 250
Autotoxin, 7
Avidity, 82

B cell, differentiation factor, 63
  factors, 76

  growth factor, 63
  growth factors, 108
  polyclonal activation, 71
  precursors, 63
  pre-existing, 254
  receptors, 64, 71
B lymphocytes, 75
  characteristics, 73
BCG vaccine, 172
Bactercidal substances, 18
Bacterial
  attachment, 127
  endocarditis, 22
  endotoxin, 38
  infection, 133
  lipopolysaccharide, 71
  structure, 128
  toxins, 135
Bacteriocins, 20
Basic polypeptides, 19
Basophils, 67
Bence-Jones protein, 244
Benjamin Jesty, 5
Benjamin Waterhouse, 6
Beta 2 microglobulin, 196
Bird fancier's lung, 292
Blocking antibody, 227, 228
Blood group distribution, 186
Blood groups, 184
  and infection, 133
  MN, 190
Blood transfusion, 185
Bone marrow, 51, 56, 63
Bordet, 6, 9
Bordetella pertussis, 38
Bradykinins, 225
Bruton type deficiency, 142, 240
Burkitt's lymphoma, 208
Burnet, 7, 9
  and Fenner, 248
Bursa of Fabricius, 63

C reactive protein (CRP), 19, 20
  test, 300
C3, 26
Caeruloplasmin, 19
Candida albicans, 292
Canine distemper virus, 263
Capsulate organisms, 132
Carcino-embryonic antigen, 211
Carcinogens, chemical, 207
Cardiolipin, 33
Carrier effect, 73
  molecule, 31

CD 4 lymphocytes, 55
CD 8 lymphocytes, 55
Cell cooperation, 1122
Cell mediated
  mechanisms, 107
  response, 106
  immunity, 6, 46
  tests, 295
Cellular defence, nonspecific, 48
CH 50, 298
Chediak-Higashi syndrome, 238
Chemiluminescence, 301
Chemotaxin, 26, 131
Chemotaxis, 29, 301
Cholera
  toxin, 134
  vaccine, 177
Chromium hypersensitivity, 237
Chronic
  granulomatous disease, 238
  infection, 132
Class 2 antigens, 113
Classical pathway, 26
Clonal selection, 7, 83, 249
Clones, 69
Coeliac disease, 61
Cold antibodies, 293
Colony stimulating factors, 52, 76, 108, 210
Colostral IgA, 105
Combined immunodeficiency, 241
Commensal organisms, 20
Complement, 6, 23
  activation, 102
  assays, 297
  components, 26
  defects, 239
  deficiencies, 30
  effects, 29
  fixation, 271, 279
  fixation test, 289
  pathways, 28
  receptors, 29
  regulation, 27
  system, 25
    evolution, 48
Complete antibody, 188
Compromised host, 120, 124
Coniosporium corticale, 164
Contrasupressor T cells, 62
Coombs, 9
  and Gell, 223
  antiglobulin test, 281
  test, 189, 247, 279
Copper, 15
Coproantibodies, 136

Cowpox vaccine, 172
Cross reacting antigens, 32
Cyclosporin A, 204
Cytokines, 10, 76, 108
Cytotoxic
  T cells, 47, 76, 111
  T lymphocytes, 152
  test, 284
Cytotoxicity, antibody mediated, 146

D region, 113
Delayed hypersensitivity, 235
Delta chain, 104
Demyelinating disease, 263
Demyelination, 263
Dendritic cells, 75
Dengue virus, 146
Di George's syndrome, 242
Diabetes, 16
  mellitus, 262
Diagnostic applications, 288
Diapedesis, 23
Diet, 16
Diphtheria toxin, 133
Directive theory, 82
Disease associations, HLA, 257
Disodium chromoglycate, 228
Domain, 94
Donor lymphocytes in graft, 198
DR, 44
Drugs, antiviral, 151
  as haptens, 251
Durham, 9

ECF, 67
Edelman, 9
Edward Jenner, 5
Ehrlich, 7, 9, 183
  and Morgenroth, 246
ELISA, 286
  assay, 290, 299
Endocarditis, 138
Endogeneous mediators, 23
Enveloped viruses, 131
Enzyme
  cascade systems, 25
  linked antibody, 286
Eosinophils, 67, 224
Epidermal growth factor, 210
Epstein-Barr
  Virus, 147, 254

Epstein-Barr (contd)
  virus receptors, 71
Erythroblastosis fetalis, 187
Erythropoietin, 52
Escape mechanisms, parasite, 163
Evasion
  by microorganisms, 120
  mechanisms, 126
Exogeneous mediators, 23
Extrinsic alveolitis, diagnosis, 292

Fab, 96
Factor, B 27
Farmer's lung disease, 163
Farr test, 269
Fatty acids, 17
Feed back regulation, 45
Fetal
  antigens, 189
  liver, 51, 63
Fibrinogen, 19
Filariasis, 156
Fluorescent antibody, 283
  labels, 282
Follicles, 58
Food hypersensitivity, 61
Forbidden clones, 83
Foreign, 246
Foreignness, 35
Forssman antigens, 32, 289
Francis Home, 5
Freund's adjuvant, 91
FTA-ABS test, 290
Fungal infections, 162

Gastric acid, 16
Gastrointestinal diseases, 61
Genetic control of immunity, 112
Germ
  free animals, 20
  theory of disease, 6
Germinal centre, 58
Glenny, 9, 76
Glomerulonephritis, 139
Glucocorticoids, 16
Gm allotype, 99, 258
Gonococcal infection, 133
Gonococci, 25
Graft
  immunosuppresion, 203
  rejection, 48
    MHC and, 155

mechanisms, 197
versus host disease, 207
Grafts
  antibody role of, 199
  immunosuppression, 201
  incompatible, 200
  kidney, 199
  lymphocyte factors, 199
  tolerance to, 201
Granulocytes, 67
Granulomatous reaction, 161
Gross agent, 213
Growth factors, 76, 108, 209
  and oncogenes, 209
Gut associated lymphoid tissue, 63

H-2 system, 195
H-2D antigens, 155
H-2K antigens, 155
Haemagglutination, 278, 290
Haemocytes, 49
Haemolytic anaemia, 230
  disease, 187
Haemopoieisis, 51
Hair dyes, 237
Hairy cell leukemia, 218
Hapten, 35
Haptens, 31, 251
Hashimoto's disease, 248
HAT medium, 79
Heavy chains, 97
Heidelberger, 9
Helminths, 160
  immunity to, 156
Helper T cells, 54
Hepatitis B, 146, 273
  vaccination, 176
  vaccine, 168
Heterophile antigens, 32
Hexose monophosphate shunt, 24
Histamine, 131, 224
Histiocytes, 21
Histocompatibility antigens, 195
HIV, 150, 210
HLA B27, arthritis, 262
HLA and disease, 256
HLA
  disease associations, 257
  locus, 195
  susceptibility, 255
HLA-D locus, 196
HTLV I, 210
HTLV III, 150
Hormonal influences, 15

Horror autotoxicus, 246
Horseshoe crab, 50
Humoral response, 86
Hydrogen peroxide, 238
Hydrolytic enzymes, 24
Hydroxyl radicals, 65
Hypersensitivity, 222
  delayed, 223
  food, 61
  immediate, 222
  inducer of, 236
  reaction, 151
  tests, 291
  to dyes, 237
  type 1, 224
  type 2, 228
  type 3, 232
  type 4, 235
Hypochlorite, 65
Hypogammaglobulinanaemia, 148
Hypothyroidism, 16

I region, 113, 196
IR genes, 44
Ia antigens, 113, 114
Iatrogenic disease, 120
Idiopathic steatorrhoea, 61
Idiotypes, 97
Ig replacement therapy, 246
IgA, 94, 99, 136, 143
  colostrol, 105
  salivary, 105
  secretion, 105
  secretory component, 105
IgD, 64, 94, 99, 104
IgE, 94
  anaphylaxis, 226
  quantitation, 291
IgG, 94, 96
IgM, 94, 99
IgM–IgG switch, 78
Immobilization tests, 271
Immune complex
  detection, 298, 300
  disease, 138, 157
Immune complexes and viruses, 145
Immune deficiency, 11
  secondary, 244
  tests for, 245, 294
Immune response
  acquired, 43
  cell mediated, 43
  cells in, 69
  control of, 112
  effector, 46

essentials of, 75
evolution of, 47
features of, 43
feed back, 45
genes, 44, 255
humoral, 43
inducer cells, 75
(IR) gene, 44
invertebrate, 47
origins, 47
primary, 43, 88
secondary, 43, 88
Immune surveillance, 211
Immune system
  cells of, 51
  tissues of, 51
  tolerance in, 76, 83
Immunity, 4, 9
  and infection, 132
  cell mediated, 106
  cellular processes, 81
  determinants of, 89
  main pathway, 115
  minor pathway, 115
  to food, 61
  to helminths, 156, 160
  to protozoa, 156
Immunization, passive, 180
Immuno-cyto-adherence, 87
Immunobiology, 7, 9
Immunochemistry, 9
Immunodeficiency, 237
  primary, 243
  secondary, 242
Immunodiffusion, 274
Immunoelectrophoresis, 273, 275
Immunogenicity, 37
Immunogens, 31
Immunoglobulin, 92, 96
  activity, 92
  allotypes, 99
  classes, 94
  classes, 26, 95
  constant regions, 96
  domain, 94, 98
  evolution, 93
  function, 100
  heavy chain, 94
  hinge region, 98
  idiotypes, 99
  J chain, 100
  production, 86
  structure, 92, 100
  synthesis, 77, 85
  transport, 104
  variable regions, 97

Immunoglobulin (*contd*)
  variation, 96
Immunoglobulins, 46
  as opsonins, 103
Immunological
  enhancement, 203
  memory, 44, 82, 88, 135
  surveillance, 111
  tolerance, 83, 90
Immunopathology, 218, 221
Immunosuppression, 10, 158, 201
Immunotherapy
  active, 216
  alpha interferon, 218
  passive, 216
  tumor, 215
Impedins, 125, 126
Incomplete antibody, 188
Incubation period, 140, 143
Inducer cells, 109
Infection
  and immunity, 119, 131
  and inflammation, 131
  diagnosis of, 301
Infections, fungal, 162
Inflammation, 21, 23
Influenza, 144
  vaccine, 168, 179
Innate
  immune defects, 238
  immunity, 13, 14, 16, 25
Interdigitating cells, 56, 62
Interferon, 98, 109, 154
  effects of, 111
Interleukin 3, 76
Interleukin 4, 76
Interleukins, 98, 109, 110
Intermolecular forces, 269
Invertebrate
  agglutinins, 49
  cellular immunity, 50
  immunity, 48
  opsonins, 49
Ir genes, 154
Isoantibodies, 184

J chains, 79, 100
Jenner, 9
Jerne, 9
  plaque technique, 87

K cells, 231
Kabat, 9

Kaposi's sarcoma, AIDS, 151
Kappa chains, 97
  genes, 85
Kidney grafts, 199
Killer (K) cells, 47, 231
  phagocytes, 47
Kitasato, 6, 9
Koch, 9
Kohler, 9, 79
Kupffer cells, 21, 22

Lactobacilli, 20
Lactoferrin, 24
Lambda
  chains, 97
  genes, 85
Landsteiner, 7, 9, 35, 183
Langerhan's cells 62, 75, 113
Latent viruses, 142
Lazy leucocyte syndrome, 238
LAV, 150
LCM Virus, 146, 148
Leeuenhoek, 6
Leprosy, 14
Leucocidins, 125
Leucotriene C, 225
Leukin, 24
Leukocyte
  antigens, 191
  grouping, 196
Light chains, 97
Localized haemolysis in gel, 87
Ly antigens, 54
Lymph node, medullary macrophages,
  70
Lymph nodes, 56, 58
Lymphocytes
  activation products, 107
  CD 4, 55
  CD 8, 55
  function, 295
  function test, 301
  long lived, 53
  recirculation of, 67
  surface markers, 55
  transformation, 296, 107
  T4, 55
  T8, 55
Lymphoid
  follicles, 70
  tissue, primary, 51
  tissue, secondary, 56
Lymphokines, 47, 110
  and type 4 hypersensitivity, 235

Lymphoma, 213
Lymphopoeisis, 52
Lysozyme, 16, 18, 19, 24

M protein, 136
M-type protein, 244
Macrophage immunity, 139
Macrophages, 21, 22, 65, 74, 75
  sinus lining, 70
  MAF, 108
Major histocompatibility, 55, 112
Malaria, 15, 16, 158
  parasites, 156
Malignant disease, 206
Malphigian bodies, 58
  corpuscle, 60
MALT, 58, 61, 62
Malt worker's lung, 164, 292
Maple bark strippers disease, 164
Marrack, 9
Mast cell mediators, 225
Mast cells, 67
Mechanical barriers, 16
Medawar, 9, 83
Meningitis, 133
Meningococcal meningitis, 14, 133,
  166
Metazoa, 50
Metchnikoff, 6, 9, 22
MHC, 112
  antigens, 72
  class II, 75
  disparity, 190
  gene complex, 155
  gene products, 114
  restriction, 148
  susceptibility to viruses, 154
Microbicidal activity, 15, 65
Micrococcus lysodeikticus, 19
Micromonospora faeni, 164, 292
MIF, 108, 236
Migration inhibition, 296
Milk protein, 61
Milstein, 9
  and Kohler, 11, 79
MNS system, 190
Moldy hay, 292
Molecular genetics, 85
Moloney virus, lymphoma, 213
Monoclonal antibodies, 11, 34, 79
Monoclonal antibody production, 80
Monocytes, 21, 65
Monokines, 109, 110
Mononuclear phagocyte system, 21

Mourant, 9
Mucosal associated lymphocytes, 58
Mucous membranes, 16, 18
Multiple sclerosis, 263
Murine encephalitis virus, 263
Myasthenia gravis, 264
Mycoses, 162
Myeloma cells, 79
Myeloperoxidase, 24

NADPH, 238
Napoleon, 6
Natural killer (NK) cells, 47, 64
NBT test, 238, 301
Neuroendocrine peptides, 10
Neutralisation of toxins, 134
  tests, 271
Neutrophils, 65
Nickel hypersensitivity, 237
NK cells, 47, 64, 111, 152
Non-secretion, 163
Non-specific defence, 13
  resistance, 140
Normal flora, 20, 120
Null cells, 64
Nutritional factors, 15
NZB mice, 253

Occupational hazards, 176
Oncogenes, 209
Opportunistic pathogens, 21
Opsonins, 23, 29
Opsonisation, 103
Optimal proportions, 271, 272
Oral polio vaccine, 144
Organ specific antibodies, 293
Owen, 9
Oxygen-dependent killing, 65
  system, 24
Oxygen-independent killing, 65
  system, 24

PAF, 67, 225
Para-aminobenzoic acid, 16
Parasite immunosuppression, 158
Parvovirus, in RA, 254
Passive immunization, 180
Pasteur, 6, 9
Patch test, 300
Paul Ehrlich, 6

Paul-Bunnel test, 289
Penicillin, 237
Pfeiffer, 6, 9
Phagocyte definition, 22
   function tests, 301
Phagocytes, 6, 24, 65
   differentiation of, 66
   function, 66
   killer cells, 47
   origin, 66
   tests of, 296
   vacuoles, 24
Phagocytin, 24
Phagocytosis, 21
   evolution of, 50
Pharmacological mediators, 224
Physical abnormalities, 15
Phytohaemagglutinins, 106
PHA, 106
PK test, 226
Pituitary peptides, 45
Plasma cell, 77, 89
Plasmodium falciparum, 15
Platelet antigens, 191
Pneumococcal polysaccharide, 32
Pneumococci, 33
Pneumocystis carini, 150
Poison ivy, 237
Polio vaccine, 144
Polyarthritis, 147
Polyclonal B cell activation, 159
Polymorphonuclear leukocytes, 21
Polysaccharide antigens, 39
Portals of entry, 128
Porter, 9
Post capillary venules, 69
Prausnitz-Küstner, 226
Precipitation, 271
Predisposing factors, 124
Premunition, 158
Prick test, 300
Primary immune response, 88
   immunodeficiency, 240
   interaction, 269
Primulin, 237
Progenitor cells, 51
Protection and immunity, 119
Protein A, 125
Protochordates, 50
Protozoa, 158
   immunity to, 156
Prozone phenomenon, 277
Pseudo-Schick response, 236
Pulmonary aspergillosis, 292
Pyer's patches, 56, 63
Pyrexia, 25

Qa antigen, 54

Rabies, 14
   vaccine, 179
Race, 9
Radial immunodiffusion, 276
Radioimmunoassay, 285, 288
Reaginic antibody, 226, 271
Receptors, 23
   B cell, 64
Recirculation of lymphocytes,
   67
Recognition, 3
   evolution of, 50
Recombinant DNA, 10, 168
Red cell lysis, 27
Regulatory circuits, 54
Replacement therapy, 245
RES, 21
Resistance to infection, 18
Respiratory viruses, 16
Reticulum cells, 21
Retroviruses, 150
   in tumours, 209
Reverse transcriptase, 131
Rhesus
   blood group, 186
   incompatibility, 187
Rheumatic fever, 138
Rheumatoid
   arthritis, 254, 261
   factor, 254, 262
   test, 294
Rhinoviruses, 129
Ring worm, 17
RNA viruses, 130
Robert Koch, 6
Rosette, 86
Rous sarcoma virus, 209, 210
Routine vaccination, 173
Rubella
   congenital infection, 149
   lymphocyte reactions, 149

Salivary IgA, 105
Salmonella, 136
SALT, 62
Sarcoma, 213
Schistosome eggs, 161
Schistosomiasis, 156
Schultz-Dale reaction, 224
Sebaceous secretions, 17

Secondary
  effects, 269
  immune response, 88
  lymphoid tissue, 56
  phenomena, 269
Secretor state, 192
  and infection susceptibility, 133
Secretory component, 105
Sedormid, 230
Selective
  theory, 82
  transport of Ig, 104
Self, 246
  — reactive clones, 83
  — markers, 248
  /non-self, 3
Sensitizing dose, 224
Sequestered antigens, 250
Serotonin, 225
Serum
  electrophoresis, 240
  sickness, 232
Shocking dose, 224
Side chain theory, 6
Sinus lining cells, 60
  macrophages, 21, 22, 70
Sjörgen's syndrome, 293
Skin, 16
  associated lymphoid tissue, 62
  test, delayed, 295
  tests in allergy, 271
SLE, 247, 253
Sleeping sickness, 159
Smallpox, 5
  vaccination, 176
  vaccine, 177
Smoking, 20
Spleen, 56, 58
  Malphigian bodies, 70
  marginal zone, 70
  red pulp, 58
  white pulp, 58
SRS-A, 67, 225
Stem cells, 51
Streptococcal cell wall, 33
Superoxide, 65
Suppressor
  T cells, 252
  cells, 54, 76
Surface secretions, 16
Susceptibility, 14
  fungal, 163
  to fungi, 162
  and non-secretion, 163
  and secretion, 192
SV40 virus, 212

Sweat, 17
Swiss type agammaglobulinaemia, 241
Synthesis of immunoglobulin, 77
Syphilis, 14, 33
  diagnosis of, 281, 289
Systemic lupus erythematosus, 253,
  247

Tat gene, 210
T cell lymphokines, 63
  receptor, 72, 75
  recognition, 72
  surface markers, 55
T cells
  autoreactive, 255
  contrasuppressor, 62
  cytotoxic, 47
T cytotoxic cells, 72
T dependent antigens, 72
T helper cells, 54, 72
  independent antigens, 72
  lymphocyte, subpopulations, 54
  lymphocytes, characteritics, 73
  suppressor cell, 54, 76
T4 lymphocytes, 55
T8 lymphocytes, 55
Tdh cells, 76
TL antigens, 54
Technical advances, 11
Temperature and innate immunity,
  24
Theories of immunity, 82
Thymic
  differentiation, 55
  dysplasia, 242
Thymosin, 52
Thymus, 53
  evolution of, 48
Tiselius, 9
Tissue
  defences, 18
  fixation of Ig, 103
  transplantation, 195
Titre, 276
Togavirus, 129
Tolerance, 76, 83
  to grafts, 201
Tonsils, 56
Toxic
  complex syndrome, 232
  complexes, 144
Toxigenic organisms, 132
Toxoid vaccines, 171
Transgenic mice, 10

Transplantation, 11
  antigens, 8, 195
  terminology, 194
Treponema pallidum, 33
Triple vaccine, 39
Trypanosomes, 159
Trypanosomiasis, 157
Tumour
  antigens, 212
  burden, 215
  immunity, 207
  macrophages, 211
  necrosis factor, 160
  shedding, 214
  therapy, 215
Tumours
  oncogenes, 209
  retroviruses, 209
Tumour necrosis factor, 108
Type 1 hypersensitivity, 224
Type 2 hypersensitivity, 228
Type 3 hypersensitivity, 232
Type 4 hypersensitivity, 235
Tyrosine, 34

Ulcerative colitis, 61
Universal donor, 185
  recipient, 186
Urinary tract infection, 133

VDRL test, 289
Vaccination, 165
  procedures, 174
  reactions, 178
Vaccine
  attenuated, 172
  autogenous, 180
  BCG, 172
  cholera, 170, 177
  contraindication, 180
  cowpox, 172
  hepatitis B, 168
  influenza, 168, 179
  killed, 171
  leprosy, 169
  live, 172
  malaria, 169
  measles, 172
  preparations, 172
  rabies, 179
  rubella, 175

traveller's, 175
  trypanosomes, 170
  veterinary, 173
  yellow fever, 172, 177
Vaccines, special, 177
Vaccinia gangrenosa, 179
  virus, 171
Vaccinof, 6
Variola, 4
Variolation, 5
Vascular endothelium, 113
Vasoactive amines, 131
Veiled cells, 62
Vibrio cholera, 136
Viral
  antigenic drift, 144
  immunity, 140
  infections complexes in, 145
  penetration of, 130
  persistence of, 144
  replication of, 129, 130
  uncoating, 130
  vaccines, 168
Virion assembly, 130
Virus
  dengue, 146
  elimination, 147
  Epstein-Barr, 147
  haemagglutination, 280
  HIV, 150, 210
  LCM, 146
  structure, 130
  yellow fever, 147
  west Nile, 147
Viruses, 129
  latent, 142
Visna virus, 263
von Behring, 6, 9
von Pirquet, 222

Warm antibodies, 293
Wasserman
  reaction, 281
  test, 289
Water in oil emulsion, 90
West Nile virus, 147
Wheat protein, 61
Widal test, 278, 288

Yellow fever, 147